DIETARY SUPPLEMENTS IN SPORT PERFORMANCE

Kimberly Mueller, MS, RD, CSSD

Lonnie Lowery, PhD

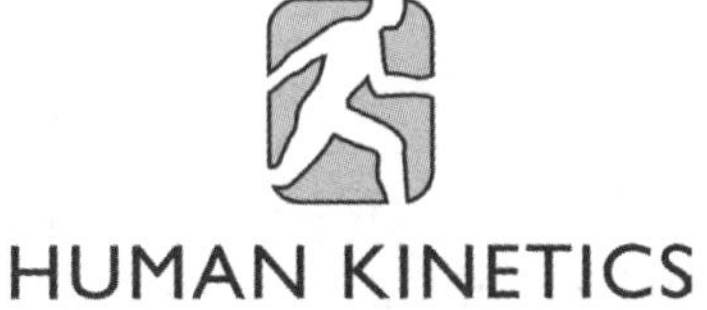

HUMAN KINETICS

Library of Congress Cataloging-in-Publication Data

Names: Mueller, Kimberly, 1976- author | Lowery, Lonnie Michael author
Title: Dietary supplements in sport performance / Kimberly Mueller, Lonnie
Lowery.
Description: Champaign, IL : Human Kinetics, 2026. | Includes
bibliographical references.
Identifiers: LCCN 2025026190 (print) | LCCN 2025026191 (ebook) | ISBN
9781718221543 paperback | ISBN 9781718221550 epub | ISBN 9781718221567
pdf
Subjects: LCSH: Athletes--Nutrition | Athletes--Health and hygiene |
Dietary supplements
Classification: LCC TX361.A8 M84 2926 (print) | LCC TX361.A8 (ebook)
LC record available at https://lccn.loc.gov/2025026190
LC ebook record available at https://lccn.loc.gov/2025026191

ISBN: 978-1-7182-2154-3 (print)

This book is a revised edition of *The Athlete's Guide to Sports Supplements*, published in 2013 by Human Kinetics.

The web addresses cited in this text were current as of April 2025, unless otherwise noted.

Acquisitions Editors: Korey Van Wyk and Diana Vincer; **Developmental Editor:** Anne Hall; **Managing Editor:** Kim Kaufman; **Copyeditor:** Heather Gauen Hutches; **Permissions Manager:** Laurel Mitchell; **Graphic Designer:** Denise Lowry; **Cover Designer:** Keri Evans; **Cover Design Specialist:** Susan Rothermel Allen; **Photograph (cover):** carlosgaw/E+/Getty Images; **Photo Production Manager:** Jason Allen; **Senior Art Manager:** Kelly Hendren; **Printer:** Versa Press

Human Kinetics books are available at special discounts for bulk purchase. Special editions or book excerpts can also be created to specification. For details, contact the Special Sales Manager at Human Kinetics.

Printed in the United States of America   10 9 8 7 6 5 4 3 2 1

The paper in this book is certified under a sustainable forestry program.

Human Kinetics
1607 N. Market Street
Champaign, IL 61820
USA

United States and International
Website: US.HumanKinetics.com
Email: info@hkusa.com
Phone: 1-800-747-4457

Human Kinetics' authorized representative for product safety in the EU is Mare Nostrum Group B.V., Mauritskade 21D, 1091 GC Amsterdam, The Netherlands.
Email: gpsr@mare-nostrum.co.uk

E9120

CONTENTS

SUPPLEMENT FINDER

Key Symbols

✔ Beneficial

? More research needed

⚠ Unverified

🏋 Master athletes

🏃 Youth athletes

♀ Female athletes

🧰 Injured athletes

💧 Diabetes

🥜 Food allergies

🥗 Plant-based

☀ Hot environment

⛰ Altitude

Supplement	Fuel usage	Cardiovascular performance		Muscular performance		Neural performance		Hydration	
		Maximal aerobic capacity: Speed	Improving aerobic capacity: Endurance	Strength and power	Endurance	Focus and cognition	Motivation and motor	Fluid balance	Electrolyte balance
Acai berry									
Acetylcysteine		?			?				
Adenosine triphosphate (ATP)	?			?					
Agmatine							?		
Alpha-GPC				?		?	?		
Alpha-lipoic acid									
Apple cider vinegar									
Arachidonic acid					?				
Arginine		?	?	?	?				
Aspartates			?						
Astaxanthin									
Astragalus									
Avocado soybean unsaponifiables									
Bacopa monnieri						?			
Beetroot		✓	✓		?	?	?		
Berberine									
Beta-alanine					✓	?	?		
Beta-carotene									
Beta glucan									
Betaine								?	
Boron (B)									

	Recovery						Weight and body composition		
	Short-term		Long-term						
	Rehydration	Glycogen repletion	Joint, tendon, bone, and muscle health	Immunity	Endocrine support	Antioxidant protection	Muscle preservation and hypertrophy	Fat loss	Special populations
						?			
						?			[mountains]
			?						
					?				
						?			[droplet]
								?	[bowl]
									[weightlifter] [medical kit]
						?			
				?					
			?						[weightlifter] [female] [medical kit]
									[bowl]
						?			[female] [bowl] [mountains]
								⚠	[bowl]
									[female] [bowl] [mountains]
						⚠			
			?	✓					
								?	
			?						[weightlifter]

Supplement	Fuel usage	Cardiovascular performance		Muscular performance		Neural performance		Hydration	
		Maximal aerobic capacity: Speed	Improving aerobic capacity: Endurance	Strength and power	Endurance	Focus and cognition	Motivation and motor	Fluid balance	Electrolyte balance
Boswellia serrata (BS)									
Branched-chain amino acids (BCAAs)				?	?		?		
Bromelain									
Caffeine --Coffee	?	?	✓	✓	✓	✓	?		
Calcium (Ca)							?		?*
Cannabidiol (CBD)							?		
Capsicum	?				?		?		
Carbohydrate (CHO)	✓	✓	✓	✓	✓	✓	✓	✓	
Carnitine	?	?		?	?				
Casein				✓					
Cat's claw									
Chia seeds									
Chitosan									
Choline		?			?	?	?		
Chondroitin									
Chromium (Cr)									
Chrysin									
Cinnamon	?								
Cissus quadrangularis									

*In deficient states

| | Recovery | | | | | | Weight and body composition | | |
| Short-term | | Long-term | | | | | | | |
Rehydration	Glycogen repletion	Joint, tendon, bone, and muscle health	Immunity	Endocrine support	Antioxidant protection	Muscle preservation and hypertrophy	Fat loss	Special populations
		?						
		?						
		?						
	✓						?	
		?					?	
		?			✓			
✓	✓		✓	✓		✓		
		?						
		?				✓		
		?						
							?	
							?	
		?						
		?						
							?	
				⚠				
		?			✓		?	
		?			?			

Supplement	Fuel usage	Cardiovascular performance		Muscular performance		Neural performance		Hydration	
		Maximal aerobic capacity: Speed	Improving aerobic capacity: Endurance	Strength and power	Endurance	Focus and cognition	Motivation and motor	Fluid balance	Electrolyte balance
Citicoline						?			
Citrulline malate (CM)	?	?	?		?		?		
Cocoa		?	?						
Coconut								✓	
Coenzyme Q10 (CoQ10)									
Colostrum			?	?	?				
Conjugated linoleic acid (CLA)									
Copper (Cu)									
Cordyceps sinensis		?			?				
Creatine				✓	✓				
Curcumin									
Deer antler (DA)				⚠					
Dehydroepiandrosterone (DHEA)									
Dendrobium							⚠		
Devil's claw									
Dimethylamylamine (DMAA)							?		
Dimethylethanolamine (DMAE)						?			
Ecdysteroids				?					
Echinacea									
Egg protein				✓					

| | Recovery | | | | | | Weight and body composition | | |
| Short-term | | Long-term | | | | | | | |
Rehydration	Glycogen repletion	Joint, tendon, bone, and muscle health	Immunity	Endocrine support	Antioxidant protection	Muscle preservation and hypertrophy	Fat loss	Special populations
		?						
		?			✓			
✓			?				?	
		?			✓			💧
		?	?	?		?	?	
						?	?	
		?						♀ 🧰
					?			⛰
		?			✓			🏋 🏃 ♀ 🥗
			?		✓			🏋 🧰 🥜
				⚠				
			?					
		⚠						
		?	?					
		✓				✓		🏋 🏃 ♀ 🧰 ⛰ 🥗

Supplement	Fuel usage	Cardiovascular performance		Muscular performance		Neural performance		Hydration	
		Maximal aerobic capacity: Speed	Improving aerobic capacity: Endurance	Strength and power	Endurance	Focus and cognition	Motivation and motor	Fluid balance	Electrolyte balance
Elderberry									
Fenugreek	?			?					
Fiber									
5-hydroxytryptophan (5-HTP)						?	?		
Flaxseed	?								
Folic acid		?				?			
Fucoxanthin									
Gamma-aminobutyric acid (GABA)						?			
Gamma-linolenic acid (GLA)									
Garlic									
Ginger									
Ginkgo biloba									
Ginseng		?				?	?		
Glucosamine									
Glucuronolactone							⚠		
Glutamine	?								
Glutathione									
Glycerol									
Grape seed						?			
Green tea extract									
Gymnema sylvestre (GS)									

| | Recovery | | | | | Weight and body composition | | |
| Short-term | | Long-term | | | | | | |
Rehydration	Glycogen repletion	Joint, tendon, bone, and muscle health	Immunity	Endocrine support	Antioxidant protection	Muscle preservation and hypertrophy	Fat loss	Special populations
		?	?		✓			(peanut)
	?					?	?	(weightlifter) (female) (blood drop)
			?				✓	(weightlifter) (female) (blood drop) (first aid)
							?	
		?		✓	✓		✓	(female) (blood drop) (bowl)
								(weightlifter) (runner) (female) (peanut)
				?	✓		?	(blood drop)
		?				?	?	
	?	?	✓	?	✓			(female) (first aid) (blood drop) (bowl)
		?	✓	✓	✓			(first aid) (blood drop) (peanut) (bowl)
					✓			(sun) (mountains)
		?		?				(female) (blood drop)
		?						(weightlifter) (first aid)
	?	?	?					(weightlifter) (first aid) (mountains)
					?			
?								(sun)
		?	?		✓			
					?	?		(bowl)
				?			?	(blood drop)

Supplement	Fuel usage	Cardiovascular performance		Muscular performance		Neural performance		Hydration	
		Maximal aerobic capacity: Speed	Improving aerobic capacity: Endurance	Strength and power	Endurance	Focus and cognition	Motivation and motor	Fluid balance	Electrolyte balance
Hoodia gordonii									
Hordenine							?		
Horny goat weed									
Huperzine A						?	?		
Hyaluronic acid (HA)									
Hydroxy-beta-methylbutyrate (HMB)				?					
Hydroxycitric acid (HCA)									
Hydroxytyrosol (HT)			?						
Inosine			⚠						
Inositol						?			
Iron		✓	✓		✓				
Isomaltulose	✓								
Ketones	?								
Leucine				✓	?				
Lutein						?			
Maca			?						
Magnesium (Mg)									✓
Medicinal mushrooms						?			
Medium-chain triglycerides (MCTs)	⚠								
Melatonin				?	?	?			
Methylsulfonylmethane (MSM)									

| | Recovery | | | | | | Weight and body composition | | |
| Short-term | | Long-term | | | | | | | |
Rehydration	Glycogen repletion	Joint, tendon, bone, and muscle health	Immunity	Endocrine support	Antioxidant protection	Muscle preservation and hypertrophy	Fat loss	Special populations
		?					?	🥣
								🥣
				⚠				🥣
								🥣
		?						🏋 🧰
		?				?		🏋 🧰
							?	
					?			🥣
		?						
			✓	✓				♀ 💧 🥣 ⛰
				✓				💧
		?				?	?	🏋 🧰 ⛰
					?			
								🥣
		?		✓				♀ 💧 ☀ ⛰
			?					
							?	
		?			✓			
		?			✓			🧰

Supplement Finder *(continued)*

Supplement	Fuel usage	Cardiovascular performance		Muscular performance		Neural performance		Hydration	
		Maximal aerobic capacity: Speed	Improving aerobic capacity: Endurance	Strength and power	Endurance	Focus and cognition	Motivation and motor	Fluid balance	Electrolyte balance
Mucuna pruriens									
Mycoprotein									
Naringin									
Nicotinamide riboside (NR)			?						
Omega-3 fatty acids						?	?		
Ornithine				?	?				
Pantothenic acid									
Phosphate salts		?	?		?				
Phosphatidic acid (PA)									
Phosphatidylserine (PS)		?				?			
Pine bark extract		?	?		?				
Piperine									
Potassium (K)								✔	✔
Probiotics						?			
Pterostilbene				?					
Pyruvate				?	?				
Quercetin		?	?						
Raspberry ketone									
Red yeast rice									
Resveratrol		?	?	?	?				
Rhodiola rosea (RR)		?	?	?	?	?			

| | Recovery | | | | | | Weight and body composition | | |
| | Short-term | | Long-term | | | | | | |
	Rehydration	Glycogen repletion	Joint, tendon, bone, and muscle health	Immunity	Endocrine support	Antioxidant protection	Muscle preservation and hypertrophy	Fat loss	Special populations
					?				🥗
							✓		
								⚠	
			?						🏋
			✓	✓				?	🏋 🏃 ♀ ⚕ 🥜
					?	?			🏃
									⛰
							?		
			?		?				🏋 🏃
			?			✓			⛰ 💧
								⚠	
	✓	✓	?						☀
				✓					♀ 🥜 ☀
						?		?	
								⚠	
		?	?	?		✓			🏋 ⚕ 💧 🥜 ⛰
								⚠	
			?						🏋
		?	?	?		✓			💧
				?					

Supplement	Fuel usage	Cardiovascular performance		Muscular performance		Neural performance		Hydration	
		Maximal aerobic capacity: Speed	Improving aerobic capacity: Endurance	Strength and power	Endurance	Focus and cognition	Motivation and motor	Fluid balance	Electrolyte balance
Riboflavin									
Ribose									
Rutaecarpine									
S-adenosyl methionine (SAMe)							?		
Salt								✓	✓
Sea buckthorn		?	?				?		
Selenium (Se)									
Sodium bicarbonate and sodium citrate		?	✓		✓				
Soy protein				?					
Spirulina		?							
Superoxide dismutase (SOD)									
Synephrine									
Tart cherry			?						
Taurine		?	?		?	?	?		
Theacrine							?		
Thiamine			?		?				
Tribulus									
Tyrosine						?			
Undenatured type II collagen (UC-II)									
Valerian									
Vanadium (V)									

| | Recovery | | | | | | Weight and body composition | | |
| Short-term | | Long-term | | | | | | | |
Rehydration	Glycogen repletion	Joint, tendon, bone, and muscle health	Immunity	Endocrine support	Antioxidant protection	Muscle preservation and hypertrophy	Fat loss	Special populations
								🏃 ♀ 🥗
		?						
							⚠	
		?						🧰
✓								☀ ⛰
		?	?	?	✓			
			?		✓			
								⛰
		✓			✓	✓		🏋 🏃 ♀ 🥗 ⛰
					?			
		?			✓			
							⚠	
		?		?	✓			♀ 🧰 ⛰
		?						💧 ☀
								🏋 🏃
				⚠			⚠	
								☀ ⛰
		?						🏋 🧰
							⚠	💧

Supplement	Fuel usage	Maximal aerobic capacity: Speed	Improving aerobic capacity: Endurance	Strength and power	Endurance	Focus and cognition	Motivation and motor	Fluid balance	Electrolyte balance
		Cardiovascular performance		**Muscular performance**		**Neural performance**		**Hydration**	
Vinpocetine						?			
Vitamin B$_{12}$									
Vitamin C									
Vitamin D		?	?	?	?				
Vitamin E									
Whey protein				✔					
Willow bark									
Withania somnifera (WS)		?		?	?	?			
Yohimbe									
Zeaxanthin									
Zinc (Zn)									
Zinc magnesium aspartate (ZMA)									

| | Recovery | | | | | | Weight and body composition | | |
| | Short-term | | Long-term | | | | | | |
	Rehydration	Glycogen repletion	Joint, tendon, bone, and muscle health	Immunity	Endocrine support	Antioxidant protection	Muscle preservation and hypertrophy	Fat loss	Special populations
						?			
			?	?		✓			
			✓	✓	✓		✓	✓	
			?	?		✓			
			✓				✓		
			?						
			?	?	?				
					?			?	
						?			
				?		✓			

PREFACE

Each year, there are a handful of athletes who defy odds and break performance barriers once believed to be impossible. In 2019, Kenyan runner Eliud Kipchoge became the first man in recorded history to break 2 hours in the marathon, a feat once deemed impossible. Although the run was not recognized as a world record because Kipchoge had pacers and received outside nutritional aid from cyclists on course, it has paved the way for other athletes to further test the limits of human performance as they experiment with their own nutrition, training, and equipment. Late Kenyan professional runner Kelvin Kiptum established himself as the men's world-record holder at the 2023 Chicago Marathon, running a blazing 2:00:35, and Kenyan runner Ruth Chepngetich became the first woman to break 2:10:00 in the marathon, establishing a new world record at the 2024 Chicago Marathon with a time of 2:09:56. At the 2024 Summer Olympics in Paris, 17 new world records were established across multiple sports, and such barriers will continue to be broken as athletes apply the latest strategies to aid human performance.

The science of training athletes has come a long way in the last 100 years. Top-level sport scientists are developing new methods of training, strategies for nutrition and supplement use, recovery protocols, and psychological tools to assist athletes in optimizing their abilities. This is in large part why performance milestones continue to be broken. This book is designed to shed light on the truths behind nutritional supplements and strategies for their use to enhance health and performance.

Chapter 1 focuses on what you—the athlete, coach, or health professional—should know about supplements. We address the history of the sport supplement industry and provide you with insight into the manufacturing practices and regulation of sport supplements. We give you the tools to assess, evaluate, and purchase supplements to fit your needs and the needs of your athletes. Common questions are addressed, especially concerning the efficacy of supplement use in sports.

Chapter 2 explores the performance variables that are often targeted by supplement industry marketing, including claims that these key performance indicators can be enhanced through supplementation with various ingredients. This chapter will give you a better understanding of how supplements might be beneficial and which areas of performance they could affect. To specifically address how a particular supplement may be ergogenic (i.e., enhance physical performance), each system is examined closely. There are also several other variables that have a profound impact on performance in sport, including hydration status, overall recovery, and body composition. Most athletes will tailor their training to focus on one or several of these performance factors depending on their specific needs.

In addition to training, athletes will often seek guidance from a sports dietitian or other health professional about nutrition strategies and supplements that may help give them a performance edge. Chapter 3 provides an alphabetical guide to some of the most popular performance-focused supplements marketed today. For each supplement, you'll find a description of the ingredient along with common supplement names and food sources, a discussion of the latest scientific research, practical applications for dosing, and, if applicable, recommended daily intake, deficiency and toxicity symptoms, and drug or supplement interactions.

As you flip through the supplement guide, you'll see that each performance variable is assigned a symbol that will serve as a quick reference tool. If a supplement has been proven to be beneficial for a particular performance variable, the supplement entry will be marked with the corresponding black symbol shown in table 3.1; if more research is needed to assess that performance variable, the entry will be marked with a gray corresponding symbol. Supplements that are applicable to special populations will also have corresponding symbols. You can also use the supplement finder located at the beginning of the book to quickly identify supplements that have demonstrated benefits based on these performance variables.

Our final chapter explores the unique nutritional challenges certain populations have to overcome in order to perform at peak and details the supplements that may help them excel. This chapter includes nutritional recommendations for the following categories of athletes:

- Master athletes
- Child and adolescent athletes
- Female athletes
- Injured athletes
- Athletes with diabetes
- Athletes with food allergies or intolerances
- Plant-based athletes
- Athletes competing in hot environments
- Athletes competing at altitude

Finally, a complete list of references and resources can be found online at https://ancillaries.humankinetics.com/DietarySupplementsInSportPerformance.

ACKNOWLEDGMENTS

When esteemed publisher Human Kinetics first approached me about taking on this project, I enthusiastically took on the monumental challenge, one that had been a prominent part of my career bucket list since becoming a registered dietitian in 2000. I will forever be grateful for this wonderful opportunity to continue to help dispel the myths and discuss the truths that exist in the nutrition and dietary supplement industry and ultimately create an important reference tool for anyone involved in the training and development of athletes.

Much like the team of people who all aid in the success of an athlete, including coaches, teammates, parents, trainers, doctors, dietitians, and others, this project could not have been accomplished without the invaluable support of several key players over the years. My undergraduate and graduate studies and athletic career at both Illinois State University and Florida State University certainly laid the groundwork for my career passion as a sports dietitian. In particular, research collaboration with professors Dr. Robert Cullen and Dr. Dale Brown as well as work on the nutrition and dietary supplement front with former team physician Dr. Bryan Barootes of Illinois State University really opened my eyes to the nutritional issues in sports and fostered my determination to help fellow athletes safely and successfully achieve peak performance. Since taking on the reins as a Registered Dietitian 25 years ago, I have been thankful for all the athletes who trusted my expertise to help them as they chased down various health and performance goals. I am thankful for the career-paving experiences and the breakthrough research my fellow sport science colleagues continue to do to help facilitate some of the mind-blowing performances that have made history in recent years. I'd also like to extend a huge amount of gratitude to my brilliant coauthors, Josh Hingst, for the thousands of hours he has put into our first edition project and Lonnie Lowery, for stepping up to help make critical updates to our second edition as well as to Korey Van Wyk, Anne Hall, and the team of editors and staff at Human Kinetics who have helped make this project a reality.

Finally, I'd like to thank my late husband, Daniel Kirby; two kids, Kaia and Kamren (aspiring athletes themselves); and family and friends for their unparalleled support, love, and encouragement to carpe diem as I have chased after my professional and athletic dreams.

—Kimberly Mueller

In 1983 my oldest sister, knowing I was enamored with my plastic-and-cement weight set, bought me a bodybuilding publication off the newsstand (back then the Internet was called magazines). She thought it was funny, but I was immediately hooked; what started as a family joke became the Big Bang of my athletic and academic career.

Forty years later, I am largely the product of that seminal passion and the friends and mentors who cultivated it. Their support led to professional and personal endeavors that necessitated the synthesis of two sometimes disparate fields—not to mention overcoming the stigma that can accompany bodybuilding. Thanks to Dr. Peter Lemon and Dr. Mike Jenkins, I received my master's degrees in exercise physiology and nutrition/dietetics, as well as my doctorate in the former and license to practice in the latter. This brought me to esteemed publishers like Human Kinetics, so I also owe many clever academic colleagues my gratitude in this regard. Admittedly, of the books, chapters, and manuscripts

"

I've coauthored, most topics—uncommon fats, antioxidants, proteins, and coffees—are too specialized for a truly broad audience. What I've long felt was really necessary was a single compendium that an athlete or coach could hold up and say, "This has our answers to all things sport supplements." This is the book you are holding in your hands. I thank editors Korey Van Wyk and Anne Hall and, of course, coauthor Kim Mueller for making this happen. Lastly, thanks in part to Rob "Fortress" Fortney, I have fond memories of placing in regional bodybuilding contests and writing for the magazines I once consumed so voraciously. No acknowledgement I could offer would be complete without The Mighty Fortress.

Now, as a bit of a veteran in more ways than one—to which my aching joints and former university students can attest—I have enormous gratitude for the family that started, and tolerated, all of this. Perhaps most importantly, I thank my mom, Gloria Whetstone, for her unwavering belief in me, and my brilliant and tolerant wife, Kelly Lowery, for doing things to support my obsession that few spouses would.

—Lonnie Lowery

Understanding Supplements and Functional Foods

Balanced, whole food nutrition is the most important factor in fueling athletic performance. However, when every second faster and every ounce stronger counts, an athlete will often do everything possible to gain that competitive edge, from using specialized gear to the latest in sport nutrition. This innate drive to succeed combined with an interest in filling nutritional gaps and maintaining overall health and wellness has made the dietary supplement industry one of the fastest-growing markets worldwide, with revenues in the United States topping off near 55 million in 2024 with expectations of growth to nearly 77 million by 2030 (United States Dietary Supplements Market Size and Outlook, 2025).

As officially defined in the Dietary Supplement Health and Education Act of 1994, a dietary supplement is a pill, capsule, tablet, powder, or liquid intended to supplement the whole food diet by providing any combination of the following nutritional ingredients: vitamins; minerals; herbs or other botanicals (excluding tobacco); amino acids; a dietary substance used to increase total dietary intake (such as carbohydrate and protein); and a concentrate, metabolite, constituent, or extract. Many sport nutritional supplements are advertised as increasing testosterone levels in the body, thereby enhancing the ability to build lean body mass (similar to anabolic steroids). Other nutritional supplements are marketed as improving energy levels or speeding postworkout recovery. There are supplements whose labels claim they facilitate body fat and weight loss, which is especially alluring to athletes competing in sports where physique is spotlighted, such as dance and gymnastics. Unlike steroids, however, which are only available in the United States with a doctor's prescription, nutritional supplements can be purchased over the counter, and they are subject to relatively scant regulations about their effectiveness and safety. With the growing popularity of nutritional supplements has come an alarming increase in the number of athletes, both amateur and professional, testing positive for banned substances, raising ethical and safety concerns. Despite the potential risks, data indicate that some 70% to 90% of collegiate and Olympic-level athletes take at least one supplement (Burns et al., 2004; Froiland et al., 2004). For this reason, it is important to be an educated consumer when using nutritional or sport supplements to enhance health and performance.

The need for consumer education extends to functional foods, which have a variety of definitions but can be described as foods that claim to extend a benefit beyond nutrition, generally as it relates to health or disease prevention, by modifying the farming of the whole food or by adding ingredients during manufacturing. Functional foods essentially offer hard-to-get dietary substances (either in type or in amount), such as phytochemicals, omega-3 fatty acids, prebiotics, probiotics, and protein, with few changes in eating habits. From a marketing standpoint, these foods capitalize on the desire to efficiently access health- or performance-enhancing nutrients though can further blur the line between whole food nutrition and dietary supplement. Athletes focusing on their training programs or with limited education of nutrition are a target market for functional foods.

This chapter will provide an in-depth look at the evolution and use of dietary supplements in sports; discuss the legalities and regulations that affect the supplement industry; and explain the keys to being an informed consumer, including safety considerations, important supplement resources, and how to read supplement labels.

Nutrition, Dietary Supplements, Functional Foods, and Performance: A Historical Perspective

As sport scientist Ronald Maughan (2001) puts it, "Without proper nutrition, the full potential of the athlete will not be realized, because performance will not be at its peak, training levels may not be sustained, recovery from injury will be slower, and the athlete may be more susceptible to injury and infection." It is well known that certain nutrients, specifically carbohydrates, fats, proteins, vitamins, minerals, and water, are essential for health and sport performance. Further, nonessential food ingredients such as peptides and phytochemicals are broadly recognized as beneficial to health. Even myconutrients (compounds from medicinal mushrooms) are getting scientific attention. The idea that various ingredients in food could enhance physical stature, health, and athletic performance is not a modern phenomenon; rather, it dates back over 4,000 years. The ancient Greeks were at the forefront of sport nutrition as they sought to optimize athletic prowess during competition. Warriors of the time were reported to use such foods as deer liver and lion heart, hoping that consumption would produce bravery, speed, or strength. Although in its infancy, the concept of ergogenic (performance-enhancing) nutrients and the sport nutrition market was beginning to bloom.

In modern times, the topic of sport nutrition has continued to evolve, with health researchers and food scientists working overtime to define and isolate nutrients that could enhance various metabolic reactions important to health and athletic performance. Current research continues to build on these nutritional discoveries and further refine the correct dosing, form, and timing of administration of each nutrient to help athletes maximize their health and performance potential.

Vitamin and Mineral Supplementation

At the forefront of the discovery of vitamins and minerals was the ancient Greek physician Hippocrates, who once stated, "Let food be thy medicine and medicine be thy food." These famous words served as a launching point for a series of research studies evaluating the impact of food ingredients on the prevention of debilitating diseases such as scurvy, which is estimated to have afflicted millions of prisoners, slaves, soldiers, orphans, and sailors over several hundred years before Doctor James Lind discovered in the mid-1700s that a diet rich in citrus juices—later known to be rich in vitamin C—helped combat the disease. Nearly 200 years later, in 1912, the term vitamin was officially coined by Polish biochemist Casmir Funk, who discovered that thiamine helped correct symptoms of beriberi, a nervous system disease caused by a thiamine deficiency in the diet.

Over the next 30 years, a total of 13 vitamins, 9 water soluble and 4 fat soluble, were isolated and named along with their associated deficiency conditions. Along with 7 major minerals and 10 trace minerals, these vitamins are known as micronutrients, or substances considered essential for health and protection against deficiency symptoms. A useful metaphor is to think of micronutrients as "metabolic spark plugs"—not the fuel itself, but a component that helps the human body to use the fuel. Beyond playing an important role in energy production, hemoglobin synthesis, maintenance of bone health, immune function, and protection of the body against oxidative damage, micronutrients assist with synthesis and repair of muscle tissue during recovery from exercise and injury. See table 1.1 for descriptions and examples of the micronutrients.

TABLE 1.1 Micronutrients

	Water-soluble vitamins	Fat-soluble vitamins	Major minerals	Trace minerals
Description	Requires the presence of water for absorption; are differently stored than fat soluble nutrients in the body, making daily intake essential. Important for energy production and antioxidant effects.	Stored within fat throughout the body and are slower to excrete from the body, making toxicity symptoms possible when supplementing with megadoses. Important for eye, skin, and bone health as well as antioxidant effects.	Needed in relatively large quantities (>100 mg daily) to form bone structure, aid enzyme function, allow muscle contraction, and balance body fluids.	Needed in small quantities to aid enzyme function, carry oxygen, serve as antioxidants, aid immune system function, and support reproduction.
Examples	B_1 (thiamine) B_2 (riboflavin) B_3 (niacin) B_5 (pantothenic acid) B_6 (pyridoxine) B_7 (biotin) B_9 (folic acid) B_{12} (cobalamin) C (ascorbic acid)	A (retinol) D (calciferol) E (tocopherol) K_1 (phylloquinone)	Calcium Chloride Magnesium Phosphorus Potassium Sodium	Iron Zinc Manganese Copper Fluoride Molybdenum Iodine Chromium Selenium

The importance of micronutrients in protection against deficiency symptoms and debilitating disease led the United States Food and Nutrition Board to establish the Recommended Dietary Allowances (RDAs) in 1941. The purpose of the RDAs is to define the daily intake level of nutrients, including vitamins and minerals, considered sufficient to meet the requirements of nearly all (97%-98%) healthy individuals in each life stage and gender group. There is still debate, however, as to whether the RDAs are sufficient to support the increased metabolic demands of an athlete. Intense exercise, in particular, can accelerate the turnover and loss of micronutrients from the body, thus suggesting increased requirements may be necessary to support building, repair, and maintenance of lean body mass in athletes.

As early as the late 1930s, vitamin and mineral supplements were being used in athletics, with front-of-the-pack Tour de France cyclists reporting that they rode better after taking supplements. In fact, the multivitamin and multimineral supplement, introduced in the 1940s, has remained one of the most commonly used supplements by athletes. Although a multivitamin can certainly serve as nutritional insurance for an athlete in combination with a balanced whole food diet, research has failed to support the correlation between supplementation and enhanced performance. The only exception is when a known dietary or blood nutrient deficiency presents itself.

Athletes at greatest risk for poor vitamin and mineral status and who may benefit from vitamin and mineral supplementation include those who restrict energy intake or follow extreme weight-loss regimens, those who eliminate one or more of the major food groups from their diet, those with food allergies or nutrient absorption issues, those completing an extraordinarily high volume of training, and those who eat mostly processed foods.

Carbohydrate Supplementation

In the 1920s, after noting that low blood glucose levels were associated with symptoms of fatigue, stupor, and inability to concentrate (collectively known as bonking), scientists started to explore the idea that carbohydrate supplementation could enhance performance. During the 1925 Boston Marathon, for instance, it was discovered that athletes who ate a high-carbohydrate diet in the 24 hours leading up to the race and who supplemented with hard candy immediately prior to and during the race were able to maintain better blood sugar levels thereby avoiding bonking, and run faster thanks to more carbohydrate fuel left in the glycogen tank. This precipitated a series of studies further evaluating the role of carbohydrate in exercise, especially in endurance performance.

In the 1960s Swedish researchers demonstrated that consumption of a high-carbohydrate diet during endurance training improved performance (Ahlborg et al., 1967). In addition, it was found that carbohydrate supplementation during exercise helped delay the onset of muscle fatigue associated with depleted muscle glycogen stores, also known as hitting the wall. To determine the optimal amount of carbohydrate needed to maximize glycogen stores, researchers manipulated the dietary carbohydrate intake of athletes in the week leading up to endurance performance. Physiologist Gunvar Ahlborg introduced the concept of glycogen supercompensation, also known as carbo-loading, which became a mainstay practice among endurance athletes in the 1970s. It continues to be used by athletes such as football, basketball, soccer, and hockey players, who participate in sports where the duration of high-intensity play can increase the risk for glycogen depletion and consequent performance decline.

The Ahlborg, or classic, method of carbo-loading entails an athlete training to exhaustion to deplete glycogen stores 1 week prior to race day and then ingesting a low-carbohydrate diet for 2 to 5 days before increasing carbohydrate intake to 70% to 85% of total caloric intake, often upward of 600 g (2,400 calories), for 1 or 2 days to facilitate glycogen supercompensation. However, this method of carbo-loading left many athletes feeling irritable and unmotivated during the depletion phase and bloated with water weight and sluggish during the loading phase. The depletion phase is now discounted by health professionals. Current carbo-loading techniques instruct athletes to follow an appropriate taper by consuming 45% to 65% of their calorie intake from carbohydrates starting 2 to 3 weeks out from race day. The final 72 hours precompetition constitute the loading phase, with athletes increasing dietary intake of carbohydrate by approximately 25%, or to a level equivalent to 3.6 to 5.5 g of carbohydrate/lb (8-12 g of carbohydrate/kg) of body weight.

Continued identification of the benefits of carbohydrate supplementation on muscle and liver glycogen stores and consequent performance during high- and low-intensity exercise inspired the creation of sport drinks; the first known sport nutrition product, Gatorade, was developed by researchers at the University of Florida in 1965 to help the performance of the Florida Gators football team. Gatorade, a mixture of glucose and sucrose in water at approximately a 6% solution, is essentially responsible for the profitable sport beverage and food market today, which includes products such as energy gels (Hammer Gel, Powergel, Gu), energy chews (Clif Bloks, Honey Stingers), and energy bars (Bonk Breaker, PureFit, PowerBar).

Current research continues to evaluate the effects of carbohydrate on exercise, with attention focused on the effects of different types and combinations of carbohydrates on carbohydrate absorption and consequent muscle performance during exercise.

Protein Supplementation

Since ancient times, proteins and their building blocks, amino acids, have been consumed to support vigorous training and enhance athletic performance. It was once reported that the legendary Greek wrestler Milo of Croton ate upward of 20 lb (9.1 kg) of meat daily to support his training regimen. Though on the excessive end of the spectrum, it is true that higher protein intakes help increase the free pool of amino acids essential for protein synthesis. Still, the perceived value of dietary protein in sport has fluctuated over time. Over the mid-1800s to the early 1900s, it became clear that protein was not a preferred fuel source during exercise and as a result, interest in the study of protein metabolism in exercise waned for decades to follow. According to noted sports nutrition researcher Peter Lemon, this led to the "over-sweeping generalization that dietary protein was not important for exercising individuals, which resulted in little interest and study of protein metabolism with exercise over the next 30 years or so" (Lemon, 2012). It was not until the 1970s, with more modern laboratory techniques such as metabolic tracers, that an understanding emerged regarding the central role of dietary protein and its component amino acids in the overall metabolic response to exercise.

A total of 20 amino acids combine in various ways to help develop muscles, bone, tendons, skin, hair, and other tissues as well as aid nutrient transportation and enzyme production. Of these, 9 are essential or indispensable, meaning they must be obtained through the diet, and 11 are nonessential or dispensable, meaning they can be synthesized by the body from other metabolism products.

As early as 1930, scientists worked to understand protein quality. This led to the development of biological value (BV), a measure of the amount of protein from food that becomes incorporated into the proteins of the body. Early work identified the egg as the gold standard of protein quality with a BV of 100. Since that time, more modern methods such as the protein digestibility-corrected amino acid score (PDCAS) and, more recently, the digestible indispensable amino acid score (DIAAS) have largely replaced BV in human nutrition. Although protein needs are slightly to moderately higher for athletes versus nonathletes, some athletes have taken these needs to extremes, consuming excessive amounts of protein daily and increasing the demand for protein supplements.

Essential (Indispensable) Amino Acids

- Isoleucine
- Leucine
- Lysine
- Methionine
- Phenylalanine
- Threonine
- Tryptophan
- Valine

Nonessential (Dispensable) Amino Acids

- Alanine
- Arginine
- Asparagine
- Aspartic acid
- Cysteine
- Glutamic acid
- Glutamine
- Glycine
- Histidine
- Proline
- Serine
- Tyrosine

The evolution of protein supplements began in the 1930s when a young pharmacist named Eugene Schiff developed a method of processing whey from milk for human consumption. Decades later, it was scientifically established that supplemental protein could facilitate increases in muscle mass and gains in strength, which led to the popularity of protein powders, including the whey protein created by Schiff. Bob Hoffman, who is considered the father of American weightlifting, referred to protein powder as a secret weapon for the athletes he trained for the 1954 World Weightlifting Championships. When scientific interest progressed and protein supplements became more readily available, particularly after the 1970s, strength athletes and bodybuilders became more interested in not just protein supplements but increased intake through consumption of such protein-rich foods as beef, eggs, chicken, fish, dairy foods, soybeans, nuts, and legumes.

Although the current RDA for protein intake is 0.36 g/lb (0.8 g/kg) of body weight for the average American, there is conflicting evidence regarding the optimal dose for athletes. Since early work on the subject in the 1970s and 1980s by the likes of Peter Lemon and Gail Butterfield, it has been known that additional protein and essential amino acids, in conjunction with an energy-sufficient diet, are critical for muscle growth, especially during the early stages of a strength-training program. It is also known that protein oxidation accelerates during cardiovascular exercise, thereby rationalizing increased protein consumption by strength and endurance-oriented athletes. Consequently, leaders from the American College of Sports Medicine (ACSM), American Dietetic Association (ADA), and Dietitians of Canada (DOC) essentially doubled the daily protein recommendations for athletes. Endurance-focused athletes, such as runners, cyclists, and triathletes, were instructed to aim for a daily intake of 1.2 to 1.4 g/kg (0.54-0.63 g/lb) of body weight; strength-focused athletes, such as football players, target a range of 1.2 to 1.7 g/kg (0.54-0.77 g/lb) of body weight. Protein intake above these recommendations, especially at the expense of other valuable macronutrients such as carbohydrates, healthy fats, and nutrient-dense fruits and vegetables, can jeopardize an athlete's performance instead of enhance it.

Because most athletes in Western countries consume plenty of protein from whole food intake, supplementation is often not necessary. However, supplements can be more practical in some settings to ensure athletes are getting adequate high-quality proteins before, during, or after exercise. In addition, there are special populations of athletes for whom protein supplementation is warranted. For example, athletes following vegetarian or vegan diets may benefit from supplemental protein due to the relatively lower quality and digestibility of plant protein sources, with factors such as fiber reducing protein absorption by as much as 10%. Supplemental protein may also help preserve muscle mass in athletes who are restricting calories or trying to lose weight.

Herbal and Botanical Supplementation

Herbals, which are derived from the leaves, bark, berries, roots, gums, seeds, stems, or flowers of plants and are rich in naturally occurring substances called phytochemicals (known to have physiologic effects), have been used to enhance health and performance for over 4,000 years. In China and Japan, for example, warriors, wrestlers, and other athletes were documented as using a variety of raw herbal concoctions and teas to help improve endurance and strength. In 200 AD, an herbal practitioner by the name of Galen created the first classification system that paired common illnesses with their associated herbal remedies, laying the groundwork for the use of herbals in the pharmaceutical world. In fact, several current medications are merely extracts of traditional herbs. Today, herbals can be consumed in teas, tinctures, energy drinks, pills, and capsules, as well as applied topically. A number of herbal constituents (phytochemicals), including the broad class of polyphenols, also appear in functional foods.

It is estimated that 1 out of 5 athletes uses some form of herbal supplement, often consumed via sport drinks or foods. For example, one of the biggest sellers worldwide is ginseng, which is believed to have anabolic qualities among other ergogenic or adaptogenic traits. Herbal supplements and functional foods that contain herbal ingredients are often marketed to help increase energy, enhance blood flow, hasten recovery, produce fat loss, promote muscle growth, or trigger other physiological or metabolic responses important for exercise performance. The body of research supporting such beneficial qualities is currently still being developed.

Some countries, including Germany, regulate herbals like medicine; the United States currently regulates most herbal supplements as dietary supplements under the Dietary Supplement Health and Education Act. As a result, safety data collection and appropriate risk assessments have not been conducted on most herbal ingredients. This reality magnifies the importance of being an educated consumer when choosing to pair whole food intake with herbal supplements.

Supplement and Functional Food Trends for the Future

Over the past century, there has been tremendous progress in our understanding of how and why various food ingredients and dietary supplements aid health and physical performance. Perhaps of greatest relevance to athletes was the introduction of sport-specific food products such as energy gels, chews, bars, sport drinks, protein powders, and recovery shakes designed to address a wide variety of performance-limiting factors, including psychomotor fatigue, muscle cramping, glycogen depletion, suboptimal muscle growth, and underrecovery. The increase in university sport nutrition programs has helped generate more studies that not only continue to evaluate how to combat limiting performance factors through proper dosing and timing of intake. Such studies have also evaluated ingredient and supplement pairings for enhanced uptake and use and gender differences in sports nutrition needs. For example, endurance athletes now can consume sports drinks that offer more than one type of sugar to enhance the uptake of carbohydrate into the muscles, thereby further delaying the onset of muscle fatigue associated with glycogen depletion. Creatine is now often offered in coordination with carbohydrate to enhance absorption. The increase in data collection on female athletes has led to the arrival of female-specific products that consider female physiology, hormonal fluxes, and recovery needs.

In response to the dramatic increase in the number of athletes competing in endurance and ultraendurance events such as marathons, ultramarathons, and Ironman triathlons, a wave of new ingredient blends and products geared specifically toward these athletes has emerged. Of course, women's involvement in strength sports is also a rising trend, bringing a newer demographic to the attention of bodybuilding and powerlifting marketers. Customization is also a hot trend; companies such as Infinit Nutrition (www.infinitnutrition. us) and YouBar (www.youbars.com) allow users to custom-blend ingredients to create products such as sport drinks, protein shakes, and energy bars specifically catering to an athlete's unique health, training needs, and performance goals.

Another emerging field of study is nutrigenomics, which evaluates how individual genetic differences can affect the way we respond to nutrients and other naturally occurring compounds in the foods we eat. Researchers at Kansas State University published an article exploring the role of specific nutrients in gene expression and how nutrients may affect the progression of disease as well as human performance (Getz, Adhikari, & Medeiros, 2010). It's believed by some that in the next 5 to 10 years, we will be able to visit our physicians to determine our genetic makeup and work with nutritional professionals to customize our diets based on our unique physiological needs and goals. Indeed, this concept is now increasingly referred to as precision nutrition.

Researchers have also pointed out that colonic microbiota may have a more significant impact than even genetics regarding certain aspects of physical fitness. Watch for functional foods from coffees to yogurts to snack bars to protein drinks that contain pre- and probiotics (the former feeding specific populations of healthy gut bacteria such as bifidobacteria, and the latter being live organisms an athlete might ingest with the hopes of influencing their specific microbiotic "fingerprint"). These pre- and probiotic manipulations and their influence in the body beyond the gut are of interest to scientists and athletes alike.

In line with the new wave of thinking that inflammation may be at the root of many health issues, a multitude of anti-inflammatory ingredients (generally extracts from plants like polyphenols and food ingredients such as uncommon lipids) are being marketed for disease protection as well as athletic recovery. For example, in the 2012 Olympic Games, several groups of athletes took 4 oz (0.12 L) of tart cherry juice twice daily to help counter inflammation and aid recovery. Other polyphenols include those from coffee extracts, blueberries, grapes, green tea, grapefruit, onions, and many others. These compounds, although not known for high bioavailability, interact with the gut microbiome and appear to act indirectly on inflammation. Omega-3 fatty acids and fish oils continue to be touted as strong anti-inflammatories—and not without substantial supporting research—and are among the most commonly used supplements. Continue to watch this trend grow over the next decade.

Prevalence of Supplement Use

Dietary supplement use continues to be widespread among U.S. adults aged 20 and over. The National Health and Nutrition Examination Survey (Centers for Disease Control and Prevention, National Center for Health Statistics, 2011) reported that between 2005 and 2008, more than 50% of the U.S. population used at least one dietary supplement, including multivitamins, minerals, and herbs, and the multivitamin and multimineral supplement was the top choice among consumers. More recently, according to the National Center for Health Statistics: "During 2017–2018, 57.6% of adults aged 20 and over reported using any dietary supplement in the past 30 days. A higher percentage of women (63.8%) reported dietary supplement use than men (50.8%). For both sexes, dietary supplement use increased with age" (Mishra et al., 2021). Dietary supplements are often perceived as quick fixes for poor lifestyle choices, including imbalanced nutrition, lack of exercise, and deficient sleep patterns. Although exercise may not be a problem for most athletes, there still remains a perception that dietary supplementation can help offset the consequences of a diet rich in nutritionally empty foods.

With a growing number of athletes using dietary supplements, many sport governing bodies are laying down ground rules to minimize health and safety risks to athletes, maintain ethical standards, and reduce liability risks. For example, the Iowa High School Athletic Association discourages school personnel, including coaches, from supplying, recommending, or permitting the use of any drug, medication, or food supplement solely for performance-enhancing purposes. Even so, in an unpublished survey of their student-athletes in grades 9 through 12, it was discovered that 96% were taking some form of supplement, with the most popular being vitamin supplements, energy-enhancing products (e.g., Red Bull), meal replacement bars and shakes, creatine (males only), and weight-loss products (females only). Friends, coaches, and parents were identified as top sources of information; doctors and registered dietitians surprisingly failed to be mentioned.

Similar results have been seen among college-aged athletes as well as professional athletes. Data have long indicated that some 80% to 90% of collegiate athletes are using some type of sports supplement (Burns et al., 2004; Froiland et al., 2004). Female athletes commonly report using multivitamins, calcium, and vitamin D supplements, whereas males typically use amino acid and protein supplements. Interestingly, at the Olympic level, recent reports have shown the use of dietary supplements dropped by 8% from 2002 to 2009 (Heikkinen et al., 2011), perhaps as a result of many athletes being stripped of their medals by the International Olympic Committee (IOC) after being testing positive for banned substances. At the professional level, surveys taken at the Olympic Games revealed 69% of athletes in Atlanta and 74% at the Sydney Games were using sport supplements, though subsequent reports suggested decreasing numbers among this population of athletes, perhaps due to concern about supplement purity (Heikkinen et al., 2011; Huang, Johnson, & Pipe, 2006). Most recently, in 2023, Myoenzono and colleagues reported data on athletes who participated in the Tokyo 2020 and Beijing 2022 Olympic and Paralympic Games. The values were fairly consistent with past data, finding that approximately 70% of Tokyo 2020 Olympians and Paralympians, 70% of Beijing 2022 Olympians, and approximately 50% of Beijing 2022 Paralympians used supplements.

It's impossible to ignore the prevalence of dietary supplement use in athletics. Thus, it's important for athletes, coaches, and sport performance professionals to be educated on how supplements are regulated and what to look for in a dietary supplement. It's also important for them to find resources providing credible evidence to support the benefits of a sports supplement.

Regulation of Dietary Supplements

Dietary supplemnents are regulated but there has been a history of confusion regarding this. According to the medical advisor for Consumer Reports, Dr. Orly Avitzur (as reported by CNN Health in 2011), "There is a false perception that supplements fall under the same regulatory umbrella as prescription drugs." In actuality, dietary supplements are treated much like foods in the United States. Although a proposed law, the Nutrition Advertising Coordination Act of 1991 would have allowed harsher penalties for making unsubstantiated drug claims on supplement labels and made it illegal to advertise nutritional or therapeutic claims on supplement labels, the health food industry not surprisingly responded with pushback over fears of revenue loss. It did not pass, and instead the regulatory power of the FDA and the Federal Trade Commission (FTC) over supplements was further limited under President Clinton with the signing of the Dietary Supplement Health and Education Act (DSHEA) in 1994.

Although many consumers had expressed concern about the possible loss of freedom to purchase dietary supplements, the results of several surveys interestingly reveal that most want just what the Nutrition Advertising Coordination Act intended: increased consumer protection. They want the government to review safety data and approve dietary supplements prior to sale. They want the government to verify all health-related claims before they can be included in advertisements and on product labels. However, the DSHEA passed instead, allowing the dietary supplement industry to turn into one of the most profitable in the world, especially with the increased availability of Internet and online mass marketing through social media. As of the time of this writing, the controversy continues. In 2024, the FDA's Deputy Commissioner lamented few barriers to entry into the dietary supplement market, a statement that brought quick rebuttal from the National Products Association.

Today the regulation of dietary supplements is truly at a crossroads, although supplement industry leaders and the FDA continue to battle. The FDA is invested in protecting consumers from fraudulent marketing and potential health risks associated with ingestion of any supplement ingredient, including those not listed on the label. The supplement industry resists more stringent regulation by the FDA, especially as it relates to safety, which would have a negative impact on profit margins. Many believe that the freedom of the consumer to access potential health- and performance-enhancing ingredients would be limited by mandatory FDA testing of all new ingredients prior to their market release. Although dietary supplements should continue to be available to consumers, most health professionals believe the purity and safety of the ingredients need to be established first.

Concerns regarding supplement safety escalated to an all-time high after the FDA's struggles to ban ephedra despite its several reported adverse side effects, including death. In direct response, the Dietary Supplement and Nonprescription Drug Consumer Protection Act was enacted in 2006, serving as a stepping stone in the right direction in regard to supplement safety. Under this Act, manufacturers of dietary supplements and nonprescription drugs are required to notify the FDA about serious adverse events related to their products, including deaths, life-threatening experiences, inpatient hospitalizations, persistent or significant disability or incapacity, birth defects, and the need for medical intervention to prevent any such problems. In addition, a telephone number or address is required on product labels so consumers can contact the manufacturer as needed.

In 2011, FDA dietary supplements chief Dan Fabricant introduced the framework for new dietary ingredients (NDI), defined as any dietary ingredient that was not sold in the United States as a dietary supplement before October 15, 1994. With the FDA's NDI notice, specific safety information for any dietary supplement containing a new dietary ingredient is required from the manufacturer prior to marketing. Although safety information is yet to be required in advance for older dietary supplement ingredients, manufacturers still have to report any adverse effects to the FDA. Much like the increased regulatory suggestions made by the FDA in the early 1990s, the introduction of the NDI notice stirred quite a bit of controversy, with dietary supplement industry leaders once again claiming that any gain of regulatory power by the FDA would be catastrophic, stifling new product development and threatening scores of products already on the market. This is likely not true, but such regulation will help ensure that the scores of new ingredients being discovered get a safety stamp of approval prior to being released to the marketplace. Readers interested in how dietary supplements interact with the Food Safety Modernization Act (FSMA) can find public information at www.fda.gov/food/food-safety-modernization-act-fsma/frequently-asked-questions-fsma.

Understanding Supplement Risks

As a result of the comparatively lax regulation of dietary supplements, athletes, coaches, and parents of athletes should understand the following risks associated with dietary supplement use.

Purity

Athletes often believe that because dietary supplements can be purchased at a store or over the Internet, they must be pure. Unfortunately, this is often untrue. Although the FDA has established quality standards for dietary supplements to help ensure their identity, purity, strength, and composition, there are many manufacturing facilities that have yet to be inspected by the FDA. As a result, athletes should be aware that some dietary supplements may list inaccurate quantities of active ingredients on the label as well as possibly contain ingredients not included on their labels.

From October 2000 until November 2001, the International Olympic Committee investigated 634 nonhormonal nutritional supplements (e.g., vitamins, minerals, proteins, creatine) obtained from 215 suppliers; the investigation found 15% to be contaminated with banned substances, mainly steroidal substances or prohormones, that were not listed on the product labels and would have caused a user to fail a doping test (Geyer et al., 2004). A 2007 investigation of over 60 dietary supplements discovered 12.5% contained banned substances not declared on the labels, specifically anabolic steroids and ephedrine (Martello, Felli, & Chiarotti, 2007). Additionally, a popular nutritional supplement for weight loss was found to contain the beta2-agonist clenbuterol, which is banned by both the World Anti-Doping Agency (WADA) and the NCAA (Geyer et al., 2008). Finally, a 2011 investigation by the California firm Anti-Doping Research revealed that 10 products purchased from the popular online store Amazon contained illegal steroids that are known to have dangerous side effects such as liver toxicity (William Reed Business Media, 2011). These cases demonstrate how easily an athlete may become the victim of inadvertent doping, exposing themselves to both health risk and potential legal and personal consequences.

Readers may also remember seven-time Tour de France champion, Lance Armstrong's history of performance-enhancing drug use coming to light in 2012, a charge that led not only to Armstrong being stripped of all his titles from 1998 on, but also to a lifetime ban from competition in all sports that follow the WADA code. A ban from sport is a legitimate risk for any athlete choosing to use a banned drug or unregulated substance during a competitive season.

Fortunately, several independent organizations, including U.S. Pharmacopeia, ConsumerLab.com, NSF International, and Natural Products Association, offer quality testing that assures the product was properly manufactured, contains the ingredients listed on the supplement label, and is devoid of harmful levels of contaminants. Athletes choosing to add dietary supplements to their performance regimen should look for these stamps of approval, though they should also be aware that such approvals do not guarantee the safety or effectiveness of the product.

Safety

It is a common misconception that if a substance is natural, it must be safe and beneficial. However, dietary supplements, including herbals and such hormones as DHEA and melatonin, can be marketed and introduced on store shelves before manufacturers are even required to submit safety information to the FDA, which essentially leaves the consumer blind when it comes to potential health risks. Although the FDA does issue warning letters and take other actions, without immediate, up-front access to safety information, they must follow up or otherwise compile information regarding adverse events, product sampling, studies in scientific literature, and other sources of evidence in an attempt to regulate the safety of dietary supplements. It is impossible for the FDA to keep up with the thousands of existing and new dietary supplements readily available in health stores, through sales reps, and on the Internet; thus, the safety of untested dietary supplements must be questioned.

Furthermore, supplement safety may be in question as a result of mislabeling. In 2010 an herbal weight-loss supplement was found to contain fenfluramine, a stimulant drug withdrawn from the U.S. market in 1997 after studies demonstrated that it caused serious heart valve damage; other potentially harmful pharmaceutical ingredients were also absent from the product label. Weight-loss supplements have frequently been on the safety hot seat. In 2004, as a result of adverse health effects such as heart attacks, strokes, and death, the FDA banned ephedrine alkaloids that were marketed for purposes other than asthma, colds, or allergies. Unfortunately, the ban was enacted after many consumers had already experienced the consequences of ephedrine toxicity.

Athletes should be aware that dietary supplements often contain active ingredients that can exert strong effects on the body and are likely to cause some side effects, especially when used as a replacement for or in combination with prescribed medications. In addition, contaminants such as heavy metals, pesticides, and microbiological toxins found within some dietary or herbal supplements are legitimate risks to the overall health of an athlete. For example, in 2019 Stanford researchers found lead in turmeric sourced from Bangladesh; lead is a neurotoxin that can cause lethargy, abdominal pain, nausea, headaches, and in serious cases seizure and coma. Cadmium, hexavalent chromium, mercury, and arsenic are often seen in herbal supplements outsourced from China, where the soil, water, and air run a greater risk of being contaminated by these metals.

Unproven Claims

Supplement companies may make claims about their products without supporting scientific evidence as long as they do not claim to prevent, treat, cure, or mitigate disease. These often take the form of structure and function claims such as "May help support a healthy [blank]." Distributors of sports supplements have the ultimate leeway because claims are generally associated with some performance variable rather than a disease state. Often, the primary support for an ergogenic claim is testimonial rather than science based. Furthermore, it is not uncommon to find advertisements suggesting that all athletes, including those consuming a well-balanced diet, are at risk for nutritional deficiencies. This is a stretch from the truth. Even when science is involved, the research study design could be poor, the number of subjects small, the statistical analyses lenient, or the research funded by a company involved with the dietary supplement, making any valid indication of proof of claim questionable. (Again, the FDA does issue warning letters against bogus claims as they become aware of them. These can be found at www.fda.gov/food/compliance-enforcement-food/warning-letters-related-food-beverages-and-dietary-supplements.) In any case, athletes and coaches should always approach supplement claims with skepticism and remember the old adage, "If it sounds too good to be true, it probably is."

Tips for Being a Supplement-Savvy Athlete

The battle for regulatory power is likely to be an ongoing one, but the hope for the future is a dietary supplement industry that provides more scientific rather than testimonial evidence for the claims being made, and more importantly, one that requires independent testing from a third party to ensure the purity and safety of the ingredients for consumers. In the meantime, the following sections offer advice for coaches, athletes, parents, and health professionals on how to be proactive and educated consumers by researching the legitimacy of claims as well as any reported risks associated with the ingredients in the supplement.

Talk With Your Health Care Provider

A single online search of dietary supplements will lead to a plethora of information, often conflicting and usually generated by unqualified parties. A trip to the gym may lead to a sales pitch, because many fitness professionals are pressured to meet a sales quota for a gym's supplement line or are merely looking for additional income through supplement sales. There are even supplement companies that offer free nutrition coaching clinics, but these are fancy ploys for their sales reps to sell products. Thus, it is important to be extremely selective about where and from whom you are gathering information. Athletes are encouraged to speak to a health care provider such as a doctor or pharmacist to establish potential risks and benefits prior to using any dietary supplements. This is especially important for athletes with pending surgeries.

For more detailed nutrition and dietary supplement advice, athletes should speak with a registered dietitian (RD), who typically possesses a bachelor's or master's degree, has completed a 6- to 12-month dietetic internship, and has successfully passed a national examination. A registered dietitian can help customize a menu plan designed to meet the nutritional demands of training and competition. The RD can also help determine the safety and efficacy of dietary supplement use by

- assessing the athlete's nutritional status to determine the likelihood of vitamin or mineral deficiency;
- evaluating the potential benefit or harm of nutrient supplementation given the athlete's nutritional and health status;
- evaluating the safety of a supplement given the form, dose, and potential for interaction with food, other dietary supplements, and over-the-counter and prescription medications;
- educating athletes as to the potential benefit of receiving nutrients through conventional and fortified foods;

- recommending nutrient supplementation when food intake is inadequate;
- evaluating research alongside scientists regarding nutrient supplementation; and
- being aware of regulatory, legal, and ethical issues involved in recommending and selling nutrient supplements.

Fortunately, it is estimated that over 50% of university athletic departments as well as professional and amateur athletic teams either have an RD on-site or contract out with one. Many of these professional RDs are members of the Collegiate and Professional Sports Dietitians Association (CPSDA), have completed a dual degree in exercise physiology or sport nutrition (a very rigorous approach), have personal experience in sport that may help provide some perspective, or are board-certified specialists in sport dietetics (CSSD). The CPSDA has coined the term sports RD to identify those dietitians working in professional, collegiate, amateur, and military performance settings. The Commission on Dietetic Registration developed a certification in sport dietetics to identify RDs with documented practical experience and successful completion of an examination in sport nutrition. Because of sports RDs' involvement in these settings and experience in working with sports supplements, they are generally the best source for information, aside from university exercise physiology or sports nutrition departments. For those wishing to pursue access, a list of sport-minded registered dietitians in the United States can be found at www.scandpg.org/search-rd.

Find Reputable Resources

All parties involved with an athlete, including the athlete themselves, should be aware of the resources available for reliable information about supplements. Table 1.2 provides a quick reference guide of credible websites for information on important issues involving dietary supplements.

Choose Supplements That Have Undergone Third-Party Testing

Training the body for peak performance is not something that happens overnight. Athletes spend hours each day preparing for competition, and coaches and families spend equal amounts of time in support of an athlete's performance endeavors. The last thing anyone wants holding them back is a failed drug test caused by a contaminated dietary supplement. Thus, any athlete thinking about using a dietary supplement should make sure it has undergone independent testing by a third-party lab.

NSF, a global, independent public health organization whose goal is to protect human health and safety, is considered the gold standard of third-party testing. NSF wrote the only accredited American National Standard (NSF/ANSI 173) that verifies the health and safety of dietary supplements. NSF Certified for Sport (www.nsfsport.com), which is recognized by the National Football League (NFL), National Football League Players Association (NFLPA), Major League Baseball (MLB), Major League Baseball Players Association (MLBPA), Professional Golfers' Association (PGA), Ladies Professional Golf Association (LPGA), and the Canadian Center for Ethics in Sports (CCES), ensure that participating sports supplement manufacturers provide confirmation of substance content and purity, compliance with regulations, and assessment of public safety and environmental concerns

TABLE 1.2 Online Resources for Dietary Supplements

Purity of dietary supplements	For the general public: ConsumerLab, www.consumerlab.com U.S. Pharmacopeia (USP), www.usp.org
	For athletes: NSF Certified for Sport Program, www.nsf.org Informed Choice, www.informed-choice.org Informed Sport, www.informed-sport.com
Safety of dietary supplements and ingredients	National Institutes of Health Office of Dietary Supplements https://ods.od.nih.gov/
Dietary supplement regulation	Food and Drug Administration, www.fda.gov Federal Trade Commission, www.ftc.gov Council for Responsible Nutrition (CRN), www.crnusa.org Natural Products Association (NPA), www.npainfo.org
Nutrition and dietary supplement information	Office of Dietary Supplements (NIH), http://ods.od.nih.gov Academy of Nutrition and Dietetics, www.eatright.org The International Society of Sports Nutrition (ISSN), www.sportsnutritionsociety.org Australian Institute of Sport (AIS), www.ausport.gov.au/nutrition Gatorade Sports Science Institute, www.gssiweb.com Sports, Cardiovascular, and Wellness Nutritionists (SCAN), https://www.scandpg.org/new-dpg-launch Sports Oracle, www.sportsoracle.com USADA Supplement Connect, www.usada.org/athletes/substances/supplement-connect/ National Council Against Health Fraud (NCAHF), https://quackwatch.org/ncahf/
Drug testing and banned substances lists	National Collegiate Athletic Association (NCAA), www.ncaa.org United States Anti-Doping Agency (USADA), www.usada.org World Anti-Doping Agency (WADA), www.wada-ama.org
Reading supplement labels	Council for Responsible Nutrition, https://www.crnusa.org/
Research	Pub Med, https://pubmed.ncbi.nlm.nih.gov/ Sport Science, www.sportsci.org *Journal of the International Society of Sports Nutrition*, www.jissn.com *International Journal of Sport Nutrition and Exercise Metabolism*, http://journals.humankinetics.com/IJSNEM *Journal of Dietary Supplements*, https://www.tandfonline.com/journals/ijds20

for products used by athletes. A link to NSF-approved supplements can be found in the References and Resources file online. Sports supplements must undergo rigorous testing and inspection to verify compliance with NSF/ANSI Standard 173, including

- label claim review (confirms the label matches contents);
- toxicology review (certifies formulation);
- contaminant review (checks for undeclared ingredients or contaminants in the product); and
- facility audits (biannual good manufacturing practices audits at the manufacturing facility, plus an on-site inspection to check for banned substances).

With the increased concern regarding athletes testing positive for banned substances, it is likely more third-party testing programs will exist in the future. Moreover, it is the hope that the products of all supplement companies will someday be mandated to undergo such testing prior to becoming available to consumers. According to USADA, in order for third-party testing to be credible, it should

- be free from conflicts of interest,
- have external accreditations,
- conduct an audit of the supplement company based on good manufacturing practices established by the US Food and Drug Administration (FDA),
- evaluate the dietary supplement for overall safety and quality, and
- have a validated and accredited method to test for prohibited substances.

Refer to table 1.2 for a list of resources of information on reputable third-party testing.

Choose Supplements That Have Scientific Evidence of Results

Although the purity of a dietary supplement can be established through independent testing, the efficacy of supplement claims cannot, which is why it is important to opt for dietary supplements that have evidence of results from well-controlled and replicated scientific research. This can be efficiently done by searching online for position statements published by the International Society of Sports Nutrition (ISSN).

UNDERSTANDING RESEARCH STUDIES

Although there are numerous scientific studies available, the majority provide less than valid results due to either poor study design or the small number of subjects. Therefore, when evaluating research associated with dietary supplements, it is important to keep in mind the following definitions:

- **Experimental versus observational studies.** Experimental studies compare an intervention group to a control group, allowing for cause-and-effect conclusions. (Ideally the groups are treated identically except for the nutrition or training intervention, making it the cause of any changes.) In contrast, observational studies are typically limited to correlations (relatedness between preexisting variables) that lack the causal conclusions of experimental trials. The value of observational or epidemiological studies is that they can examine great numbers of participants and suggest hypotheses for future experimental models (preclinical or clinical).

- **Double-blind.** In this type of clinical study, both the subjects participating and the researchers are unaware of when the experimental medication or procedure has been given or followed.

- **Placebo-controlled.** In this method of research, an inactive substance (placebo) is given to the control group, and the treatment being tested (e.g., dietary supplement) is given to the experimental group. The results obtained from the two groups are then compared to see if the treatment being tested is more effective than the placebo. When conducted as a double-blind study, this type of research is considered the gold standard of clinical research.

- **Randomized control trial (RCT).** This is a study in which subjects are selected according to relevant characteristics and then randomly assigned to either an experimental group or a control group.

- **Preclinical studies.** Often research begins in vitro ("in a dish") or in animal models. Not only do such models allow for greater control than when examining free-living persons, they may be the only ethical way to answer key questions. They can also provide pilot data that can help human researchers properly "power" a study with an appropriate number of subjects.

- **Clinical trial.** This is an experimental study with human subjects. Gold-standard clinical trials are double-blind, placebo-controlled studies that use random assignment of subjects to experimental or control groups.

- **Internal and external validity.** Internal validity is the degree to which researchers are measuring what they intend to measure, using appropriate methodology and conclusions. External validity refers to how well the findings from a sample of subjects extrapolate to the overall population of interest.

- **Large number of subjects.** In general, the larger the number of subjects, the more reproducible the research results (increased statistical power).

- Replicated research. When results of a study have been replicated, they gain more clout.

- **Statistical significance.** Typically, a result is considered statistically significant when it has a p-value (probability value) of less than 5% ($p < 0.05$), which means that the result would occur by chance less than 5% of the time . This is a probability standard used by many researchers. However, more statistically compelling levels of significance are $p < 0.01$ and $p < 0.001$, meaning the result would occur by chance less than 1% of the time.

- **Conflicts of interest.** One ethical challenge in research is to account for any bias that may occur as a result of pressure on investigators to produce significant findings for a commercial funding source. This is often done with a disclosure statement in abstracts, posters, and manuscripts, allowing the reader to take such knowledge into account.

Learn How to Read Supplement Labels

The dietary supplement label (see figure 1.1) lists essential information about the product in the bottle. Prior to using any supplement, it is critical to always read the label and follow directions for use.

How to read a supplement facts label

Dietary supplements are required by law to feature a supplement facts label. If a product is missing supplement facts or any other required label information, the product is subject to enforcement by FDA and could be deemed as misbranded.

1. Supplement facts is the name given to the nutrition information panel of a dietary supplement product.

2. Serving size is the manufacturer's suggested serving expressed in the appropriate unit (tablet, capsule, softgel, packet, teaspoonful, etc.).

3. Servings Per Container tells the net content of the dietary supplement.

4. Amount per serving heads the listing of dietary ingredients in the supplement and the quantity of each.

5. Percent daily value (DV) tells what percentage of the recommended daily intake for each nutrient is contained in each serving. The DVs are for adults and children ages 4 and up, unless otherwise indicated.

6. All dietary ingredients contained in the supplement are identified by their common or usual name. A dietary ingredient can be a vitamin, mineral, botanical, amino acid, or other dietary substance, as well as a concentrate, metabolite, constituent, extract, or combination of any of the above.

7. The amount of dietary ingredient in each serving is declared in metric units. Milligram (mg) and microgram (mcg) are common units.

8. A symbol, such as an asterisk, placed under the % Daily Value heading indicates that the Daily Value has not been established for that dietary ingredient.

9. A footnote contains explanations for symbols, such as the asterisk, placed under the % Daily Value heading. Explanations may include "Daily Value not established."

10. The list of all ingredients in the supplement, including any ingredient that is the source of a dietary ingredient, in decreasing order by weight.

www.crnusa.org

[1] Supplement Facts

[2] Serving Size 1 Tablet
[3] Servings Per Container 100

	[4] Amount Per Serving	[5] % Daily Value
Vitamin A (50% as beta-carotene)	900 mg	100%
[6] Vitamin C	[7] 250 mg	278%
Vitamin D	20 mcg	100%
Vitamin E	75 mg	500%
Vitamin K	120 mcg	100%
Thiamin	1.2 mg	100%
Riboflavin	1.3 mg	100%
Niacin	16 mg	100%
Vitamin B6	1.7 mg	100%
Folate	400 mcg DFE (240 mcg folic acid)	100%
Vitamin B12	2.4 mcg	100%
Biotin	30 mcg	100%
Pantothenic Acid	5 mg	100%
Choline	550 mg	100%
Calcium	260 mg	20%
Iron	18 mg	100%
Phosphorus	250 mg	20%
Iodine	150 mcg	100%
Magnesium	210 mg	50%
Zinc	11 mg	100%
Selenium	25 mcg	45%
Copper	0.9 mg	100%
Boron	150 mcg	[8] *

[9] * Daily Value not established.

[10] Other Ingredients: Choline bitartrate, calcium carbonate, ascorbic acid, dicalcium phosphate, magnesium oxide, microcrystalline cellulose, dl-alpha tocopherol acetate, ferrous fumarate, niacinamide, zinc oxide, magnesium stearate, d-calcium pantothenate, vitamin A acetate, pyridoxine hydrochloride, potassium iodide, boron citrate, phylloquinone, thiamin mononitrate, copper sulfate, d-biotin, sodium selenate, cholecalciferol, and cyanocobalamin

FIGURE 1.1 Before choosing a supplement, it's important to understand the information on the supplement label.

Used with permission from the Council for Responsible Nutrition, www.crnusa.org.

Know How to Report Fraudulent Supplements or Adverse Reactions

Any athlete who experiences an adverse reaction to a dietary supplement should immediately contact their health care provider, then report the problem directly to the FDA by calling the FDA's MedWatch hotline at 1-800-FDA-1088 or submitting a report by fax to 1-800-FDA-0178.

DANGERS OF SUPPLEMENT CONTAMINATION

Olympic swimming hopeful Jessica Hardy tested positive in 2008 for the banned substance clenbuterol, later discovered to be the result of a contaminated supplement she was taking leading up to the Beijing Olympic Games. Although unknowingly taking the banned substance, Hardy was still required to serve a one-year suspension and missed the Beijing Olympics. She was allowed to compete in the 2012 London Games, where she earned a bronze medal in the 4 × 100 m freestyle relay and a gold medal in the 4 × 100 m medley relay. Hardy's situation should bring awareness to the risks associated with sports supplements.

Summary

Over the past 100+ years, many nutritional ingredients have been found to play vital roles in health, well-being, and performance. The year 2012 marked the 100th anniversary of the official coining of the term vitamin, with Casmir Funk leading the way through his discovery of the B vitamin thiamine. Soon after, vitamin supplements made their way into athletics based on the idea that they might enhance performance. In the 1920s scientists determined that inadequate carbohydrate intake was associated with an inability to concentrate as well as premature muscle fatigue, leading to the theory that carbohydrate supplementation may help enhance performance. In the 1930s protein supplements were introduced and later became popular among weightlifters when it was scientifically established that supplemental protein could facilitate increases in muscle mass and gains in strength. There has also been interest in herbals, which have been used to enhance health and performance for over 4,000 years in Asian culture. However, the full benefits of supplementation with nutritional ingredients have yet to be proven, with much of the research still in its infancy. Even so, several recent surveys of athletes demonstrate a majority use at least one supplement ingredient for performance or health purposes.

Unfortunately, a legitimate risk to an athlete is a failed doping test caused by contaminated nutritional supplements, despite ongoing efforts to improve regulatory and manufacturing guidelines. Reviews of supplements available online have revealed that some products are laced with steroids and stimulants, which are prohibited for use in sports. Although it has been suggested that athletes avoid dietary supplements altogether, this approach is unrealistic and unnecessary. There are a variety of legitimate reasons for an athlete to use supplements in coordination with a well-balanced diet. Furthermore, over the past decade, there has been an influx of data from clinical trials demonstrating a variety of health and performance benefits with the use of certain dietary supplements. Fortunately, more supplement manufacturers are having their products rigorously tested by third-party testing facilities to minimize risks, although it is important to question whether these watchdog groups have conflicts of interest of their own.

Athletes choosing to pair their performance diet with dietary supplements are encouraged not only to choose supplements that are tested by facilities such as NSF, but also to speak to a doctor, pharmacist, exercise physiologist, or registered dietitian about supplements prior to use. Lastly, in instances of adverse events or contamination, athletes should contact organizations such as the FTC and FDA, as well as the Better Business Bureau (BBB) and National Council Against Health Fraud (NCAHF).

2

Keys to Peak Performance

Tapping into athletic potential and unlocking the door to peak performance require a dedicated focus on a myriad of cardiovascular, muscular, psychological, and health-centered variables that are largely influenced by smart physical training and proper nutrition. To gain a competitive advantage, athletes often go beyond whole food nutrition and use dietary supplements marketed to address specific components of performance, such as muscle strength or endurance. The purpose of this chapter is to discuss the science behind these performance variables and how they may be affected by popular dietary supplements.

Each performance variable discussed in this chapter, including related subcomponents, is assigned a symbol in table 3.1 on page 40 that will serve as a quick reference tool in the A-to-Z supplement guide presented in chapter 3.

Fuel Usage

Watch an image of an athlete in motion, and it is easy to see how dynamic the human body is. Each intricate movement is driven by billions of microscopic units, each with its unique function, fueled by a molecule called adenosine triphosphate (ATP). The human body carries enough ATP within the muscles (~100 g) to support 1 to 4 seconds of intense activity before needing to tap into its triple-line system of energy production to fuel sport performance (see table 2.1). All lines of the energy system work together, yet the intensity of sport activity dictates the proportion of energy supplied by each (see figure 2.1).

ATP-Phosphocreatine Energy System

The smallest fuel tank, called the ATP-phosphocreatine (ATP-PC) or alactic energy system, operates without oxygen and uses phosphocreatine (PC) in the muscles to generate ATP for 5 to 10 seconds of explosive activity, making it a commonly used and important fuel system for athletes engaged in sports that incorporate quick, all-out bursts of energy (e.g., jumping, sprinting, blocking). Because creatine is stored in limited capacity (~120 g), creatine supplements have become popular among power- and speed-oriented athletes wanting to enhance performance.

TABLE 2.1 Primary Metabolic Demands of Various Sports

Sport	ATP-Phosphocreatine Energy System	Anaerobic-Lactate Energy System	Aerobic Energy System
Baseball	High	Low	—
Basketball	High	Moderate to high	—
Boxing	High	High	Moderate
Diving	High	Low	—
Fencing	High	Moderate	—
Field events	High	—	—
Field hockey	High	Moderate	Moderate
Football (American)	High	Moderate	Low
Gymnastics	High	Moderate	—
Golf	High	—	—
Ice hockey	High	Moderate	Moderate
Lacrosse	High	Moderate	Moderate
Marathon	Low	Low	High
Mixed martial arts	High	High	Moderate
Powerlifting	High	Low	Low
Skiing:			
Cross-country	Low	Low	High
Downhill	High	High	Moderate
Soccer	High	Moderate	Moderate
Strength competitions	High	Moderate to high	Low
Swimming:			
Short distance	High	Moderate	—
Long distance	--		High
Tennis	High	Moderate	—
Track (athletics):			
Short distance	High	Moderate	—
Long distance	--	Moderate	High
Ultraendurance events	Low	Low	High
Volleyball	High	Moderate	—
Wrestling	High	High	Moderate
Weightlifting	High	Low	Low

Note: All types of metabolism are involved to some extent in all activities.

Reprinted by permission from N.A. Ratamess, "Adaptations to Anaerobic Training Programs," in *Essentials of Strength Training and Conditioning*, 3rd ed., by National Strength and Conditioning Association, edited by T.R. Baechle (Human Kinetics, 2008), 95.

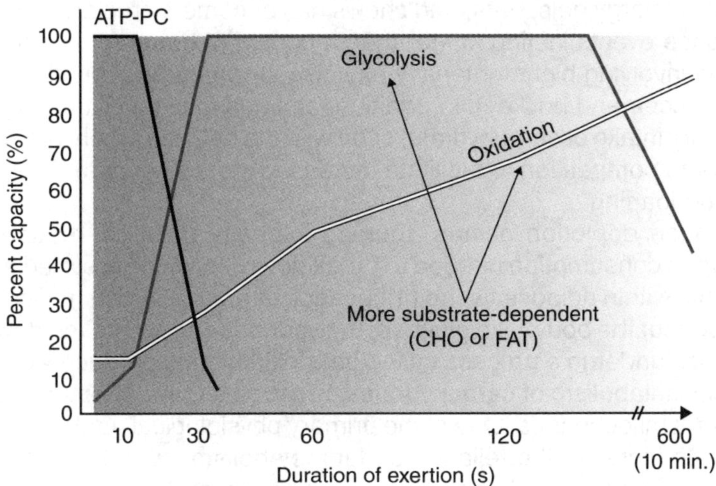

FIGURE 2.1   Anaerobic-aerobic exercise spectrum.

* Grey shading indicates primarily anaerobic capacity; percentages vary by training status.

Adapted from McArdle et al. (2015); Lowery et al. (2023).

Anaerobic-Lactate Energy System

More sustained, moderate- to high-intensity efforts lasting up to 3 minutes (e.g., 800 m dash) or repeated explosive periods of activity (e.g., boxing) rely on the midsize fuel tank, called the anaerobic-lactate (or lactic acid) energy system. Without an immediate need for oxygen, this system quickly breaks down glucose (carbohydrate) into pyruvic acid through a series of enzymatic reactions to help generate ATP. This metabolic process is called anaerobic or fast glycolysis; it results in the formation of fatigue-inducing hydrogen ions that impair muscle contraction through a number of mechanisms. Several popular supplements claim to buffer hydrogen ions, thus helping protect against premature muscle fatigue caused by acidosis, allowing an athlete to perform longer with greater power and speed.

Aerobic Energy System

The final and largest energy tank, called the aerobic energy system, breaks down carbohydrates (stored in the body as glycogen), fats, and at times protein in the presence of oxygen to more slowly generate a plentiful amount of ATP; it plays an important role during endurance sport activity as well as aiding recovery between periods of heightened exertion (e.g., interval training). Unlike anaerobic metabolism, where hydrogen ions can build up and potentially limit performance, the byproducts of aerobic metabolism, carbon dioxide and water, are easily disposed of through respiration, making it easier to sustain an aerobic effort for a longer time.

During aerobic metabolism, glucose (carbohydrate), stored as glycogen in limited amounts within the liver and muscles, is broken down via glycolysis. This is the same pathway seen in anaerobic (fast) glycolysis but is slower and coupled to the Krebs cycle and electron transport chain. The human body is capable of storing enough carbohydrate energy to fuel up to 2 hours of moderate- to high-intensity training before depletion is inevitable, and the onset of low blood sugar and muscle fatigue ensue (known as bonking or hitting the wall). This is why the use of carbohydrate supplementation from sources like sport drinks, energy gels, bars, and chews has become a crucial practice for athletes during endurance events lasting longer than a couple of hours (e.g., marathon) as well as team sports involving higher-intensity exercise for prolonged durations (e.g., basketball, football, soccer, and hockey). In addition, athletes may taper training volume while increasing dietary intake of carbohydrate, often with the help of carbohydrate supplements, for 3 days prior to competition to facilitate increased storage of carbohydrate, a practice known as carbo-loading.

When glycogen depletion occurs, training intensity must be reduced to facilitate increased oxygen consumption needed to break down fat, which is stored as triglycerides in large amounts within adipose tissue (thousands of grams) and in muscular oil droplets (~300 g) throughout the body. Like glucose, triglycerides can be broken down to form free fatty acids, which undergo a process called beta-oxidation to produce ATP. This process, like the aerobic metabolism of carbohydrates, is coupled to the Krebs cycle and electron transport chain in mitochondria. One of the primary physiological goals of an aerobic training program is to increase the reliance on fat metabolism, even when generating more power or speed, thus helping to spare glycogen stores and extend endurance. Several nutritional ingredients, including caffeine, have been explored for their potential role in boosting fat metabolism.

As the last-resort source of energy, protein can be broken down into amino acids (building blocks of protein), deaminated, and converted into either glucose or other metabolic intermediates to generate ATP. Although most aerobic activity uses minimal amounts of protein for energy, during times of low glycogen availability, such as in the later stages of an ultraendurance event, protein can contribute as much as 18% of total energy requirements, thus having implications for recovery. This is one reason protein supplementation has been researched as a plausible addition to intense or high-volume training regimens. The use of protein supplements before, during, and after training has been explored by sports scientists for the purpose of sparing muscle glycogen, thereby enhancing endurance performance, stimulating protein synthesis, preventing protein breakdown, and aiding recovery from sport activity.

Cardiovascular Performance

All athletes, regardless of sport, depend on the ability of the heart, blood vessels, and lungs to supply oxygen and energy to working muscles. During training and competition, these demands grow, causing the heart to beat more rapidly and with greater force, the rate of blood flowing through the heart and to the muscles to increase up to 20-fold, and the lungs to fill up with more oxygen-rich air. Cardiovascular performance is limited by the ability to keep up with these increased demands and, more specifically, the body's ability to consume oxygen. The need for oxygen is dependent on two key physiological parameters: (1) maximal aerobic capacity and (2) anaerobic threshold.

Maximal Aerobic Capacity: Speed

Maximal aerobic capacity, also known as $\dot{V}O_2$max, is defined as the highest rate of oxygen consumption attainable during exhaustive exercise. This rate is supported by the maximum pumping capacity of the heart as well as the ability of the muscles to resist fatigue.

Because the body ultimately requires oxygen to convert food into energy, the ability to consume large amounts of oxygen facilitates increased energy production for enhanced speed and endurance. Therefore, having a high $\dot{V}O_2$max is like being equipped with the powerful engine of a race car, making it an important performance variable for endurance sports such as the triathlon, cycling, rowing, distance running, cross-country skiing, and swimming as well as team sports requiring endurance such as soccer, basketball, and hockey.

$\dot{V}O_2$max is often expressed as an absolute rate in liters of oxygen per minute (for example, to obtain caloric expenditure) but is more accurately represented as milliliters of oxygen per kilogram of body weight per minute, especially when evaluating differences between men and women. Values of aerobic capacity vary greatly between individuals and even between athletes competing in the same sport as a result of sex and body composition differences as well as other factors such as genetics, age, and training status. For example, male athletes tend to have $\dot{V}O_2$max values 15% to 30% higher than female athletes, in part due to differences in body composition. Depending on baseline fitness, physical training can boost aerobic capacity by as much as 20%. Genetics alone has been shown to account for 25% to 50% of the variance in $\dot{V}O_2$max seen between individuals.

$\dot{V}O_2$max numbers typically range between 2.5 and 6.0 L/minute—or 25 and 94 mL/kg/minute—with untrained females and trained elite male endurance athletes falling on the low and high end of the spectrum, respectively. The highest $\dot{V}O_2$max ever recorded was by elite male Nordic skier Bjorn Daehlie at 94 mL/kg/minute, which towers over the average athlete's $\dot{V}O_2$max by 30% to 40%. The highest $\dot{V}O_2$max recorded for a female was by U.S. cross country runner Joan Benoit Samuelson with a measured $\dot{V}O_2$max of 78.6 mL/kg/minute. Table 2.2 displays the aerobic capacities of athletic groups based on sex.

$\dot{V}O_2$max is affected by altitude. Even after allowing for full acclimatization, athletes living, training, or competing at an altitude of sea level to 5,000 feet (1,524 m) should expect about a 5% to 7% loss in aerobic capacity when they travel to higher elevations: for every 1,000 feet (305 m) of elevation gain above 5,000 feet (1,524 m), expect a 2% drop.

Improving Aerobic Capacity: Endurance

Athletes wanting to improve maximal aerobic capacity should focus on increasing the rate of oxygen delivery to and consequent uptake by the muscles. It is well known that training has a profound impact on both. Recently, several nutritional ingredients and supplements, often marketed as oxygen enhancers, have shown promise in providing additional benefit. Research evaluating the impact various nutritional ingredients have on oxygen consumption, both via delivery and uptake, generally looks at one or several of the following five variables:

1. Cardiac output
2. Blood volume
3. Hemoglobin
4. Mitochondrial density and enzyme levels
5. Capillary density

TABLE 2.2 $\dot{V}O_2$max (mL/kg/minute) in Various Athletic Groups

Sport	Age (years)	Males	Females
Baseball/softball	18-32	48-56	52-57
Basketball	18-30	40-60	43-60
Canoeing	22-28	55-67	48-52
Cycling	18-26	62-74	47-57
Football	20-36	42-60	—
Gymnastics	18-22	52-58	36-50
Ice hockey	10-30	50-63	—
Jockey	20-40	50-60	—
Orienteering	20-60	47-53	46-60
Racquetball	20-35	55-62	50-60
Rowing	20-35	60-72	58-65
Skiing, alpine	18-30	57-68	50-55
Skiing, Nordic	20-28	65-94	60-77
Ski jumping	18-24	58-63	—
Soccer	22-28	54-64	50-60
Speed skating	18-24	56-73	44-55
Swimming	10-25	50-70	40-60
Track and field, discus	22-30	42-55	—
Track and field, running	18-39 40-75	60-85 40-60	50-75 35-60
Track and field, shot put	22-30	40-46	—
Volleyball	18-22	—	40-56
Weightlifting	20-30	38-52	—
Wrestling	20-30	52-65	—

Adapted by permission from W.L Kenney, J.H. Wilmore and D.L. Costill, *Physiology of Sport and Exercise*, 6th ed. (Human Kinetics, 2016).

Cardiac Output

During exertion, an athlete's heart becomes a powerful pump, allowing for more blood, oxygen, and nutrients to be delivered to the working muscles and aiding the elimination of carbon dioxide and other metabolic waste products that can exacerbate muscle fatigue and negatively affect performance. The actual amount of blood pumped by the heart each minute is known as cardiac output and is influenced by both stroke volume (the amount of blood that the heart pumps each time it beats) and heart rate (the number of times the heart beats in a minute). At rest, cardiac output for adults averages about 5 to 8 L/minute, but for elite-level endurance athletes competing in cross-country skiing, this can increase to an amazing 40 L/minute.

NUTRITION AND CARDIAC OUTPUT

Following a healthy diet that is low in saturated fats and rich in whole grains, fruits, and vegetables can help protect against plaque buildup in the arteries, which leads to blockages and restricted blood flow and negatively affects cardiac output. In addition, several ingredients, such as nitric oxide (found in beetroot), can help dilate the blood vessels and allow for greater blood flow to the working muscles during exercise.

Blood Volume

Defined as the total volume of fluid that circulates through the heart, arteries, and capillaries, including red blood cells, white blood cells, and plasma, blood volume is closely regulated by the kidneys. A boost in blood volume, naturally seen with physical training and further enhanced with heat and altitude acclimatization, occurs as a result of increases in antidiuretic hormones, aldosterone, and the plasma protein albumin. The primary benefits are enhanced oxygen transport abilities and consequent improvements in endurance performance and muscle recovery. A typical adult maintains a blood volume of 4.7 to 5.0 L, with levels slightly lower for women. An elite-level endurance athlete may have blood levels as much as 30% higher than those of the average adult.

BANNED SUBSTANCE ALERT

EPO (erythropoietin) and some plasma expanders, which help boost blood volume and red blood cell production, are prohibited substances in athletic competitions worldwide. Testing positive would immediately disqualify the athlete and lead to a temporary ban from competition.

Hemoglobin

Hemoglobin is a protein in red blood cells that carries oxygen. Healthy levels fall between 13.8 and 17.2 g/dL for men and between 12.1 and 15.1 g/dL for women. Slightly lower levels in athletes, especially those engaged in endurance training and competition, are common and generally are caused by sport anemia, or pseudoanemia, which occurs when the expansion of plasma volume resulting from aerobic training reduces the concentration of red blood cells that carry hemoglobin. Despite a reduced concentration of red blood cells, the rise in plasma volume actually aids oxygen delivery to the muscles to some extent. Levels significantly lower than the norm, however, may indicate excessive fluid intake or a nutritional deficiency in iron, folate, vitamin B12, or vitamin B6, all of which can negatively affect cardiovascular performance.

Mitochondrial Density and Enzyme Levels

Deep inside muscle fibers are microscopic structures called mitochondria, also known as powerhouses due to the role they play in energy production. The number of mitochondria present within the muscle, or mitochondrial density, increases in response to calcium ion levels rising during muscle contraction and ATP levels failing to keep up with demands in skeletal muscle cells during exercise. Training, especially endurance-focused activity, not only helps to improve mitochondrial density but also facilitates an increased number of oxidative enzymes available to break down glucose, fat molecules, and certain amino acids to produce ATP for muscle contraction and other cellular functions. This adaptation in trained muscle allows for more fats to be used to generate ATP, thereby helping to spare muscle glycogen, critical for reaching peak endurance potential.

Capillary Density

Improving capillary density, the number of tiny blood vessels within each muscle, aids the distribution of oxygen- and nutrient-rich blood to the muscles; doing so also aids the clearance of lactate from the fast-twitch (type IIa and type IIb) muscle fibers and into the slow-twitch (type I) muscle fibers and the liver, thereby reducing muscle fatigue, aiding muscle recovery, and maximizing endurance potential.

Anaerobic Capacity

Thought to be a better predictor of performance than aerobic capacity, anaerobic capacity refers to the ability of an athlete to sustain a submaximal level of work with limited amounts of oxygen. Anaerobic capacity is a relevant performance variable for stop-and-go sports requiring intense bursts of energy (e.g., soccer, basketball, football, tennis, boxing, and hockey); it also applies to certain styles of weightlifting when the goal is to keep the time between sets as short as possible. It becomes a relevant factor for endurance athletes competing in events such as cycling or running races where a response to an opponent's attack needs to be quickly countered (e.g., sprint to the finish line).

During anaerobic activity, which involves rapid contraction of fast-twitch muscle fibers, the demand for oxygen and fuel exceeds the rate of supply, triggering a shift of focus from aerobic to anaerobic metabolism. For the first 10 to 20 seconds of anaerobic activity, energy is generated from stored ATP and the ATP-PC energy system; beyond that, muscle glycogen breakdown and fast glycolysis provide additional energy. Unlike the aerobic fuel tank, however, whose energy supply can last hours, the faster but limited anaerobic fuel tank can only supply enough energy for physical exertions lasting up to a few minutes before the fuel runs out or clearance of byproducts, specifically lactate, fails to keep up with their production, a state known as anaerobic threshold (AT).

Recreational athletes typically hit their AT near 65% to 80% of their $\dot{V}O_2max$, whereas elite and world-class endurance athletes may peak near 85% to 95% of their $\dot{V}O_2max$. This allows professional athletes to hold a strong pace for longer distances, such as the marathon.

NUTRITION AND ANAEROBIC CAPACITY

There are several dietary supplements that have demonstrated promise in aiding anaerobic capacity, including creatine, which helps build total body creatine stores, and buffering agents such as bicarbonate, phosphate, and more recently beta-alanine. These ingredients can help increase cellular and blood pH by countering the effects of hydrogen ion accumulation and consequent muscle fatigue during high-intensity training and competition.

Improving Anaerobic Capacity

To improve anaerobic capacity, an athlete should focus on increasing (1) the amounts of ATP and PC on hand, (2) the amount of glycogen available for breakdown, and (3) lactate shuttling and clearance ability of the muscle. These can be achieved through incorporation of interval training (e.g., 100 m sprint repeats) into any exercise or training program. Such high-intensity efforts help improve the activity of glycolytic enzymes such as hexokinase (HK) and phosphofructokinase (PFK), which are important for better muscle-force generation and sustained contractions during exertion.

Muscular Performance

Many sports require an athlete to be explosive and powerful. Athletes are required to accelerate and decelerate rapidly, change direction quickly and efficiently, jump maximally, swing or throw as hard as possible, and maintain this maximal performance for an extended period. Strength, power, and endurance are key variables that can influence an athlete's ability to perform all of these tasks.

Strength and Power

Muscle strength can be defined as the maximal amount of force (newtons, N) that a muscle or muscle group can generate. It is not to be confused with muscle power (watts, N-m/s), which is derived from force and the speed or velocity at which force can be generated. A common misconception is the idea that the strongest athlete will be the fastest or most explosive. Although this is not the case, it is true that a physically stronger athlete will be a faster and more explosive athlete. Therefore, developing strength is an essential performance variable. Many athletes engage in structured weight-training programs in the off-season to maximize strength before the competitive season begins.

Power is the ability to generate force quickly. As the speed of movement increases, the amount of force that the muscle is capable of producing decreases, and vice versa—thus maximal force is produced at slower speeds. This is the disconnect between strength and power. Strength and power are developed through physiological and neurological changes to the motor unit. Through training, the entire muscle can increase in size, including the cross-sectional area of the muscle and the density of muscle fibers within. A larger, denser muscle results in an improvement in strength and power. These changes are largely influenced by the endocrine system. During exercise, a cascade of hormonal events takes place, with stress and catabolic hormones increasing to meet the demands of training. These hormones—cortisol, epinephrine, and norepinephrine—break down carbohydrate, fat, and protein stores; they also act on the nervous system to increase motor unit and muscle fiber recruitment. Activation of more motor units, and consequently more muscle fibers, will increase the number of active fibers contributing to the development of muscle contraction and force. Build-up of these catabolic hormones is followed by a response of anabolic hormones, including testosterone, growth hormone, and IGF-1 (insulin-like growth factor 1), which act on the muscle to initiate or otherwise enhance anabolic and recovery responses. Anabolic hormones and nutrients spark increases in the rates of protein synthesis, or muscle building. This process of creating a larger, denser muscle, known as hypertrophy, elicits improvements in the muscle's strength and power capabilities. Hypertrophy is related to body composition that will be discussed in more detail later in the chapter.

A common misconception is that the only way to have stronger and more powerful muscles is for them to get bigger; in fact, a significant portion of changes in strength and power are actually the result of neurological changes. Each muscle in the body is made up of thousands of muscle fibers and several motor units (nerves and the muscle fibers they innervate). The speed at which these motor units are activated, the number of muscle fibers innervated within each motor unit, and the synchronization of motor units within the same muscle and other muscles working together all affect muscle performance. Some of the neurological changes that take place through training include the following:

- An increase in the number of muscle fibers that contract simultaneously. Based on neurological signals, one's brain recruits and activates more muscle fibers to contract. By applying resistance and requiring the muscle to develop more force, the body will adapt neurologically and signal more muscle fibers to contract.

- Increase in the rate of contraction of muscle fibers. The faster the muscle is able to contract and develop force, the more power it will produce.

- Improved efficiency and synchronization of firing muscle fibers. Through adaptation to training, the muscle fibers become more efficient and operate in sync.

- Decreased inhibition of antagonistic muscle fibers. During a leg extension where the quadriceps are the primary moving muscle, for example, the hamstrings contract and inhibit leg extension. Training lessens this degree of inhibition.

- Improved efficiency of stretch reflexes controlling muscle tension. The muscles are like a rubber band: The farther they are stretched, the faster and more forcefully they contract in the opposite direction. It's not just passive tension—this stretch reflex can be trained, improving its efficiency and the amount of force and speed at which muscle fibers contract.

- Improved conduction velocity and excitation threshold of nerve fibers. This involves the speed at which neural signals activate motor units and the amount of muscle fibers activated with each signal.

A muscle performance icon will be used in chapter 3 to identify certain sports supplements that target improving these neurological functions and produce gains in power and strength.

Endurance

Athletes who engage in sports requiring repetitive periods of maximal or submaximal effort—such as sprinting to defend a goal, sliding defensively in a basketball game, resisting an opponent in a wrestling match, or even performing as many curl-ups or push-ups as possible within a fixed amount of time—require muscular endurance. An athlete's ability to sprint repeatedly during a football game or soccer match requires metabolic efficiency and fitness. Athletes must be capable of clearing the fatigue-inducing byproducts of high-intensity muscle contraction, such as hydrogen ions, during recovery sessions and rest periods. In addition, athletes require a well-trained neuromuscular system that is capable of resisting fatigue and maintaining muscular force and power. Because lowered muscle glycogen levels negatively affect the neuromuscular system, athletes in endurance sports must maximize glycogen before competition and prevent its depletion during competition to ensure peak performance. Dietary supplements such as caffeine and the amino acids taurine and tyrosine are thought to prevent neuromuscular fatigue and improve endurance.

Psychometric Neural Performance

When evaluating the dynamics of sport performance, the focus is often on the cardio-vascular and muscular systems. Yet it's the athlete's brain that acts as the control center for many of the processes that propel performance, making it an essential component of athletic success. Feeding the brain with specific nutrients and supplements can help enhance alertness, reaction time, balance, dexterity, focus, memory, visual acuity, speed, strength, endurance, mood, and motivation. If we simply define "neural" as the measurement of such central nervous system-related characteristics, we can investigate whether nutrients or products have an impact in this broad category. For example, some supplements with purported memory and cognitive-enhancing effects contain an ingredient known as citicoline (CDP choline), which itself contains a combination of cytidine and choline. Choline has a role in the production of acetylcholine, an important neurotransmitter that affects the peripheral nervous system (muscle contraction) and the central nervous system (arousal and sensory perception). Other dietary supplements such as Ginkgo biloba also claim to improve cognitive performance. The mechanisms of ginkgo are less understood but may involve a neural protective effect on the central nervous system. Tyrosine, which is a nonessential amino acid, may also affect the central nervous system and the brain's perception of fatigue and motivation. For sports requiring a high level of hand–eye coordination and quick decision making, including baseball, basketball, and tennis, these types of supplements are appealing and potentially offer a competitive advantage.

Hydration

When it comes to performance decline in athletes, dehydration—defined as the excessive loss of body fluid, including both water and electrolytes—is a common culprit. With 60% to 70% of total body mass and 70% to 75% of muscle mass comprising fluid, it is not hard to understand why. Because disruptions can alter physical performance by reducing blood volume, decreasing skin blood flow, decreasing heat dissipation, increasing core body temperature, and increasing the rate of muscle glycogen use, maintenance of fluid balance is key to optimal functioning. A mere 2% loss of body weight can start to negatively affect performance with such symptoms as cessation of sweating, muscle cramps, nausea, vomiting, lightheadedness, weakness, heart palpitations, and decreased urine output, with urine color a dark yellow to burnt orange.

Armstrong and colleagues (1985) evaluated the impact dehydration has on athletic performance and found that just a 1% change in body mass correlated with adding 0.17, 0.39, and 1.59 minutes to 1,500, 5,000, and 10,000 m finish times in comparison to performance when the runners were in a state of fluid balance. A 2% decline in body mass led to a further reduction in speed, ranging from just over 3% for the 1,500 m to well over 6% for the 5,000 and 10,000 m. As losses start to approach and then exceed 5%, the capacity for work can decrease by as much as 30%. Dehydration becomes life threatening when 10% to 20% of body weight is lost. Although endurance athletes and team sport athletes engaged in training and competition for 2 or more hours are at greatest risk for the performance detriments associated with dehydration, there is evidence that the capacity to perform high-intensity, short-duration exercise (e.g., sprinting) can drop by as much as 4% to 5% with prior dehydration equivalent to only 2.5% of body weight (ACSM et al., 2007). The cumulative impact of dehydration can be devastating for any athlete, but is especially relevant for athletes competing in several short-duration events over a period of several hours to several days. Imagine reaching the 100 m final of an important track meet only to experience a 45% decline in performance capacity!

Monitoring Hydration

The simplest and most common method to monitor acute changes in hydration status is to calculate sweat rate by comparing the athlete's pre- and postexercise weight while also taking note of fluid intake and loss via urination (see figure 2.2). Although this method fails to account for small losses from substrate oxidation, calculating sweat rate allows the athlete's team of coaches and trainers to devise a drinking protocol to help minimize the health and performance detriments of dehydration. To protect against performance and health declines associated with disturbances in important physiological functions, athletes should target drinking fluids at the same rate losses occur via sweating. It is estimated that during exertion, the average athlete will lose 1 to 2 lb (0.45-0.90 kg) of body weight each hour. During exertion in extreme environmental conditions, such as heat and humidity, sweat rate can easily double. Consuming 0.4 to 0.8 L of fluid each hour of exercise seems to be an acceptable amount for most athletes to achieve fluid balance in optimal conditions, with additional electrolytes (particularly 460-690 mg/L of sodium and 80-195 mg/L of potassium) recommended when exercise exceeds 2 hours or when exerting in hot and humid climates. Unfortunately, research has shown that the volume of fluid that most athletes voluntarily choose to drink during exercise replaces less than half of their fluid losses, making dehydration, especially during prolonged training and competition, a legitimate concern. Furthermore, extreme environmental conditions may produce a rate of loss that exceeds what can be tolerably consumed by an athlete or physically absorbed by the body.

Testing Protocol

1. Measure preexercise nude weight.
2. Measure fluids consumed (in ounces) during exercise.
3. If possible, measure urine volume (in ounces) during exercise.
4. Measure postexercise nude weight.
5. Make note of total exercise time in hours (e.g., 0.5 hour, 1.5 hours) and any other relevant data such as exercise intensity and environmental conditions.

Calculation

1. Subtract postworkout weight from preworkout weight (in pounds/kilograms) and multiply by 16 ounces.
2. Subtract total volume of urine (ounces).
3. Add total volume of fluids (ounces) consumed during exercise.
4. Divide by exercise time to determine hourly sweat rate in fluid ounces.

An online calculator is available at www.triharder.com/THM_SwRate.aspx, which can be used with English or metric equivalents.

FIGURE 2.2   Sweat rate calculation.

Preventing Dehydration

Continual access to fluid during training and competition can sometimes present a challenge, and certain environmental factors—heat, humidity, and altitude—can often increase fluid needs to a level beyond what the body can physically absorb. As a result, many athletes practice heat acclimatization and use nutritional strategies to help maximize fluid uptake, improve hydration status, and protect against the undesirable performance and health declines of dehydration.

Heat Acclimatization

Dehydration increases risk for heat illness, which refers to a group of disorders that result from a disruption of thermoregulation due to heat stress caused by environmental heat exposure, exertion, or a combination of these two factors. This risk is compounded by lack of acclimatization. Signs of heat-related illness, which begin as muscle cramps, rash or flushed face, edema, and fainting, can arise with just 3% loss of body weight and quickly progress into heat exhaustion followed by potentially life-threatening heat stroke. Consistent exposure to heat and humidity through training or living promotes several physiological adaptations that can be extremely advantageous to the athlete (as well as comforting to parents and coaches who may be concerned about an athlete's risk for heat illness). These positive adaptations include a boost in blood volume, which assures that the body can meet the demand for blood supply, and enhanced sweating ability, which includes a faster onset of sweating, greater distribution of sweat over the body, and an increase in sweat rate. To help conserve fluid, the body also becomes more efficient in retaining sodium, thereby lowering the concentration of the mineral in sweat. Full acclimatization takes about 10 to 14 days to complete, although some benefits are seen as soon as 4 to 5 days.

Nutritional Strategies

Enhancing fluid uptake is dependent on the rate at which fluid is emptied from the stomach into the small intestine for absorption into the bloodstream. Carbohydrates and electrolytes are two key ingredients that help increase fluid uptake, which is one reason health professionals often recommend sport drinks as a better fluid choice than water during longer training sessions and competition. The concentration of carbohydrates, however, is important, with optimal levels for uptake at 4% to 6%; this means that the drink should contain approximately 15 to 20 g of carbohydrate/8 oz of fluid (15-20 g of carbohydrate/240 mL of fluid). The inclusion of electrolytes, especially sodium and potassium, facilitates intestinal absorption of water. Finally, the osmolality, or the total concentration of nutrients in a sport drink, including carbohydrate and electrolytes, plays a role in fluid uptake. Levels that are equal to (isotonic) or marginally lower than (hypotonic) those of blood (275-299 milliosmoles/kg) are ideal for fluid uptake. Some sport drink companies even provide an osmolality calculator to help an athlete create a custom blend that is optimal for fluid uptake and performance.

In the lead-up to as well as during competition, especially when battling heat or humidity, many athletes practice salt loading, or increasing sodium intake using liquids such as broth or pickle juice with electrolyte supplements. The goal is protection against the muscle cramping and fatigue associated with dehydration. One study found that supplementation with a highly concentrated sodium beverage prior to running to exhaustion at 70% of $\dot{V}O_2$max in a hot environment helped athletes maintain a higher blood volume, lower core body temperature, and lower level of perceived exertion than when they consumed a low-sodium beverage before running (Sims et al., 2007). Because sodium affects the osmolality of a solution, extremely high levels of sodium are generally not recommended for consumption during training and competition. Precompetition salt-loading protocols entail consuming 0.5 to 1 g of sodium/hour with fluids in the 2 to 3 hours prior to starting an event. (Note that it is important not to consume 2 g in one acute dose.) This can easily be achieved through high-sodium food or sipping on a sport drink with added electrolytes prior to competition.

A final practice used by many athletes to aid hydration during competition is hyperhydration; this may include glycerol plus water but is most commonly achieved through a simple intake of large volumes of fluid in the days and hours leading up to competition. Although this practice does indeed speed the release of fluid from the gut into the small intestine for absorption, drinking excessive amounts of any type of fluid can be dangerous if fluids consumed beyond absorption cause blood sodium levels to drop, triggering a potentially fatal condition known as hyponatremia, or water intoxication. This condition most commonly affects female endurance athletes and is marked by one or several of the following symptoms: clear urine, muscle fatigue, pressure headache, dizziness, confusion, nausea, vomiting, irritability, and drowsiness.

Recovery

Athletes use various types of stressors to elicit specific adaptations in the body, such as changes in strength, power, speed, anaerobic threshold, or oxidative capacity. Although the actual training (or stress) is important, the often-overlooked aspect is rest and recovery. The recovery process is complex and involves many body systems working together, including the neuromuscular, metabolic, endocrine, immune, antioxidant, and joint systems. Without adequate recovery the body is unable to adapt to the training stress; the athlete does not improve and ultimately becomes overtrained—a state all athletes must work hard and train smart to avoid.

Neuromuscular System

The functioning of the neuromuscular system—the number of muscle fibers and motor units recruited, in addition to the speed of contraction and amount of force the muscle can produce—are dependent on adequate recovery of this system, yet it is one of the least understood. There are ways to measure neuromuscular function, but research related to the impact of nutritional supplements or other recovery modalities has been limited. Also of note in the neural recovery space is the relatively recent trend to indirectly measure the autonomic nervous system (sympathetic versus parasympathetic drive) via heart rate variability (HRV). This fine-scale fluctuation in beat-to-beat cardiac activity is a valid method of monitoring training stress and recovery and is done via smart watches, rings and other biosensors. For example, global HRV scales from these devices may show a decrease in arbitrary units, indicating too much sympathetic drive and underrecovery.

Metabolic System

Muscles also undergo depletion of fuel stores; those stores must be restored before adequate performance can be ensured in the next training session or event. Carbohydrates or glycogen stores are the only fuel that can be used anaerobically by muscle; therefore, sports that require lots of high-intensity movement (e.g., sprinting, jumping, changes of direction) will tap into and quickly deplete glycogen and phosphocreatine. Because the production of ATP is influenced by the form of exercise an athlete engages in as well as the availability of these energy substrates, their restoration is another key component of optimal recovery. Muscle glycogen is also important for the endurance athlete because low glycogen stores limit performance. Certain supplements enhance the restoration of muscle glycogen and phosphocreatine stores, therefore speeding recovery. Supplements containing special formulations and types of carbohydrates are becoming popular; in addition, many supplement companies manufacture specialized formulations of creatine that the companies claim are superior to those of other competitors. See the creatine entry in chapter 3 for more information.

Endocrine System

The endocrine system is a complex system of glands that secrete a variety of hormones in response to exercise and recovery. The catabolic hormones cortisol, epinephrine, and norepinephrine drive the breakdown of fat, glycogen stores, and protein in response to the stressful demands of exercise. More stressful exercise or training sessions will elicit greater release of these catabolic hormones. The anabolic hormones testosterone, growth hormone, and IGF-1 are also released during exercise and throughout the recovery phase; they can initiate protein synthesis, begin the restoration of carbohydrate stores, and signal the adaptation of muscle and the neuromuscular system to training. The balance between catabolic and anabolic hormones is an important concept for athletes to understand. Constant exposure to stressful training (high volumes of work at high intensities) will drive up a catabolic response. If an appropriate period of recovery is not allowed, these hormones will dominate and push the body into an overtrained state in which increased risk of injury and poor performance persists. However, if adequate nutrients, sleep, and rest are provided, the anabolic response will dominate, giving the body time to recover; adapt to the training stress; and become stronger, more powerful, and develop greater resistance to fatigue.

Supplements such as branched-chain amino acids, protein powders, and specialized carbohydrates are claimed to affect muscle recovery in the early recovery window following training (1-4 hours). Others, including the amino acids arginine and ornithine, herbal supplements, flavonoids, and ecdysteroids, are claimed to naturally increase levels of anabolic hormones. Another group of minerals and hormones that includes zinc and amino acids (e.g., melatonin, GABA) are claimed to improve the quality of sleep or to enhance the release of anabolic hormones or improve neuromuscular recovery during sleep.

Immune System

Within the past 20 years, it has become more evident that the immune system plays a role in development, recovery, and health of athletes. In general, exercise in moderate duration and intensity enhances immune function. However, exercise of longer duration and higher intensity negatively affects and suppresses immune function. As a result, athletes must do everything possible to limit this suppression and keep the immune system functioning. Colds, flu, and upper respiratory tract infections will negatively affect training, hinder progress, and result in poor performance. In addition, the immune system has a role in the recovery process of muscle. Both white blood cells and proteins of the immune system known as cytokines can be catabolic or assist in the anti-inflammatory and healing process of muscle, providing another reason for athletes to do everything possible to maintain healthy immune function. A variety of herbal ingredients, vitamins, minerals, and amino acids are promoted as strengthening or providing support to the immune system.

Antioxidant Defense System

Antioxidants are another group of nutrients that have been given much media attention in recent years. All types of stress, exercise included, produce free radicals, which damage healthy cells throughout the body. Antioxidants are the nutrients, enzymes, and other compounds that neutralize and dispose of free radicals before they can damage cells. A common misconception is that dietary sources of antioxidants are the only defense against free radicals, but this is not true; in fact, our bodies are equipped with built-in antioxidant defense systems, and our most powerful defenses are naturally built into the cell. However, the added physical stresses of training will expose athletes to higher levels of free radicals, and supplements are marketed to protect athletes against them. Vitamins A, E, and C; minerals such as selenium and zinc; and natural components in foods and spices such as resveratrol, quercetin, curcuminoids, ginger, and cinnamon are all touted as powerful antioxidants thought to further protect athletes and their cells from free radicals.

Joint Support

Maintaining healthy joints and avoiding chronic joint pain or injury is important for athletes of all ages. Nothing can disrupt training and alter improvements in performance more than chronic pain or a lingering injury that prevents an athlete from training at 100%. One of the most common issues seen in athletes is arthritis, or joint inflammation. Athletes involved in sports requiring repetitive throwing or swinging—baseball, softball, and tennis, among others—often experience arthritis of the elbow, shoulder, or wrist; athletes in sports requiring lots of running and changes of direction often experience inflammation of the knees or hips. Degeneration of the cartilage, or connective tissues within joints, is a common cause of inflammation that can result in joint pain.

A branch of the supplement industry has targeted athletes, as well as those who are older and inactive, with promotional materials for popular supplements such as collagen and glucosamine suggest these nutrients can assist in preserving cartilage, preventing degeneration, and ultimately limiting pain and dysfunction. Unique forms of proteins that comprise joint tissue such as hyaluronic acid and undenatured type II collagen (UC-II) are also sold as supplements with the claim they will improve the production of tissue within the joint. In addition, foods, particularly healthy fats and fatty fish or fish oil supplements, provide some powerful anti-inflammatory effects that are postulated to benefit joint pain and potentially provide relief. Nutrients found in fruits, vegetables, herbs, and spices, such as bromelain (a component of pineapple), turmeric, and ginger root, also have anti-inflammatory effects and can be found as supplements in pill and powdered form. The protection of healthy joints is multifaceted and requires athletes to train smart: avoid overtraining, eat right, and optimize rest and recovery.

Weight and Body Composition

If a group of athletes were asked what they would most like to change about themselves to improve performance, chances are one of the most popular answers would involve losing body fat or improving body composition. However, a common misperception among certain athletes is that leanest is always best. Of course, fat loss or maintenance and gain of lean mass doesn't always equate to improved performance—with the possible exception of bodybuilders. All athletes are genetically different in terms of body types and body composition. There is no single equation for altering or determining body composition. Altering body composition is dependent on energy and nutrient intake, with consideration to partitioning—that is, which body compartment receives them. For some athletes, severe calorie restriction is required to reach and maintain a lean body composition, but this type of restriction will negatively affect performance. Athletes must be wise about making attempts to lose body fat. Body composition, whether it be fat loss or muscle gain, should be a focus during off-season training when peak performance is not required.

Fat Loss

A decrease in body fat essentially means that an athlete will be running, jumping, swimming, and changing direction with less mass or weight to move. For example, a male athlete who weighs 165 lb (74.8 kg) and has 10% body fat carries 16.5 lb (7.5 kg) of adipose tissue, or body fat. If the athlete reduces his body fat to 7%, he has lowered his fat mass to approximately 11.5 lb (5.2 kg); his body is more efficient with 5 lb less body fat to move. A leaner, lighter athlete moving with less body fat will be more efficient and expend less energy doing the same task as someone who is carrying more body fat (or even excess muscle mass). In addition, athletes such as high jumpers or sprinters want to maximize their strength-to-mass ratio in order to optimize their performance. However, maintenance of strength and power is key while minimizing body weight or mass. If strength is lost along with mass, improvements in performance will not be realized.

The desire for athletes to be leaner, along with a need for many nonathletes to lose weight, has created an explosion of fat-burning and weight-loss supplements. These supplements are one of the most popular types of products on the market, with nearly 200 names and brands of so-called fat burners currently available for purchase online. Unfortunately, fat burners and weight-loss supplements are also some of the most dangerous: They can contain potent stimulants that can affect cardiovascular function and even result in death, and they are often adulterated with ingredients or pharmaceuticals not listed on labels that may have powerful, often harmful effects on the body. Extreme caution should be used when choosing these products.

Most fat burners and weight-loss supplements can be assigned to one of three categories:

1. Stimulants. These contain stimulants such as caffeine, synephrine, guarana (containing caffeine plus other compounds), and many others. Some ingredients, such as ephedra and 1,3-dimethylamylamine, are now banned by the FDA. Product claims include the ability to speed up resting metabolic rate and burn fat.

2. Appetite suppressants. These include Hoodia gordonii and others that assist in controlling appetite and limiting calorie intake.

3. Fat malabsorptives. These ingredients limit the amount of fat absorbed during digestion, resulting in lowered calorie intake. Chitosan, which is a structural element found in the shell of crabs, shrimp, and lobster, is a popular ingredient found in weight-loss supplements due to its purported ability to bind fat and prevent its absorption. These types of products can have some undesirable side effects such as loose stools and diarrhea. In addition, their use will also limit the absorption of fat-soluble vitamins, healthy fats, and essential fatty acids need for optimal function.

Muscle Preservation and Hypertrophy

Muscle mass and hypertrophy are part of the broader category of body composition change. The typical textbook estimation that it takes approximately 2,700 kcal of surplus energy intake, along with additional protein, suggests that gains take weeks to months to be noticeable, even in an exercise physiology laboratory. Muscle mass and quality are important considerations for athletes and for general health. Curtis and colleagues (2015) point out that as one ages, "factors underpinning muscle quality come into play, including muscle composition, aerobic capacity and metabolism, fatty infiltration, insulin resistance, fibrosis and neural activation." A number of these characteristics, although typically considered in the context of avoiding sarcopenia (muscle loss with aging), help underscore the fact that building quality muscle mass with a combination of resistance exercise and surplus nutrient intake is of critical importance. Of course, some sports such as bodybuilding focus almost entirely on muscle aesthetics as opposed to function—indeed, the development of sports supplements has been strongly influenced by bodybuilding. Although many sports supplements are targeted toward bodybuilders, they are also used by other athletes hoping to build lean body mass. Conversely, athletes of some endurance events seek to optimize—rather than maximize—muscle mass, because extra weight could decrease their performance.

Summary

Each performance variable must be optimized for an athlete to reach their potential. Balancing and managing these variables through proper training, rest and recovery, nutrition, and the use of appropriate sports supplements when recommended is key. Chapter 3 addresses many of the supplements and ingredients available to athletes. This information will assist athletes in understanding how each supplement works—or doesn't—to enhance the performance variables discussed in this chapter.

A-to-Z Supplement Guide

The symbols listed in table 3.1 help the reader easily identify the supplements that have been supported to be beneficial for the corresponding performance variables. If there is scientific consensus that a supplement is beneficial for a particular performance variable, the supplement entry is marked with a black symbol; if additional research is needed on the benefits of a supplement for a specific performance variable, the entry is marked with a gray symbol. If the supplement is applicable to a special population, the entry will be marked with that symbol, as well.

TABLE 3.1 Performance Variables Reference Guide

Performance variable	Components included	Symbol
Fuel usage	ATP-Creatine Phosphate Energy System Anaerobic-Lactate Energy System Aerobic Energy System	
Cardiovascular performance	Maximal Aerobic Capacity: Speed Improving Aerobic Capacity: Endurance	
Muscular performance	Strength and Power Endurance	
Neural performance	Focus and Cognition Motivation and Motor	
Hydration	Fluid Balance Electrolyte Balance	

Short- and long-term recovery	Short-term:
	    Rehydration
	    Glycogen Repletion
	Long-term:
	    Joint, tendon, bone, and muscle health
	    Immunity
	    Endocrine support
	    Antioxidant protection	

Weight and body composition	Fat Loss Muscle Preservation and Hypertrophy	

Performance variable	Components included	Symbol
Special populations	Master Athletes	
	Youth Athletes	
	Female Athletes	
	Injured Athletes	
	Athletes With Diabetes	
	Athletes With Food Allergies or Intolerances	
	Plant-Based Athletes	
	Athletes Competing in Hot and Humid Environments	
	Athletes Competing at Altitude	

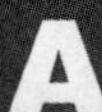

Aaron's Rod

(see *Rhodiola rosea*)

Acai Berry 

aka *Euterpe oleracea, acai d'Amazonie, acai extract, acai fruit, acai palm*

What it is: Displaying a deep purple hue, yellow flesh, and large seeds, acai berries are found on the acai palm tree (*Euterpe oleracea)*, which grows in Central and South America. The fruit contains approximately 70 kcal/99 g serving and consists of protein (9.1%); lipids (42.3%); carbohydrates (43.4%); vitamins B_1, C, and E; minerals such as iron, phosphorus, calcium, and potassium; starch; and fiber (Laurindo et al., 2023). Because their skin is tough, acai berries are traditionally soaked and blended before eating in whole form. They are more commonly sold in the consumer market as frozen pulp or juice or as a dietary supplement in tablet or capsule form.

Function: Bioactive phenolic compounds found within the leaf, pulp, fruit, skin, and seeds of an acai berry possess antioxidant and anti-inflammatory properties that, in vitro, have shown to exert cardioprotective, gastroprotective, hepatoprotective, neuroprotective, renoprotective, antilipidemic, antidiabetic, and antineoplastic activities (Laurindo et al., 2023).

Performance benefit: It is suggested that acai can protect against metabolic stress induced by oxidation, inflammation, vascular abnormalities, and physical exertion. Theoretically, acai may help reduce markers of muscle damage after intensive exercise and enhance immune function, thereby helping an athlete recover more efficiently and maintain health during intense cycles of training.

Research: Research evaluating the impact acai has on human health and performance is limited. Data from an athlete-specific population is even more sparse but has focused on the antioxidant qualities of acai and its impact on muscle damage, performance, and recovery. A 2023 placebo-controlled study found a daily supplementation protocol of 40 g of dehydrated acai over 7 days increased antioxidant activity by 11% over 24 hours and facilitated a significantly faster recovery after 24 and 72 hours in 12 healthy men completing 10 sets of 10 countermovement jumps (Dos Reis et al., 2023). Another study conducted in 2015 demonstrated a similar increase in antioxidant activity in 7 healthy junior hurdlers after 6 weeks of consuming a 100 mL acai juice blend; there was also significant attenuation of exercise-induced muscle damage as well as an improved serum lipid profile after completing a 300 m running time trial at the end of the supplementation protocol compared to the beginning. There were no differences in performance noted (Sadowska-Krępa et al., 2015).

Another 2015 study showed that consumption of an acai beverage containing 27.6 mg of anthocyanins per dose before a maximal treadmill test significantly reduced the metabolic stress induced by exercise, significantly reduced perceived effort, and significantly enhanced cardiovascular responses while increasing the time to exhaustion in 14 elite athletes completing three separate maximal treadmill tests (one baseline, one acai beverage, and one placebo beverage) (Carvalho-Peixoto et al., 2015). The small subject size and lack of control for external elements, such as training impact and diet, in many of the available studies make it hard to draw any definite conclusions. Therefore, although consumption of the acai berry provides antioxidant qualities that can help support overall health, the current consensus by health experts is that there is not enough evidence to make practical recommendations for use of acai as an ergogenic aid.

Common usage: Acai supplements are currently not recommended due to lack of scientific support. Antioxidants are better absorbed by the body through the pulp and juice of the acai plant and can be included as part of a healthful diet rich in fruits and vegetables.

Health concerns: Acai berry consumed in whole fruit form is likely safe, though the long-term safety of supplement use has yet to be confirmed and thus is not recommended if pregnant or nursing. Drinking unprocessed acai juice has been linked to outbreaks of Chagas disease and should be avoided (Nóbrega et al., 2009). Because acai is sometimes used as an oral contrast for gastrointestinal MRIs and large doses have been noted to affect the results of MRI scans, athletes should check with their doctor regarding use of acai prior to an MRI (Córdova-Fraga et al., 2004).

Acetate Replacing Factor

(see *alpha-lipoic acid*)

Acetylcysteine 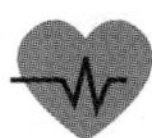 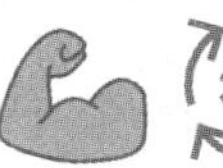 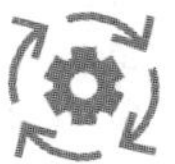 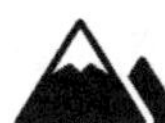

aka *N-acetylcysteine (NAC)*

What it is: A derivative of the amino acid L-cysteine, which is produced naturally by the body, acetylcysteine is marketed as an antioxidant that may protect an athlete against skeletal muscle fatigue.

Function: Production of reactive oxygen species (ROS), often called free radicals, during muscle contraction is associated with muscle fatigue and damage in the short term as well as favorable adaptive responses, specifically a stronger natural antioxidant defense system, in the long term. However, this positive adaptation may not be great enough to offset the accumulation of ROS during heavy periods of training and competition, especially for athletes just returning to training or the so-called weekend warrior who accumulates the bulk of training over 1 to 3 days. It is thought that supplementation with acetylcysteine increases the body's antioxidant capacity within the muscles, in particular the antioxidant compound glutathione, thereby protecting against muscle fatigue and damage that can otherwise hurt performance and recovery (Mason et al., 2020).

Performance benefit: Athletes may benefit from enhanced protection against muscle fatigue, helping extend endurance during both high- and low-intensity training and competition.

Research: There is conflicting evidence on the efficacy of antioxidant supplementation, especially at high doses over the long term, for trained athletes who have natural antioxidant defense systems that are thought to be sufficient to offset the potential detriments of ROS (Fernández-Lázaro et al., 2023). However, short-term supplementation may present some benefit across the fitness spectrum. A randomized, placebo-controlled study evaluating the impact of short-term (7 days) supplementation with a daily total of 1,200 mg of NAC showed that untrained subjects benefited from significant improvements in maximal oxygen uptake ($\dot{V}O_2$max) and total antioxidant capacity as well as reduced lactate production and levels of muscle fatigue during a graded exercise test (Leelarungrayub et al., 2011). Similarly, a 6-day supplementation protocol with NAC was shown to maintain higher levels of performance in recreationally trained men during repeated periods of intermittent exercise; this result led study investigators to conclude that NAC may benefit athletes during short-term competitive situations when adaptation is inconsequential, such as tournament play or track and field events in which an athlete is engaged in multiple performances over a few days (Cobley et al., 2011). Acute supplementation may also aid the performance of well-trained athletes, according to a small, double-blind, crossover study that found an intravenous infusion of NAC extended exercise time to exhaustion by 26.3% compared to placebo (Medved et al., 2004). These results, however, have been refuted in two different studies of similar design with an acute oral dose of 1,800 mg or 1,500 mg of NAC taken prior to maximum-effort cycling sessions demonstrating no significant impact on $\dot{V}O_2$ kinetics and exercise time to exhaustion or repeat-effort performance in well-trained athletes as compared to a placebo (Christensen & Bangsbo, 2019; Wicker et al., 2008). Additional research is needed to establish the merit of NAC supplementation for highly trained athletes as well as the ideal duration of use during a competitive season.

Common usage: Available in tablet and capsule form as well as in solutions at a potency of 10% to 20%, NAC is generally supplemented at doses of 600 mg taken 1 to 3 times/day. Research suggests a short-term supplementation protocol of up to 14 days is preferable over long-term use (Rhodes & Braakhuis, 2017). Findings of Ferreira and colleagues (2011) suggests a threshold oral intake of 70 mg/kg to avoid adverse effects in individuals undertaking exhaustive exercise, though tolerance has been reported to improve with flavored effervescent formulations (Greene, 2016). Of important note is that intravenous infusion greater than 100 mL/12-hour period is banned as of 2020 by the World Anti-Doping Agency (WADA).

Health concerns: Nausea, vomiting, diarrhea, rashes, and headache have been reported with oral delivery of NAC. Additionally, while rare in occurrence, formation of cysteine stones in the kidneys have occurred.

⚠ SUPPLEMENT WARNING

Loading the cell with high doses of antioxidants, especially over the long term, may interfere with the positive adaptation effects of exercise training and hinder important ROS-mediated physiological processes, including vasodilation, which helps enhance oxygen and blood flow to working cells, and insulin signaling, which promotes the uptake of glucose into muscles for energy use.

Acetyl-11-Keto-Boswellic Acid (AKBA)

(see *Boswellia serrata*)

Acetylformic Acid

(see *pyruvate*)

Adenosine Triphosphate (ATP)  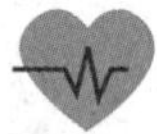

What it is: Adenosine triphosphate is the "energy currency of the cell." Present in living tissues, it is an adenosine molecule bonded to three phosphate groups. Energy is released by breaking a phosphate linkage (to form adenosine diphosphate, ADP, or still further to adenosine monophosphate, AMP) for physiological processes such as synthesis, transport, and muscular contraction. ATP is mostly "recharged" (rephosphorylated) during oxidative phosphorylation in the mitochondria, but also rapidly by substrate-level phosphorylation in the cytosol.

Function: Although ATP concentration is controlled within cells, increasing this concentration via direct supplementation may provide energy of anabolism and muscular performance.

Performance benefit: Despite discrepancies in findings over the past decade, some scientists have showed a renewed interest in the potential of ATP for increased blood flow, reduced fatigue, increased strength and power, and improved body composition. This appears to be dependent on the form ingested.

Research: Although athletes have sought to increase cellular energy production by various means, including by consuming phosphagens like creatine monohydrate (indeed likely to be effective for repeat explosive performance), direct ATP supplementation does not share the same kind of historical consensus. For example, Arts and colleagues (2012) stated "A single dose of orally administered ATP is not bioavailable, and this may explain why several studies did not find ergogenic effects of oral ATP supplementation." These researchers did point out that some supplementation studies were nonetheless suggestive of benefits. They observed increases in uric acid after release of ATP in the proximal part of the small intestine, suggesting ATP or one of its metabolites is indeed absorbed and metabolized. Whether uric acid itself may have ergogenic effects requires further study. In contrast to earlier work and skepticism, a review by Jager and colleagues (2021) emphasized that ATP acts in a way that goes beyond powering cellular processes; the presence (or absence) of intracellular ATP can "communicate signals across cells once released into the extracellular space." These researchers also pointed out that the supplemental form ATP disodium may be superior, inducing a wide range of benefits such as reduced fatigue, increased strength and power, and improved body composition. Still, they conclude, "the divergent findings surrounding ATP supplementation and an unidentified mechanism of action continue to preclude stronger conclusions from being made."

Common usage: Based on early work (Arts, 2012), recommended dosages for energy enhancement, such as those sold on the Internet, usually range from 100 to 250 mg/day. Based on the recent review by Jager and colleagues (2021), 400 mg ATP disodium, taken before exercise, may be preferred.

Health concerns: Hyperuricemia (excess uric acid) is a risk factor for gout. However, reaching serum levels this high would require chronic high doses of ATP. Those prone to gout should avoid these supplements or discuss them with their physician.

African Ginger

(see *ginger*)

Agaricus Blazei Murrill

(see *medicinal mushrooms*)

Agmatine 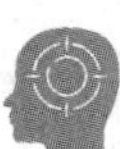 

aka *4-aminobutyl-guanidine*

What it is: Agmatine is a metabolite of the amino acid L-arginine.

Function: Agmatine blocks nitric oxide synthesis in astroglial cells and macrophages. It also modulates neurotransmitter receptor function and may indeed be a novel brain neurotransmitter itself. It may directly participate in learning and memory processes.

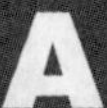

Performance benefit: Agmatine shows promise for alleviating neuropathic pain, may support cognition, and has purported antidepressive activity. These potential benefits need data to support them in athletes.

Research: A 2010 study by Keynan and colleagues (1.335 g/day for 10 days, 2.670 g/day for 10 days, 3.560 g/day for 10 days, and 3.560 g/day for 21 days) concluded that agmatine sulfate is a safe and efficacious treatment for alleviating pain and improving quality of life in lumbar disc–associated radiculopathy (pinched nerve). More research on efficacy and applications is needed in athletes.

Common usage: A recommended dose is 1,000 mg (1 g) per serving.

Health concerns: In the Keynan and colleagues (2010) investigation, three participants in the highest dose cohort had mild-to-moderate diarrhea and mild nausea during treatment, which disappeared upon treatment cessation. No other events were observed. More research on safety is needed in human athletes.

Albumin

(see *egg protein*)

Alpha-Linolenic Acid (ALA)

(see *omega-3 fatty acids*)

Allium Sativum

(see *garlic*)

Alpha-GPC 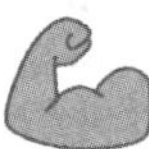 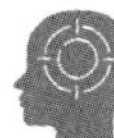 

aka *alpha-glycerylphosphorylcholine (see also choline)*

What it is: Alpha-GPC is a precursor of the neurotransmitter acetylcholine (ACh), a neurotransmitter that affects brain activity (e.g., learning and memory) and is responsible for the action potential that stimulates muscle contraction.

Function: Alpha-GPC is converted to phosphorylcholine in the body and can then serve as a source of choline for ACh synthesis. Alpha-GPC also plays a role in dopaminergic and serotonergic systems that may affect mood or motivation.

Performance benefit: Multiple ergogenic mechanisms have been proposed. It has been suggested that an alpha-GPC-induced increase in ACh could result in a greater signal for muscle contraction and thus the production of increased muscular force. Supplementation may also help prevent exercise-induced reductions in choline levels, increase endurance performance, and enhance growth hormone secretion. Taken chronically (400 mg/day for 2 weeks), alpha-GPC may also increase motivation (Tamura et al., 2021)—a key factor in many sports.

Research: A wide range of doses have been studied, from 150 to 1,000 mg, with 600 mg being most common. Both acute and chronic dosing have been examined. Such variation makes interpretations challenging. Marcus and colleagues (2017) reported improved power output during countermovement jumps as well as increased free serum choline concentrations but also cited research showing no effect. A dose–response phenomenon may be at work, and a 600 mg dose has been suggested for ergogenic effects (Marcus et al., 2017).

Common usage: Although the scientific literature is still developing, hopeful athletes ingest 200 to 1,200 mg daily.

Health concerns: Alpha-GPC appears to be safe, with no serious side effects or toxicities when human subjects were orally administered alpha-GPC (1,200 mg/day) for 6 months (Tamura et al., 2021).

Alpha-Keto Acid, Alpha-Ketopropionic Acid

(see *pyruvate*)

Alpha-Lipoic Acid  

aka *acetate replacing factor, dihydrolipoic acid, lipoic acid, lipolate, pyruvate oxidation factor, thiotic acid*

What it is: A naturally occurring compound found within the body and also derived from consumption of such foods as organ meats, spinach, and yeast, alpha-lipoic acid plays a key role in the conversion of nutrients, especially glucose, into energy. It also has antioxidant qualities of potential benefit to the endurance, strength, and immunity of an athlete.

Function: Animal research has demonstrated alpha-lipoic acid to activate GLUT4, a protein important for the uptake of glucose by muscles, as well as a molecule called PGC1-α, which seems to enhance the cell's ability to synthesize mitochondria. Both are key factors in enhancing muscle endurance. GLUT4 also serves as a proposed mechanism of action because of its apparent ability to increase uptake of creatine by the muscles, which may facilitate gains in muscle strength. Additionally, as an antioxidant that is both water and fat soluble, alpha-lipoic acid protects all the cells of the human body; in particular, it can help dispose of increased metabolic waste products produced during exercise that may otherwise damage cells, hurt overall immune function, and hinder recovery from intense training.

SUPPLEMENT FACT

Alpha-lipoic acid occurs in nature in two mirror image forms, labeled R and S, with only the R form being used by the body. Look for supplements containing the R label versus the R/S label.

Performance benefit: Athletes may benefit from enhanced muscle endurance and strength as well as improved recovery times.

Research: Much of the current research evaluating alpha-lipoic acid is animal focused. One study of rats demonstrated a 45% increase in glucose uptake by muscles after 15 days of supplementing with alpha-lipoic acid at a dose of 30 mg/kg of body weight (Saengsirisuwan et al., 2004). When supplementation was combined with 60 minutes of treadmill running, glucose uptake by the muscles increased an impressive 124%, signaling the profound impact training has on glucose uptake dynamics. Nonetheless, supplementation with alpha-lipoic acid did significantly enhance this effect. Because the study was conducted on obese animals, however, it is difficult to draw conclusions for a fit, athletic human population. One human study did determine that a daily supplementation protocol with 600 mg of alpha-lipoic acid over 8 days to reduce oxidative damage in the muscles of healthy trained and untrained men after completing a weighted exercise test, suggesting potential applications from a recovery perspective (Zembron-Lacny et al., 2009). Another human study, of double-blind, randomized, crossover design—albeit with only 17 well-trained male athletes—demonstrated moderate inhibition of muscle damage and inflammation with a supplementation protocol consisting of 150 mg alpha-lipoic acid consumed 2 hours before a maximal strength test and then again immediately after (total of 300 mg alpha-lipoic acid) over a period of 6 days compared to a placebo group. The alpha-lipoic acid–supplemented group were also able to maintain their performance significantly longer over the 6-day intensive training protocol versus the placebo group (Isenmann et al., 2020). Additional research, particularly on human athletes, needs to further investigate the antioxidative function of alpha-lipoic acid before practical recommendations for supplementation can be made.

Common usage: The oral dosage of alpha-lipoic acid given in numerous clinical trials range from 200 to 1,800 mg daily.

Health concerns: Though infrequent in occurrence, reported side effects include allergic skin reactions such as rashes, hives, and itching as well as gastrointestinal disturbances such as stomachaches, nausea, vomiting, and diarrhea.

Alpha-Tocopherol, Alpha-Tocotrienol

(see *vitamin E*)

Amanita Muscaria, **Amavadin**

(see *vanadium*)

American Ginseng

(see *ginseng*)

Ananas Comosus, Ananase

(see *bromelain*)

Anhydrous Caffeine

(see *caffeine*)

Antiberiberi Vitamin

(see *thiamine*)

Antiscorbutic Vitamin

(see *vitamin C*)

Apple Cider Vinegar 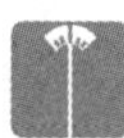 

aka *acetic acid, apple phenols*

What it is: Apple cider vinegar is an old home remedy of fermented sugars made from crushed apples. The main volatile compound in vinegars is acetic acid, which gives them a strong, sour flavor and aroma. Apple cider vinegar also contains chlorogenic acid, a major phenol in the liquid and potentially a further contributor to any benefits.

Function: Relevant to athletes, apple cider vinegar may modestly enhance fat loss, perhaps through increased satiety or effects on blood sugar and insulin action. Inhibition of lipogenesis (fat creation and storage), mediated by decreases in gene expression of fatty acid synthase and acetyl-CoA carboxylase, may also be a mechanism.

Performance benefit: Apple cider vinegar is not likely to directly enhance performance. It may be supportive by reducing body fat and overall body mass, which could theoretically lead to lower physical work requirements in sport, but this is highly speculative. Sports relying on low body fat or body mass (bodybuilding, weight class sports) may benefit directly, however.

Research: Perhaps surprisingly, some Japanese research does support reduced fat and body weight in obese subjects (Kondo et al., 2009). Healthy participants, too, have exhibited a dose–response effect on blood glucose and insulin (increasing reductions with higher doses of acetic acid) to a white bread meal, as well as increased subjective rating of satiety (Ostman et al., 2005). More research is needed, particularly given the potential for some side effects.

Common usage: Those interested in controlling hunger, decreasing fat mass, or reducing the glycemic effect of carbohydrate meals may consume 15 to 30 mL (1-2 tbsp) mixed into a large glass of water. Sensitive individuals may also rinse with more water after ingestion to avoid caustic effects.

Health concerns: Vinegar ingestion may exacerbate tooth enamel erosion. Although it may reduce quantitative and subjective measures of appetite, this also may be a result of a higher nausea rating (Darzi et al., 2014).

Arachidonic Acid 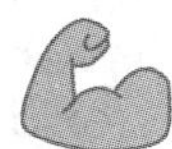

aka *eicosatetraenoic acid*

What it is: Arachidonic acid is a 20-carbon polyunsaturated omega-6 fatty acid and a substrate in cells for cyclooxygenase (COX) enzymes and prostaglandin E2 (PGE2), an inflammatory eicosanoid. It is produced in the body from linoleic acid, the common omega-6 fatty acid.

Function: Despite being a precursor to proinflammatory eicosanoids, arachidonic acid supplementation does not appear to be detrimental in this regard. It is known to affect cell membranes and cellular pathways related to inflammation and immune function.

Performance benefit: Arachidonic acid may increase anaerobic power. More research is needed, given the complex nature of fatty acid–eicosanoid metabolism and the seemingly contradictory fact that Western populations already consume a disproportionately high amount of its precursor, linoleic acid.

Research: According to Roberts and colleagues (2007), supplementation with arachidonic acid during resistance training "may enhance anaerobic capacity and lessen the inflammatory response to training. However, [it] did not promote statistically greater gains in strength [or] muscle mass." This investigation used 1.1 g compared to a similar amount of corn oil (a rich linoleic acid source) over 50 days. Importantly, the choice of placebo is very challenging in dietary fat research, as all fatty acids have biologic activity.

Common usage: Like a number of other dietary fats, athletes may consume 1 to 3 g/day over a period of several weeks in hopes of effects.

Health concerns: In the dose studied (1.1 g/day), arachidonic acid is unlikely to present health concerns in healthy athletes. Because of its fundamental effects on cell physiology, those with preexisting conditions related to tissue inflammation, hypertension, or depression should consult their physician.

Arctic Root
(see *Rhodiola rosea*)

Arginine 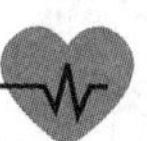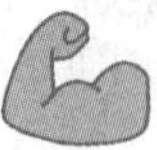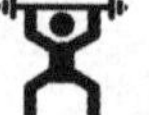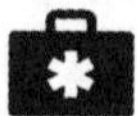

aka *L-arginine*

What it is: Arginine is a conditionally essential single amino acid, meaning that the human body can synthesize or obtain it from foods, but in certain conditions such as disease, trauma, or extreme stress, additional amounts may be needed (Campbell, La Bounty, & Roberts, 2004). The average dietary intake of acids like arginine is 3 to 6 g (Paddon-Jones, Borsheim, & Wolfe, 2004). Arginine is found in such foods as nuts, seeds, beans, fish, and chicken.

Function: Arginine plays a number of roles in the body. It can be metabolized into glucose for energy during exercise and is important in the production of nitric oxide and creatine. It can exhibit pharmaceutical and nutraceutical effects. At sufficiently high doses of 12 to 30 g, when medically administered intravenously, arginine is also known to stimulate growth hormone, a powerful anabolic hormone. This fact and other data have led to reviews by exercise physiologists that examine its ergogenic potential as a dietary supplement (Campbell, La Bounty, & Roberts, 2004). Growth hormone-stimulatory results with oral administration prior to exercise are less consistent than in medical settings. Rather, the vasodilatory effect via nitric oxide may be most promising.

Performance benefit: Arginine is thought to benefit athletes because of its role as a precursor to nitric oxide as well as its involvement in the production of growth hormone, synthesis of creatine, and interaction with the Krebs cycle, influencing aerobic energy systems. Nitric oxide is a vasodilator, which increases blood flow to the muscles and promotes superior delivery of oxygen and other nutrients, potentially enhancing performance. Growth hormone aids protein synthesis, which is critical for muscle recovery and building. Current data are not convincing that supplemental arginine-stimulated growth hormone release is adequate for increasing muscle protein synthesis, but the known effects of this sometimes-doped (injected) drug are intriguing. Any potential impact of arginine on growth hormone and nitric oxide production is therefore encouraging for both strength and power-oriented athletes as well as endurance athletes.

Research: Results of a 2021 systematic review and meta-analysis by Rezaei and colleagues indicated that L-arginine supplementation increased $\dot{V}O_2$max by 0.07 L/minute compared to controls. Nitric oxide production and vasodilation were a potential mechanism. The findings of Rezaei and colleagues (2021) are consistent with another meta-analysis from Viribay and colleagues (2020), which revealed favorable results for both aerobic ($\leq\dot{V}O_2$max) and anaerobic ($\geq\dot{V}O_2$max) performance tests with arginine supplementation. Further, acute dosing patterns should be adjusted to 0.15 g/kg of body mass, consumed 60 to 90 minutes before exercise. Chronic supplementation should include 1.5 to 2.0 g/day for 4 to 7 weeks in order to improve aerobic performance or 10 to 12 g/day for 8 weeks to enhance anaerobic performance (Viribay et al., 2020). In a study of 17 male professional water polo players, a lower dose of 5 g/day over 4 weeks was also shown to be effective in ameliorating oxidative metabolism through a mechanism of enhanced mitochondrial function, shown by the statistically significant lower lactate-to-speed ratio observed in placebo-treated controls (Gambardella et al., 2021). Interestingly, however, this did not translate to any impact on their maximal speed or muscle strength in a 200 m swimming test, but this might change if the dose and duration of supplementation matched that suggested by Viribay and colleagues (2020). There may also be subtle differences in impact seen in amateur versus professional-level athletes. Although arginine supplementation has shown promise for both aerobic and anaerobic performance, more research is needed to clarify dosages and timing as well as further evaluate the differences seen in recreational versus elite athletes. For now, it is not broadly considered a supplement with strong evidence.

Common usage: Based on current data, acute dosing patterns have been indicated at 0.15 g/kg of body mass taken 60 to 90 minutes before anaerobic or aerobic exercise. Chronic dosing patterns have been indicated at 1.5 to 2.0 g over 4 to 7 weeks for aerobic performance and 10 to 12 g/day over 8 weeks for anaerobic performance. Note the per-kg doses from Viribay and colleagues (2020). Oral doses much beyond this may lead to osmotic diarrhea in some persons.

Health concerns: Reported side effects include nausea and diarrhea. A No Observed Adverse Effect Level (NOAEL) for diet-added arginine (added mostly in the form of dietary supplements) has been reported at 30 g/day (Cynober et al., 2016), although it is not advisable to take this all at once due to diarrhea risk in susceptible persons.

Ascorbate, Ascorbic Acid

(see *vitamin C*)

Ashwagandha

(see *Withania somnifera*)

Aspartates 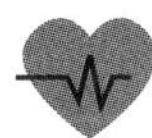

aka *aspartate salts, aspartic acid, D-aspartic acid (DAA), L-amino succinate, L-aspartate, L-aspartic acid*

What it is: As salts of the amino acid aspartic acid, aspartates are commonly bound to the minerals magnesium, potassium, calcium, and zinc in dietary supplements to facilitate enhanced absorption. Beyond being naturally produced in the body (i.e., nonessential), aspartates can be obtained from the diet through sugar cane, molasses, dairy, and meat. Their effects on human performance were discovered in the late 1950s when human trials demonstrated that magnesium and potassium aspartate supplements reduced muscle fatigue, helping to extend endurance.

Function: During physical training, especially high-intensity training, the exhaustion of ATP causes lactate and ammonia levels to rise, which is postulated to contribute to the onset of muscle fatigue and reduced endurance capacity. It is thought that aspartates reduce muscle fatigue by accelerating the conversion of ammonia to urea, thereby lowering levels of ammonia in the muscles and allowing more ATP to be produced for enhanced endurance. Furthermore, it is hypothesized that aspartate salts promote a faster rate of glycogen resynthesis during exertion, helping to protect against the fatigue-inducing glycogen depletion commonly known in sports as hitting the wall or bonking.

SUPPLEMENT FACT

Closely related to aspartic acid is asparagine, a nonessential amino acid first isolated from asparagus juice back in the early 1800s. Together, asparagine and aspartate play a role in the production of oxaloacetic acid, which helps produce energy within the mitochondria as a key intermediate in the Krebs metabolic cycle.

Performance benefit: Athletes may benefit from reduced fatigue during training and competition, resulting in enhanced endurance. Aspartates may also stimulate the immune system, potentially helping athletes stay healthy during training and competition, although this needs further study.

Research: In a 2017 randomized control trial, Melville and colleagues tested the effects of 3 months' supplementation of D-aspartic acid (DAA, 6 g/day) on the testosterone concentrations of 22 resistance-trained men. They reported no change in basal total or free testosterone but did observe a 16% reduction in estradiol across the study ($p <$ 0.01). They concluded that DAA supplementation is ineffective at changing testosterone levels or positively affecting training outcomes. Preliminary research favored aspartate supplementation for enhanced endurance, but those studies were primarily animal based and used aspartates bound to other nutrients such as magnesium and potassium or arginine, making it hard to draw conclusions regarding what impact, if any, was due to the aspartate salt and if applications could be made to a human population (Abel et al., 2005; Colombani et al., 1999; Olney, Labruyere, & de Gubareff, 1980). In fact, human data have not been favorable on the performance front. A 2007 double-blind, placebo-controlled study of 15 trained athletes, for example, failed to demonstrate any metabolic benefit (glycogen sparing) or improved endurance performance in trained athletes taking an isolated amino acid blend containing 7 g of asparagine and 7 g of aspartates before completion of an exercise-to-exhaustion test (Parisi et al., 2007). Thus, it is evident that additional large-group human studies using an isolated supplementation protocol are needed before any recommendations can be made for use in athletics.

Common usage: Not enough sound scientific data is available to establish dosing recommendations, though supplement manufacturers often recommend 4 to 5 g of aspartates, available in capsule or powdered form, in the 24-hour period leading up to competition as a means of boosting performance. To reduce fatigue, daily doses of 250 mg of both potassium and magnesium aspartate have been indicated.

Health concerns: L-aspartate is currently listed on the FDA's Generally Recognized as Safe (GRAS) list. Adverse effects have not been reported for doses of up to 10 g of aspartates over 24 hours. Doses above this may cause gastrointestinal irritation, including diarrhea.

Astaxanthin 

What it is: Astaxanthin, a metabolite of zeaxanthin and canthaxanthin, is a red fat-soluble pigment that belongs to the carotenoid group; however, it does not have provitamin A activity as do other carotenoids. Natural sources include algae, yeast, salmon, trout, krill, shrimp, and crayfish. According to Ambati and colleagues (2014), astaxanthin products are available as capsules, softgels, tablets, powders, creams, energy drinks, oils, and extracts.

Function: As an antioxidant, astaxanthin may protect cell membranes from free radical damage. Rodent data suggest that supplementation could potentially improve indices of exercise metabolism, performance, and recovery, but human data are lacking (Brown et al., 2018).

Performance benefit: As an antioxidant, astaxanthin may help reduce free radical damage in mitochondria (postulated to improve carnitine system function and fatty acid transport), which may support fat burning. It may also decrease reactive oxygen and nitrogen species that are present after eccentric (muscle lengthening) exercise, which would possibly hasten recovery. There is no consensus among human studies that these are measurably true, however.

Research: Aside from some existing data on astaxanthin's reduction of LDL (i.e., bad cholesterol) oxidation, there is speculation from animal models that astaxanthin improved mitochondrial fatty acid metabolism and even muscle recovery (because eccentric exercise induces microtrauma, including increased free radical production and sarcolemmal disruption). However, Bloomer and colleagues (2005), using an algae extract with 4 mg astaxanthin and 480 mg lutein for 3 weeks prior to damaging exercise, reported no favorable effect on markers of skeletal muscle microtrauma following eccentric loading in resistance-trained men. Further, antioxidant effects may actually be detrimental to muscle remodeling following such exercise, perhaps depending on the type of antioxidant. More controlled, scientifically rigorous research in exercising humans is necessary.

Common usage: A common dose of astaxanthin is 4 to 12 mg, co-ingested with dietary fat to enhance uptake.

Health concerns: The European Food Safety Authority (EFSA) has established an acceptable daily intake (ADI) of 0.034 mg/kg of astaxanthin (2.38 mg/day for a 70 kg individual). This is relatively low; a brief review of acute and chronic safety data by Brown and colleagues (2018) concluded that it may be possible to advocate substantially greater intake.

Astragalus 

aka *astragalus membranaceus, astragalus membrane root (AMR), astragalus mongholicus, huang qi, Radix astragali (RA)*

What it is: An herbal plant with yellow roots native to China, astragalus is also known as *huang qi,* meaning *yellow qi* (energy). Astragalus is purported to provide a wide array of medicinal benefits, especially relating to immune function. Although over 2,000 species of astragalus exist, *Astragalus membranaceus* and *Astragalus mongholicus* are the types primarily used. They are often found in soups, teas, extracts, and capsules or in combination with other herbs such as ginseng and echinacea.

Function: Intense physical training can suppress immune function and increase an athlete's risk of contracting an infection, especially in the acute postcompetition period. Astragalus contains antioxidants, which help protect cells, including those important to immune function, against damage caused by free radicals. In addition, studies have shown astragalus to carry antiviral properties, stimulating the immune system and thereby helping to protect against illness such as the common cold and upper respiratory tract infections.

Performance benefit: Astragalus may help support and enhance immune function, thereby protecting against illness that can sideline an athlete from competition.

Research: Preliminary evidence suggests astragalus taken in isolation or with other herbs may aid immune function, though well-designed trials on humans, particularly on healthy athletic populations, have been minimal. A small, double-blind, placebo-controlled study of healthy humans identified a protocol using *Astragalus membranaceus* at a dose of 2 g taken along with three medicinal mushrooms over 6 weeks to elicit a favorable immune response, significantly lowering the incidence of colds, influenza, or secondary infections (Clark & Adams, 2007; Clark, 2007). More recently, a double-blind study discovered a significant boost of immune system response to maximal physical exertion in 18 members of the Polish rowing team taking 500 mg/day of Astragalus membrane root (AMR) over 6 weeks of intensive training (Latour et al., 2021). Study investigators evaluated immune parameters for a number of cytokines, leukocyte subsets, and lactate immediately after and again 24 hours after a 2,000 m rowing time trial prior to supplementation on day 1 of

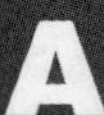

the study and again at the end of the 6 weeks. Compared to the placebo, AMR supplementation was able to restore immunological balance through stabilization of natural killer cells and subpopulations of T-regulatory lymphocytes. This study concluded that AMR shows promise as a supplement to bolster immune function and protect against infection during intensive training. Additional human trials, particularly on athletes, are warranted to draw definitive conclusions about practical guidelines for use in this population.

Common usage: In the human trials explored, a daily dose of 500 to 2,000 mg of astragalus was used over a period of 6 weeks.

Health concerns: Use of astragalus is considered safe for most adults, but because it is commonly used in conjunction with other herbal concoctions, possible secondary side effects are currently unknown.

Avocado Soybean Unsaponifiables (ASU)

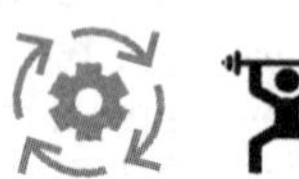
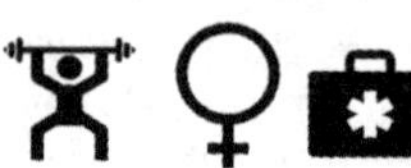

aka *Piascledine (brand name)*

What it is: Avocado soybean unsaponifiables (ASU) are natural components of avocado and soybean oils. ASU has become a popular addition to many joint supplements that promise to relieve pain and improve the symptoms of arthritis. The two types of unsaponifiables from avocado and soy appear to work synergistically in a ratio of 1:2 (Altinel et al., 2007). In France ASU is prescribed as a pharmaceutical drug known as Piascledine.

Function: ASU has been shown to inhibit the inflammatory cytokine interleukin-1β and its negative effects on synovial cells and chondrocytes, potentially preventing joint degeneration and improving joint function and health. ASU can also stimulate the growth of and prevent breakdown of cartilage. These mechanisms may prevent inflammation and degeneration of connective tissue in healthy joints (Salehi et al., 2020).

Performance benefit: Athletes commonly experience joint injuries resulting in pain, inflammation, and degeneration. ASU could prevent these negative effects, thereby lessening chronic joint strain and improving recovery from injury. Beyond its use to treat inflammatory conditions such as osteoarthritis (OA), ASU has shown potential as a natural therapeutic alternative to hormonal replacement therapy for menopausal women, making it of special interest for female master athletes entering this stage of their athletic careers (Salehi et al., 2020).

Research: One relevant, albeit skeptical, review of human literature was published by Liu and colleagues (2018), who concluded that, among six other supplemental osteoarthritis interventions, avocado soybean unsaponifiables "revealed statistically significant improvements on pain, but were of unclear clinical importance." Further, these authors suggested that the quality of existing evidence was very low and that a variety of related supplements "had no clinically important effects on pain and function at medium-term and long-term follow-ups." This is in some contrast to a meta-analysis by Christensen and colleagues reviewing the results from four randomized control trials (RCTs) in humans using ASU in the treatment of OA was also positive, showing reductions in pain and improved joint function as assessed by the Lequesne index, a validated questionnaire commonly used in research studies on arthritic conditions. Similar results were reported in a 2019 meta-analysis of randomized, placebo-controlled trials evaluating the effect of orally administered ASU on symptomatic knee OA, with a significant reduction in pain and OA symptoms using the Lequesne index and visual analog scale—though interestingly, the favorable results did not translate to patients suffering from hip OA (Simental-Mendía et al., 2019). Another double-blind, randomized, placebo-controlled, crossover trial on 40 patients with OA revealed significantly lower levels of oxidative stress as well as positive changes in serum antioxidant levels after 3 months of treatment with ASU compared to baseline and placebo levels, which study investigators conclude is a valid reason to consider ASU in the treatment of osteoarthritis (Jangravi et al., 2021). Additional research, particularly on master-level athletes who are more prone to suffer from such inflammatory conditions as OA, is warranted to establish practical recommendations for use.

Common usage: A dose of 300 mg/day is recommended. The benefits of ASU are not improved with higher doses. Further scientific trials should continue to clarify best-use supplementation strategies.

Health concerns: Reported adverse drug reactions related to ASU are rare, and its use appears safe and nontoxic.

Bacopa Monnieri 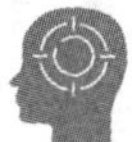 

aka *brahmi (not to be confused with gotu kola), herb of grace, Indian pennywort, thyme-leafed gratiola, water hyssop*

What it is: *Bacopa monnieri*, an adaptogen herb used in traditional Ayurvedic medicine, is common to the marshy areas of southern and Eastern India, Australia, Europe, Africa, Asia, and North and South America.

Function: The herb's collection of bacosides are thought to protect nerve cells, enhancing attention, memory, and the processing of visual information as well as supporting motor function.

Performance benefit: The herb is potentially memory enhancing and may support fatigue resistance or a reduction in anxiety, which could be helpful to athletes in pre-game scenarios.

Research: In a 2019 review of the effects of phytochemicals on cognitive function related to sport performance, David Kennedy stated "Bacopa monnieri [has] been shown to enhance relevant aspects of cognitive function and alertness. More data in exercising humans are needed" (Kennedy, 2019).

Common usage: As a standardized extract (50% bacosides), 200 to 400 mg/day is a common dose.

Health concerns: *Bacopa monnieri* is reportedly safe when consumed in doses up to 600 mg/day for up to 12 weeks. Common side effects include dry mouth, stomach cramps, nausea, and diarrhea. Bacopa might slow heart rate and gastrointestinal transit, as well as increase gastrointestinal, urinary, and pulmonary fluid secretions. Its potential to increase thyroid hormone concentrations suggest persons with thyroid issues should speak to their physician.

Baking Soda

(see *sodium bicarbonate* and *sodium citrate*)

Balaton Cherry

(see *tart cherry*)

B-Complex Vitamin

(see *thiamine*)

Beetroot 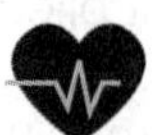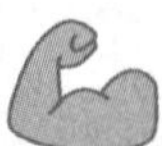

aka *beet, beetroot juice, garden beet, red beet, table beet*

What it is: Containing powerful antioxidants called anthocyanins that contribute to its distinctive reddish-purple flesh and skin, beetroot is a plant in the amaranth family whose root and leaves can be served raw, baked, steamed, pickled, or as a juice. Beetroot has been touted as a natural source of potentially performance-enhancing and recovery-facilitating dietary nitrates—nearly 300 mg per 100 g serving.

Function: Once ingested, dietary nitrates from beetroot are converted into nitric oxide. Nitric oxide serves as a vasodilator, opening up the blood vessels to allow more blood and oxygen to be delivered to the muscles, thereby lowering the oxygen cost of exercise and making aerobic exercise less tiring. Although this performance benefit may not extend to power athletes, antioxidant and vasodilatory effects may facilitate some aspects of recovery.

SUPPLEMENT FACT

The physiological effects of beetroot kick in 30 minutes postconsumption, peak after 90 minutes, and stay elevated for approximately 6 hours. Overall health and performance benefits may last as long as 2 weeks postconsumption.

Performance benefit: Athletes may benefit from reductions in the oxygen cost of exercise, improving endurance and tolerance to high-intensity training. They may also experience decreased muscle soreness and quicker recovery of performance.

Research: A 2021 systematic review and meta-analysis of 17 studies by Wong and colleagues on high-intensity interval training (HIIT) concluded that "beetroot supplementation at a dose of <12.9 mmol/day for 6 days offers no significant improvement to peak or mean power output during HIIT or SIT [sprint interval training]" but that future research should explore the efficacy of beetroot at higher doses (>12.9 mmol/day for 6 days). The authors expounded that chronic supplementation protocols with higher beetroot doses (>12.9 mmol/day for 6 days) are recommended. Regarding markers of exercise-induced muscle damage and recovery, a 2022 systematic review of nine studies and meta-analysis of six studies by Jones and colleagues concluded that beetroot juice accelerated isometric strength recovery 72 hours postexercise ($p = 0.01$) and countermovement jump performance 24 to 72 hours postexercise ($p < 0.03$). Further, pressure–pain threshold (necessary pressure required to evoke muscle soreness) was greater with beetroot juice 48 hours ($p = 0.03$) and 72 hours postexercise ($p = 0.02$). However, these authors reported that beetroot juice had no effect on markers of oxidative stress and creatine kinase release ($p > 0.05$), and that the inflammation marker C-reactive protein was actually higher versus placebo at 48 hours postexercise ($p = 0.03$). These findings suggest that nitrate-rich beetroot juice may attenuate some markers of exercise-induced muscle damage but some markers were unchanged or worsened.

In 2009, scientists at the University of Exeter in England published a series of well-designed studies evaluating the effects of a 500 mL dose of organic beetroot juice on overall performance in healthy men. The initial study found that a 6-day supplementation protocol with beetroot juice extended cycle-to-exhaustion time by 92 seconds, representing a 2% decline in the time needed to cover a set distance, compared to a placebo control beverage of black currant juice (Bailey et al., 2009). The same 6-day supplementation protocol helped reduce the oxygen consumption in trained runners during moderate- and high-intensity running, thereby extending their time to exhaustion by 15% (Lansley et al., 2011b). A follow-up study looking at the impact that beetroot juice has when taken 2.5 hours before both a 4 km and a 16.1 km time trial, separated by 3 days, replicated the initial results with trained male cyclists, improving performance by 2% to 3% compared to the placebo trials (Lansley et al., 2011a). The benefits of beetroot, however, seem to diminish a bit over longer-distance time trials: A small 2012 study failed to demonstrate a significant benefit to performance during a 80 km bike time trial for trained cyclists who consumed the same 0.5 L dose of beetroot juice 2.5 hours before beginning (Wilkerson et al., 2012).

Common usage: The research-supported dose for performance benefits is 500 mL of juiced beetroot taken 2.5 hours before a short, high-intensity period of exercise.

ATHLETES' TIP

Athletes can make their own homemade beetroot juice using the following steps. To yield the research-recommended dose of 500 mL, eight small or four large beetroots will be needed.

Step 1: Cut off green tops as needed. Scrub any dirt off the outside of the beets with a produce brush and rinse. Leave the skin intact for added nutrition.

Step 2: Cut the beetroots into halves or quarters and throw into a juicer. Because beetroots are a very hard vegetable, be sure to allow some time for juicing to occur.

Tip: Add other fruits and vegetables to adjust the flavor to desired taste.

Health concerns: There have been a few reports of abdominal cramps, diarrhea, and a temporary and harmless purple coloring of the urine known as beeturia. Of special note, the World Health Organization (WHO) has an established daily upper limit of 222 mg for dietary nitrates and nitrites due to previous links to gastrointestinal cancer and blood disorders in infants. This limit is well below the research-supported performance dose of beetroot juice. However, as refuted in research by registered dietitian Norman Hord of Michigan State University, these detrimental effects are associated with the dietary intake of nitrates and nitrites from processed meat and well water, not from vegetables such as beetroot (Hord et al., 2009).

Berberine 

aka *berberine alkaloid, berberine complex*

What it is: Berberine is a bitter yellow chemical found in plants such as European barberry, tree turmeric, goldenseal, goldthread, and Oregon grape.

Function: Some studies have shown that berberine may improve insulin sensitivity and reduce blood glucose levels in nonathletic populations, though research is not conclusive.

Performance benefit: Optimizing blood sugar is a trend among athletes, but because this population is known to already have heightened glucose tolerance—in part due to increased glucose transporter (GLUT4) activity—the addition of a phytochemical that has been shown to reduce blood glucose is unlikely to provide further benefit.

Research: A recent meta-analysis of berberine's effects on metabolic disorders by Ye and colleagues (2021) stated "Berberine can improve obesity and hyperlipidemia by reducing TG [triglycerides], TC [total cholesterol], and LDL [low-density lipoprotein] and increasing HDL [high-density lipoprotein]; reduce insulin resistance to improve type II diabetes." It is currently uncertain what benefit an athlete may obtain from such effects, given the fact that training already improves cardiometabolic health.

Common usage: A common dose is 500 mg 3 times/day, typically before meals.

Health concerns: Potential side effects for healthy persons may include diarrhea, constipation, gas, and upset stomach. The phytochemical also interferes with specific liver enzymes that are responsible for the breakdown of various medications. There is some indication of reduced intestinal glucose uptake in the intestines, which would likely be counterproductive to athletes.

Beta-Alanine 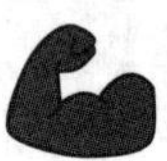 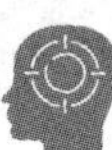   

aka β-*alanine, carnosine precursor, 3-aminopropanoic acid*

What it is: Beta-alanine is an amino acid that is naturally synthesized in the body and thus not an essential component of the diet. It does not play a role in the biosynthesis of any major proteins or enzymes as many amino acids do, but it does aid the synthesis of carnosine, an acidity-buffering, antiglycating, antioxidant, and potentially "antiaging" dipeptide found within both type I (slow-twitch) and type II (fast-twitch) muscle fibers (Hoffman et al., 2018; Wang et al., 2000). Many scientists believe the pH-buffering role to be the primary contributing factor to beta-alanine's ergogenic qualities: Studies have shown increased intramuscular levels of carnosine to be associated with reductions in muscle fatigue and enhancements of overall work capacity.

Function: The bulk of research on beta-alanine has evaluated its impact on intramuscular levels of carnosine (β-alanyl-L-histidine), a dipeptide essential for maintaining an optimal pH within the muscle. During exertion, especially during high-intensity efforts, the breakdown of carbohydrate for fast energy production triggers an increase in hydrogen ions and consequent drop in muscle pH. This process is known as acidosis, commonly described by athletes as a burning sensation that leads to extreme muscle fatigue, reduced power output, and eventual muscular failure. Carnosine serves as an effective buffer, naturally absorbing hydrogen ions, allowing the muscle to continue firing, and enabling overall strength and endurance to remain at peak levels.

Performance benefit: Possible benefits of beta-alanine supplementation include a boost in anaerobic performance or overall high-intensity work capacity, thus allowing an athlete to train harder for longer (e.g., high-repetition sets).

Research: Randomized control trials have confirmed that supplementation with beta-alanine has the potential to significantly increase carnosine levels within the muscle, especially in type II fibers, which provides an efficient buffering system for fatigue-inducing hydrogen ions that can negatively impact anaerobic performance, especially in efforts lasting from 60 to 240+ seconds (Hobson et al., 2012). For example, daily beta-alanine supplementation of 5 g/day over 7 weeks corresponded with a 45.3% and 28.2% increase in carnosine levels within the soleus and gastrocnemius muscles, respectively, in elite rowers. This result yielded a 4.3-second improvement over 2,000 m of rowing (Baguet et al., 2010). Furthermore, a 2012 meta-analysis of 15 published manuscripts including a total of 360 subjects confirmed a median performance improvement of 2.85% when a median total of 179 g of beta-alanine was supplemented across the overall dosing regimen (Hobson et al., 2012). More recently, Saunders and colleagues (2017) analyzed 40 individual studies using 65 different exercise protocols and totaling 70 exercise measures in 1,461 participants and found that "A significant overall effect size . . . was shown." Exercise duration significantly moderated effect sizes ($p = 0.004$), as did exercise type in subgroup analysis. Training status of the participants and intermittent-versus-continuous exercises did not moderate effects. These researchers concluded that "Beta-alanine had a significant overall effect while subgroup analyses revealed a number of modifying factors." Even more recently, in a review of the effects of beta-alanine and other ergogenic aids on women, Murphy and colleagues (2022) reported that, based on nine studies, "Evidence suggests that beta-alanine may lower the rate of perceived exertion and extend training bouts in women, leading to greater functional adaptations." The impact of beta-alanine hasn't uniformly yielded favorable results—again, especially when the effects are evaluated across all sport activities. Indeed, Smith-Ryan and colleagues (2012) failed to discover any performance benefit when evaluating the effect of two 800 mg tablets taken 3 times/day, or a total of 4.8g/d of beta-alanine (split into three 1.6-g doses) on anaerobic running capacity or total time to run exhaustion for short bursts at 90% to 110% peak velocity or speed lasting 1.95 to 5.06 minutes. It appears that still more research is needed on specific athletic events to confirm the potential buffering and consequent anaerobic benefits.

Common usage: To achieve the research-supported increase in muscle carnosine levels, between 3.2 and 6.4 g/day are recommended for up to 12 weeks; performance benefits begin occurring in as little as 2 weeks, with more dramatic results occurring after 4 weeks of continuous supplementation. Taking beta-alanine in coordination with carbohydrate may facilitate a quicker performance response, likely as a result of an increase in insulin, a hormone responsible for transporting amino acids into cells. It is also theorized that timing beta-alanine intake immediately before and after a workout may facilitate increased uptake into the muscles, likely because blood flow is increased during exertion. In addition to supplementation, at least some amount of beta-alanine can be obtained from such dietary sources as chicken, beef, pork, and fish.

Health concerns: Supplementation with the research-supposed dose of beta-alanine for up to 12 weeks appears to be safe, but there have been reports of paresthesia (skin irritation, flushing, and tingling, which is not considered dangerous) with doses above 10 mg/kg of body mass. Varanoske and colleagues (2019) compared 28 days of slow- versus rapid-release beta-alanine formulations (6 g daily) on changes in carnosine content of the vastus lateralis and muscle fatigue in 39 recreationally active men and women and concluded "Symptoms of paresthesia were significantly more frequent in rapid-release compared to slow-release [formulas], the latter of which did not differ from placebo." Beyond this side effect, there is concern that high doses, especially taken for 4 or more weeks, can interfere with taurine uptake and negatively affect cardiac function.

Beta-Carotene

aka *provitamin A*

What it is: Beta-carotene belongs to a class of red, orange, and yellow pigments called carotenoids and is found in abundance in many fruits and vegetables containing these colors. It readily converts to vitamin A to support normal growth and development, immune function, and vision, and as a fat-soluble antioxidant, it helps protect the integrity of cell membranes. It is stored in the liver and fatty tissues.

Function: Intense physical training triggers an increase in the production of free radicals and other reactive oxygen species (ROS), often at rates that surpass the strengthened antioxidant defenses of even the fittest athletes. This can lead to irreparable damage to lipids in cell membranes as well as the genetic material in cells, causing a plethora of health and performance concerns for the athlete. In particular, the inflammatory response brought on by lipid peroxidation, a type of free radical reaction, can suppress immune function and increase susceptibility to infection, especially of the upper respiratory tract. Beta-carotene is capable of fighting off free radical reactions within the cell membrane, thereby making the cells less vulnerable to viral attack; it may further strengthen immunity by increasing the number of T-helper cells and stimulating the activity of natural killer cells.

Performance benefit: Beta-carotene may help protect athletes, especially those engaged in ultraendurance events, from nagging illnesses that can put a damper on training and hinder performance. There is some evidence that beta-carotene's role in protecting the cell membrane from damage induced by lipid peroxidation may be effective for reducing symptoms associated with allergies and asthma, especially those symptoms that are exercise induced, as well as other inflammatory-based conditions such as osteoarthritis.

Research: Although an abundance of well-designed studies confirm a positive relationship between supplemental and whole food intake of beta-carotene and plasma levels of the antioxidant, results evaluating its impact on markers of oxidative stress and immune function are conflicting, especially among an athletic population. For instance, a small study on elite kayakers demonstrated that enhanced blood levels of beta-carotene, along with several other antioxidants, did little to protect the athletes against the detriments of exercise-induced lipid peroxidation and inflammation (Teixeira et al., 2009). However, another double-blind, placebo-controlled study demonstrated that a 7-day supplementation protocol with a popular antioxidant cocktail containing 18 mg of beta-carotene, 900 mg of vitamin C, and 90 mg of vitamin E significantly enhanced plasma antioxidant levels as well as neutrophil enzyme activity after trained athletes completed a 2-hour aerobic run (Robson, Bouic, & Myburgh, 2003). Tauler and colleagues (2006) also found significantly elevated plasma levels of vitamin C, vitamin E, and beta-carotene and consequent blood cell antioxidant enzyme defenses in amateur trained athletes after daily supplementation with 500 mg/day of vitamin E and 30 mg/day of beta-carotene with 1 g/day of vitamin C added for the final 15 days. However, according to previous research evaluating the impact of a similar antioxidant mix on upper respiratory infections in ultramarathoners, this result is likely due to vitamin C rather than beta-carotene (Peters et al., 1994). Some studies have shown that beta-carotene, when taken exclusive of other antioxidants at daily doses of 15 to 50 mg, can significantly increase the number of T-helper cells and boost natural killer cell activity in healthy individuals of a wide age spectrum, suggesting immune-supportive qualities (Ross, 2012; Wood et al., 2000). Of special note, however, are results of a 2022 meta-analysis of randomized control trials revealing potential harmful effects of low-dose, high-dose, and single-use of beta-carotene supplements on overall risk for and mortality from cardiovascular disease (CVD), making the safety of daily supplemental use of beta-carotene, particularly among those with CVD histories, questionable (Yang et al., 2022). Additional research should further evaluate if these risks translate in an athletic population.

Common usage: The research-supported daily dose of beta-carotene for general health is currently 15 to 50 mg (25,000-83,000 IU), with water-based supplements generally being recommended over oil-based for optimal absorption.

Health concerns: There are some reports of skin discoloring (turning a yellow-orange hue) at doses above 100,000 IU or 60 mg/day. Expectant mothers should take extra precautions as large doses of beta-carotene can be harmful to the fetus.

Beta-Carotene

Beta-D-Ribofuranose

(see *Ribose*)

Beta-Ecdysterone

(see *ecdysteroids*)

Beta-Glucan 

aka *beta-1,3/1,4-glucan, beta-1,3/1,6-glucan, oat bran, oat-derived beta-glucan, yeast-derived beta-glucan*

What it is: A polysaccharide or complex chain of glucose molecules that is often regarded for its immunostimulant properties, beta-glucan can be derived from a variety of sources, including whole grains (especially oat and barley); certain fungi such as baker's yeast; and the medicinal mushrooms reishi, maitake, and shiitake. The chemical makeup often dictates the biological activity of the compound.

Function: Intense physical training can challenge the immune system, with declines in such key immune markers as neutrophils, natural killer cells, T cells, and B cells often culminating in upper respiratory tract infections (URTIs). Beta-glucan activates key immune cells to help trap and consume various viral, bacterial, protozoan, and fungal invaders that can cause infection.

Performance benefit: For up to 2 weeks after intense exercise, especially endurance exercise, an athlete is at heightened risk for infection, which can slow the recovery process and cause unwanted physical and mental stress. Beta-glucan may provide a boost to immune function and help an athlete stave off infection as well as sustain the energy levels and vigor needed to train and compete at peak. Because increasing macrophage and immune cell activity promotes the breakdown and removal of damaged tissue, supplementation with beta-glucan may also aid recovery from athletic injury and facilitate faster wound healing.

Research: One double-blind, placebo-controlled study discovered a significant reduction in URTI-related symptoms such as sore throat, stuffy or runny nose, and cough as well as better overall health and a more positive mood in runners who followed a daily supplementation protocol of either 250 mg or 500 mg of yeast-derived beta-glucan for 4 weeks after completing a marathon (Talbott & Talbott, 2009). The higher dose provided only a slightly greater protective effect, indicating that more isn't necessarily better. A similar study of 357 participants racing the 2017 Austin Marathon found daily supplementation with 250 mL of a dairy beverage containing 250 mg of baker's yeast beta-glucan for 45 days prior to and after the marathon (91 days total) yielded significantly lower severity ratings for URTI symptoms, including sore throat and nasal discharge, as well as significantly quicker recovery period and fewer days down due to URTI than those subjects drinking the calorie-matched placebo ($n = 225$) (Mah et al., 2020). A shorter double-blind, randomized, crossover study found a shorter 13-day supplementation protocol, also with 250 mg of a yeast-derived beta-glucan, to promote favorable changes in cytokine markers of inflammation after completing a prolonged session of heated treadmill exercise (Zabriskie et al., 2020). Additionally, Bobovcak and colleagues (2010) showed a mere 100 mg dose of a mushroom-based beta-glucan (*Pleurotus osteratus*) each day for 2 months was essentially able to eliminate the decrease in natural killer cell activity and the overall natural killer cell count seen in elite athletes after intense exercise, thereby supporting immune system integrity. Where the beta-glucan is derived, however, may play a role in purported immunobenefits, as daily supplementation with an oat-derived beta-glucan over 18 days failed to alter resting- or exercise-induced changes in immune function or URTI incidence in trained cyclists completing a 3-hour cycle test at 57% maximal watts (Nieman et al., 2008).

Common usage: According to research, a range of 100 to 500 mg of beta-glucan taken daily throughout a heavy training cycle is an effective dose for enhanced immune protection. To aid absorption, beta-glucan should be taken on an empty stomach. Beta-glucan derived from yeast or mushroom seems to yield the most promising benefits for immune function.

Health concerns: The FDA has given beta-glucan the Generally Recognized as Safe (GRAS) rating, meaning there are no known side effects or adverse reactions associated with its intended use.

Betaine 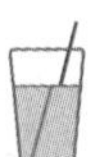 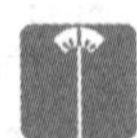

aka *glycine betaine, trimethylglycine (TMG)*

What it is: Betaine is a derivative of the nonessential amino acid glycine and is synthesized naturally within the body as well as obtained from such dietary sources as wheat, beets, spinach, and shellfish. Although traditionally used as a dietary supplement for animals, betaine has appeared as a sports supplement with the claim that it may help facilitate hydration, increase strength gains, enhance endurance, and improve recovery.

Function: Betaine has several physiological functions of potential benefit to athletic performance. One is its role as an osmolyte, helping to increase water retention by cells and thereby protecting against dehydration. Another role is as a methyl group donor, a quality that could affect multiple physiologic systems, although betaine's mechanism of action for specific benefits is still being studied. Betaine has been shown to exhibit cardio-, hepatic-, and neuroprotective effects (Arumugam et al., 2021) as well as enhance vascular health, helping to increase blood and oxygen flow to working tissue, which may benefit endurance as well as strength gains. It is also hypothesized that betaine can enhance strength and power performance by increasing skeletal muscle creatine concentration. In both endurance- and resistance-type exercise, conflicting results have been reported (Cholewa et al., 2014).

Performance benefit: Athletes may benefit from better hydration status during training and competition as well as potentially achieve enhanced strength and endurance gains. There is some evidence that supplementation with betaine enhances fat metabolism, which could spare muscle glycogen and aid endurance performance. Early speculation that betaine may help improve body composition, however, has been questioned. In a systematic review and meta-analysis, Ashtary-Larky and colleagues (2022) concluded that betaine supplementation does not show any beneficial effects on body composition indices, including body weight, body mass index, fat mass, or fat-free mass.

Research: The potential benefits of betaine as it relates to athletic performance appear to be multifaceted—though, again, results of well-designed human studies have been mixed to date. For example, a well-designed study found supplementation with 2.5 g of betaine mixed into 500 mL of Gatorade sport drink and taken daily over 14 days elicited a moderate, though statistically insignificant, improvement in muscle endurance compared to a placebo (Trepanowski et al., 2011). On the other hand, a similar protocol consisting of 2.5 g of betaine taken in two split doses along with 300 mL of Gatorade sport drink over 14 days yielded significant increases in the vertical jump power and isometric squat force of trained males compared to baseline (Lee et al., 2010). However, there were no performance improvements reported for jump squat power or the number of bench press and squat repetitions.

In another study, the same split protocol taken with 240 mL of a sport drink significantly increased the number of repetitions performed by recreationally trained athletes at 90% or greater of peak power in a squat exercise protocol after 1 and 2 weeks of supplementation compared to placebo (Hoffman et al., 2009). Of particular interest to athletes, Armstrong and colleagues (2008) discovered that rehydration with fluids containing betaine (water with 5 g of betaine/L of fluid or 6.5% carbohydrate-electrolyte solution with 5 g of betaine/L of fluid) significantly improved the plasma volume, oxygen consumption, plasma lactate concentration, and thermal sensation of runners completing a 75-minute aerobic treadmill test followed by a sprint to exhaustion compared with a comparable placebo of either water or sport drink. Although the benefits to sprint performance to exhaustion after the aerobic run were statistically insignificant and likely irrelevant for the recreational athlete, the result may indeed be consequential for the elite-level athlete. Nonetheless, with inconsistent and often statistically insignificant results, it is evident further human studies are warranted before valid conclusions for use of betaine as an ergogenic aid can be made.

Common usage: Manufactured as a byproduct of sugar beet processing, betaine supplements are available in powder, tablet, and capsule form. According to Cholewa and colleagues (2014), the ergogenic and clinical effects of betaine have been investigated with doses ranging from 500 to 9,000 mg/day. The doses typically supported by research range from 2,500 to 5,000 mg/day, generally taken in split doses, for up to 2 weeks before competition.

Health concerns: Reported side effects are generally mild and include stomach upset, nausea, and diarrhea. Athletes with cardiovascular risk factors should be aware that betaine has been shown to increase total cholesterol levels, although overall it may be cardioprotective via reductions in homocysteine when consumed at less than 4 g/day (Ashtary-Larky et al., 2022).

Beta-1,3/1,4-Glucan, Beta-1,3/1,6-Glucan

(see *beta-glucan*)

Beta-Tocopherol, Beta-Tocotrienol

(see *vitamin E*)

Bifidobacterium

(see *probiotics*)

BioPerine

(see *piperine*)

Bitter Orange

(see *synephrine*)

Black Currant Seed Oil

(see *gamma-linolenic acid*)

Black Ginger

(see *ginger*)

Black Pepper

(see *piperine*)

Borage Oil

(see *gamma-linolenic acid*)

Boron (B) 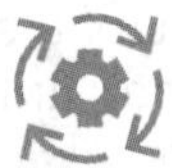 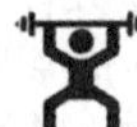

aka *boric acid, boron oxide, calcium fructoborate*

What it is: An essential mineral found in plants, boron plays a key role in many biological processes and can be found abundantly in fruits and vegetables as well as legumes.

Function: Boron plays an important role in bone growth, cognitive performance, inflammatory response, and immune health. Adequate intake has been shown to promote optimal health (Khaliq et al., 2018), whereas low boron status has been tied to poor immune function, increased risk of mortality, osteoporosis, and cognitive deterioration. Boron deficiency has also been shown to affect inflammation-regulating cytokines and chemokines, as well as decrease bone volume and the number of osteoblast (bone-forming) cells (Nielsen, 2008).

Performance benefit: Boron is speculated to benefit athletes through its ability to promote bone growth and development and provide protection against inflammation induced by injury or training stress.

Research: A supplemental dose of 3 mg/day of boron (alone or with other nutrients) has demonstrated efficacy in supporting bone health by halting bone loss and maintaining bone density (Rondanelli et al., 2020). In addition, a double-blind, placebo-controlled study found supplementation with boron (as calcium fructoborate) at a dose of 1.5, 3, or 6 mg/day over 2 weeks to significantly reduce inflammatory markers (C-reactive protein, fibrinogen) in 60 participants aged 59 to 68 who were suffering from osteoarthritis (Scorei et al., 2011). Results from animal studies have also demonstrated an association between adequate dietary intake of boron nd improved responses to antigen-induced arthritis. Further research is needed to clarify the benefits of boron in humans, particularly athletes, and if these benefits apply when dietary intake and boron status is sufficient or just when deficiencies are present. Currently, it seems as if the benefits are only experienced in boron-deficient states induced via suboptimal dietary intakes of 0.045 to 0.062 mg/day. Because boron is found so abundantly in a variety of foods, deficiency is rare.

Common usage: Most boron supplements sold contain 1.5 to 11.6 mg.

Health concerns: Intakes of 1 to 13 mg of boron/day are considered to be within an acceptable, safe range (Nielsen, 2008).

Boswellia Serrata (BS) 

aka *acetyl-11-keto-boswellic acid (AKBA), frankincense, olibanum*

What it is: *Boswellia serrata* (BS) is a species of deciduous tree commonly found in India and Arabia. The gum resin of BS has a long history dating back to biblical times. It has a wide variety of uses, including for medicinal purposes, religious ceremonies, and perfume production.

Function: The gum resin of BS contains more than 12 boswellic acids (BAs), which have anti-inflammatory properties. According to Ammon (2016), "the anti-inflammatory actions of BAs are caused by different mechanisms of action. They include inhibition of leukotriene synthesis and to a lesser extent prostaglandin synthesis." They also suppress inflammatory cytokines. As a result, BS has been used as a beneficial treatment for various inflammation-related diseases such as bronchial asthma, Crohn's disease, and arthritis (Ernst, 2008).

Performance benefit: Anti-inflammatories are commonly used by athletes to limit inflammation and pain resulting from muscle injury, arthritic joints, or muscle soreness from heavy, intensified training. Because of these effects, BS is a likely candidate for athletes looking for an alternative to nonsteroidal anti-inflammatories (NSAIDS) such as ibuprofen.

Research: Clinical studies involving BS are encouraging but scant. According to a review on osteoarthritis by Cameron and Chrubasik (2014), "extracts of Boswellia serrata show trends of benefits that warrant further investigation." Toward this end, Rudrappa and colleagues (2022) studied the analgesic effect of a formulation of turmeric and Boswellia extracts in sesame oil (266 mg curcuminoids and 10 mg acetyl-11-keto-boswellic acid [AKBA]) in reducing a wide variety of exercise-induced acute musculoskeletal pains in healthy participants. Although the combination makes BS-specific conclusions difficult, the authors concluded that exercise-induced acute musculoskeletal pain can be relieved by the intervention in about 3 hours, "signifying its strong analgesic activity." Although these studies suggest promise, they are not extensive, are limited in subject number, and are commonly found in complementary medicine journals, which rarely publish negative results. As noted, studies related to osteoarthritis of the knee have found BS to be effective in reducing pain and improving function compared with a placebo (Sengupta et al., 2011). Again, the gum resin of BS contains boswellic acids (BAs), of which AKBA is perhaps the main active component (Gong et al., 2022). Unfortunately, most gum resins of BS only contain 2% to 3% AKBA. The bioavailability of BS is also poor and known to be a limiting factor. Currently, scientists are looking to improve the effective use of BS by increasing the concentration of AKBA and improving its bioavailability.

Common usage: The common usage for BS is 600 to 3,000 mg/day (Ernst, 2008).

Health concerns: A major target of BAs is the immune system. BS extracts have been shown to decrease production of proinflammatory cytokines including IL-1, IL-2, IL-6, IFN-γ and TNF-α (Ammon, 2016). BS's suppression of this response is generally considered beneficial at the time of this writing. According to Ammon (2016), the number and severity of side effects is extremely low, with the most reported complaints being gastrointestinal symptoms. Further, allergic reactions are rare.

⚠ SUPPLEMENT WARNING

Although decreasing inflammatory cytokines may be helpful for an inflamed athlete, suppressing parts of the immune system through supplement use such as BS may not always be healthy for certain populations. People with certain infections, cancer, or other medical conditions that affect the immune system should use caution when considering taking such anti-inflammatory supplements.

Bovine Colostrum (BC)

(see *colostrum*)

Branched-Chain Amino Acids (BCAAs) 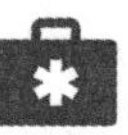 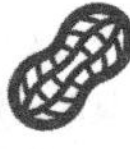

aka *isoleucine, leucine, valine*

What it is: Branched-chain amino acids (BCAAs) include the amino acids leucine, isoleucine, and valine. All three are considered essential amino acids; they cannot be made in the body and must be consumed in the diet from protein-rich foods. BCAAs account for 35% of the essential amino acids found in muscle proteins.

Function: BCAAs are key stimulators of protein synthesis (muscle building) and also play a role in the prevention of muscle breakdown. Although other essential amino acids are mainly catabolized (broken down) in the liver, BCAAs are unique in that they can be oxidized in the muscle for fuel (Shimomura et al., 2004).

Performance benefit: Because of the role BCAAs have in the regulation of protein synthesis and protein breakdown, it is believed that they can be used to prevent the catabolic, muscle-damaging effects of exercise when supplemented before or during training; they may also be used to enhance muscle building or protein synthesis when supplemented after exercise. In addition, many believe that BCAAs can have performance-enhancing effects due to their ability to be oxidized and used for fuel by the muscles. This belief has prompted many endurance athletes to supplement with BCAAs before and during competition or training.

Research: There is evidence that BCAA supplementation can reduce the level of muscle soreness and muscle damage biomarkers, such as creatine kinase and lactate dehydrogenase, following muscle-damaging exercises, particularly in resistance-trained athletes (Doma et al., 2021; Martinho et al., 2022). However, there have been inconsistencies on such favorable outcomes in endurance-trained, master-level, and untrained athletes (Manaf et al., 2021; Negro et al., 2008; Watson, Shirreffs, & Maughan, 2004). Furthermore, the reductions seen in muscle damage biomarkers have not consistently translated to enhanced recovery times and muscle performance, nor has supplementation been shown to elicit any favorable body composition changes. It is thought that differences in supplementation protocols and dietary intake of protein are likely linked to the difference in outcomes (Martinho et al., 2022). A 2017 meta-analysis revealed BCAA supplementation to be efficacious on outcomes of exercise-induced muscle damage provided the extent of muscle damage was only low to moderate and the supplementation protocol combined a high daily BCAA intake (>200 mg/kg/day) with a long duration (>10 days) (Foure et al., 2017). Additional randomized, placebo-controlled clinical trials would be needed to support the beneficial effects of this strategy, as only one study in the meta-analysis was rated as positive regarding the quality of reported beneficial events and the sample size was small. Another application of BCAAs in athletes is during recovery from injury. Early research appears positive that BCAAs can limit muscle wasting or atrophy associated with immobilization and decreases in physical training (Bajotto et al., 2011). In addition, BCAAs appear to limit immune suppression resulting from exercise. BCAAs limit reductions of serum glutamine, an important nutrient for immune health often lowered as a result of intense and prolonged training (Negro et al., 2008). Even so, questions still remain in terms of the effectiveness of BCAAs over the use of whole proteins. Because whole proteins, most notably whey protein and leucine, contain sufficient quantities of BCAAs, it does not appear that supplementation with BCAAs before or after training provides additional benefits if adequate amounts of high-quality whole proteins are consumed (Master et al., 2021).

Common usage: A variety of supplementation protocols have been used with BCAAs. Most protocols use a higher dosage of leucine and smaller dosages of valine and isoleucine. Protocols have ranged from 6 to 14 g of BCAAs/day in a ratio of 2 or 3:1:1 of leucine, valine, and isoleucine. Emerging data have shown use of omega-3 fatty acids in conjunction with BCAAs may enhance the potential recovery-focused benefits of BCAAs (Tsuchiya et al., 2022).

 Branched-Chain Amino Acids (BCAAs)

ATHLETES' TIP

Because of its singular effects on muscle protein synthesis, leucine is often dosed and sold separately from the other two BCAAs. However, *the general consensus among experts is that taking all three BCAAs (leucine, valine, and isoleucine) together is best. For further information, see the separate entry on leucine.*

Health concerns: No adverse effects of BCAA toxicity have been reported in relation to exercise and sport. Single doses of 10 g/kg have been used in mice and did not result in death. No toxic effects of BCAAs have been observed from an intake of 2.5 g/kg/day for 3 months or 1.25 g/kg/day for 1 year (Shimomura et al., 2004).

Bromelain  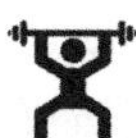 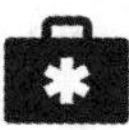

aka *Ananas comosus, Ananase (brand name), bromelainum*

What it is: A proteolytic (protein-digesting) enzyme derived from the stem and juice of the pineapple plant, bromelain quickly gained popularity as a natural anti-inflammatory and painkiller upon its release as a therapeutic supplement in 1957. It is currently used to help reduce edema, bruising, and healing time following trauma, including sport injuries and surgery.

Function: Swelling and inflammation, which manifest as redness, heat, bruising, and pain, cause collagen fibers to form adhesions that can inhibit muscle lengthening and consequent functionality of the injured tissue. Without treatment, the injury can lead to time away from training, decreased fitness, and poor performance. Bromelain's proteolytic characteristics facilitate the breakdown of adhesions in the circulatory system and connective tissue such as muscles; improve the delivery of nutrients and oxygen-rich blood to the injured tissue; and remove metabolic waste that can exacerbate inflammation. Additionally, it has also been proposed that bromelain halts the production of bradykinin, a chemical responsible for mediating the inflammatory response, and controls the number of white blood cells that accumulate within the blood vessels at the site of inflammation. Similar to other nonsteroidal anti-inflammatories (NSAIDs) such as Aspirin, Motrin, Aleve, and Celebrex, bromelain inhibits COX-2, an enzyme responsible for inflammation and pain (Hikisz & Bernasinska-Slomczewska, 2021).

Performance benefit: The anti-inflammatory and painkilling qualities of bromelain are purported to help aid the recovery of sore, inflamed muscles and joints after training and facilitate the healing of athletic injuries, especially those involving heavy bruising and hematomas. Bromelain may also provide relief for other inflammation-based conditions such as asthma, sinusitis, osteoarthritis, ulcerative colitis, and irritable bowel syndrome (Kumar et al., 2023).

Research: Although double-blind, placebo-controlled research evaluating the impact of bromelain have confirmed significant decreases in edema, inflammation, and pain in a variety of clinical cases involving trauma and surgical procedures, the evidence as it relates specifically to muscle injury and recovery is either lacking or inconsistent (Fitzhugh et al., 2008; Leelakanok et al., 2023; Maurer, 2001; Muller et al., 2012; Pereira et al., 2023). For example, one small, double-blind, placebo-controlled study failed to confirm the benefit of bromelain for treating delayed-onset muscle soreness (DOMS), with no improvements being found in pain levels, range of motion, or overall functionality of the muscle (Stone et al., 2002). Similarly, Shing and colleagues (2016) found that even though 1,000 mg/day of bromelain decreased perceived fatigue on the fourth day of a 6-day stage cycling race, it had no effect on indices of muscle injury. However, it is important to note that because bromelain acts as a protease (enzyme that regulates clot formation and resorption after an injury), its effectiveness may fail to show for any exercise that does not induce a significant membrane injury resulting in fibrin clot formation. On the favorable end, another small, randomized, placebo-controlled study found a mixed supplement cocktail containing 5.83 g of three proteolytic enzymes—bromelain, papain, and fungal proteases—consumed daily over 21 days helped reduce the damaging impact of downhill running and reduce muscle strength losses by regulating leukocyte (white blood cell) activity and inflammation; however, it's hard to draw conclusions due to the combined supplementation protocol (Buford et al., 2009). Further standardization is needed to establish doses, supplementation time, and which inflammatory condition is being addressed before practical recommendations can be made (Pereira et al., 2023).

Common usage: Recommended therapeutic doses of bromelain range from 200 to 2,000 mg over 3 to 16 weeks depending on the type and severity of the condition. For traumatic injuries, a dose at the high end of the spectrum, 2,000 mg, is recommended; it should be split into four doses and consumed on an empty stomach. For joint inflammation and pain, a range of 500 to 2,000 mg can be taken in two split doses on an empty stomach as well. As a digestive aid, a lower dose of 500 mg split into four doses and taken with meals is recommended.

Health concerns: The most commonly reported side effects include indigestion, nausea, and diarrhea. Less frequently reported are vomiting, increased heart rate, drowsiness, and heavier bleeding during menstruation. Those with an allergy to pineapple may develop breathing problems, tightness in the throat, hives, rash, or itchy skin. Women who are pregnant or nursing, children under 18 years old, individuals with kidney or liver dysfunction, and those taking blood thinners and other medications should check with a physician before supplementation.

Cacao

(see *cocoa*)

Caffeine

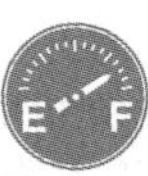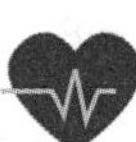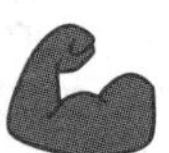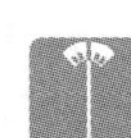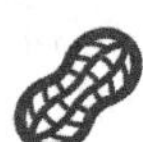

aka *anhydrous caffeine, caffeine citrate, theine*

What it is: First discovered by a German chemist in 1819, caffeine is an alkaloid compound found in over 60 species of plants, including coffee beans, tea leaves, cocoa beans, guarana, and kola nuts. With "stimulant properties that increase brain, cardiovascular, endocrine, neuromuscular, and metabolic activity" (Antonio et al., 2024), caffeine is one of the most well researched and used ergogenic aids in the world, providing beneficial effects for both physical and mental performance. Indeed, it has been reported that 76% of postcompetition urine samples of elite athletes contained measurable concentrations of caffeine (Aguilar-Navarro et al., 2019).

Function: Caffeine is absorbed within the stomach and intestine. Blood levels of caffeine peak 45 to 60 minutes after ingestion, triggering a number of physiological responses in the body that may aid performance for as long as 4 hours. Through its stimulant effects on the brain and central nervous system, caffeine allows an athlete to feel more alert with a clearer flow of thought, increased focus, and perhaps better general body coordination. In fact, when consumed as coffee, its biological and psychological effects are quite sweeping, according to a new position paper from the International Society of Sports Nutrition (Lowery et al., 2023). The primary ergogenic mechanism of action is adenosine antagonism. Through its metabolic activity, caffeine mobilizes fatty acids from fat tissue in the bloodstream and increases fat oxidation, which may help to spare muscle glycogen—although this is not likely its mechanism of action regarding performance. Still, this metabolic effect, in concert with other impacts, may help body composition over time.

Performance benefit: Athletes may be able to be more explosive, as well as better sustain exercise intensity, in addition to enjoying enhanced concentration, focus, reaction time, and tactical decision making. According to Guest and colleagues (2021):

> Supplementation with caffeine has been shown to acutely enhance various aspects of exercise performance in many but not all studies. Small to moderate benefits of caffeine use include, but are not limited to: muscular endurance, movement velocity and muscular strength, sprinting, jumping, and throwing performance, as well as a wide range of aerobic and anaerobic sport-specific actions.

Research: There is an abundance of solidly designed studies demonstrating a wide spectrum of performance benefits associated with caffeine ingestion. Among other determinations, the International Society of Sports Nutrition Position Stand on caffeine (Guest et al., 2021) concluded:

> Aerobic endurance appears to be the form of exercise with the most consistent moderate-to-large benefits from caffeine use, although the magnitude of its effects differs between individuals . . . Caffeine has consistently been shown to improve exercise performance when consumed in doses of 3-6 mg/kg body mass. Minimal effective doses of caffeine currently remain unclear but they may be as low as 2 mg/kg body mass. Very high doses of caffeine (e.g. 9 mg/kg) are associated with a high incidence of side-effects and do not seem to be required to elicit an ergogenic effect.

In relative agreement, earlier evidence suggested that caffeine ingestion at a dose of 1.3 to 4.0 mg/lb (0.59-1.82 mg/kg) provides significant enhancement of endurance exercise performance, with studies demonstrating a 20% to 50% increase in exercise time to fatigue in cyclists and runners (Burke, 2008; Cox et al., 2002; Ganio et al., 2009; Hogervorst et al., 2008). Early research attributed this effect, in part, to an approximate 30% increase in fat oxidation during exercise and thus a desirable glycogen or carbohydrate sparing effect (Costill et al., 1978; Ivy et al., 1979) but this is not the current consensus. Other mechanisms of action, mainly as they relate to central nervous system fatigue, have shown caffeine to play a role in reducing ratings of perceived effort and pain intensity, thwarting fatigue, and enhancing the physical and mental performance of athletes. For instance, male soccer players who consumed a total of 3.7 mg of caffeine/lb (1.68 mg/kg) in the form of a sport drink 1 hour before and in 15-minute intervals during a 90-minute exercise protocol not only improved sprinting performance and countermovement jumping ability but also rated the workout as more enjoyable, compared to a placebo group (Gant et al., 2010). Similarly, consumption of a caffeine-containing energy drink in a dose equivalent to 1.36 mg/lb (0.62 mg/kg) 60 minutes before exercise increased the ability to repeatedly sprint the distance covered during a simulated soccer game at a high intensity; it also enhanced jump height—a result of merit, considering how often team sport athletes are up in the air competing for a ball (Del Coso et al., 2012).

Common usage: Most research has demonstrated positive performance effects at caffeine doses of 1.4 to 2.7 mg/lb (3-6 mg/kg) (Guest et al., 2021); however, doses as low as 0.45 mg/lb (0.20 mg/kg) have shown to be beneficial as well, signaling the fact that more is not necessarily better. Caffeine can be taken all at once or split into two doses taken 60 minutes before and during competition. Because an athlete may develop a tolerance to caffeine (debatably blunting some of its effects), a conservative approach may include a washout period of 7 to 10 days when no caffeine is consumed. Withdrawal symptoms, such as headaches, can be avoided by slowly reducing caffeine consumption leading up to the washout period.

SUPPLEMENT FACT

The following list provides the caffeine content of some common food and drink:

12 oz (0.35 L) cola: 35-55 mg

12 oz (0.35 L) iced/flavored tea: 25-30 mg

8 oz (0.24 L) brewed tea: 40-60 mg

8 oz (0.24 L) green tea: 15 mg

8 oz (0.24 L) hot cocoa: 15 mg

8 oz (0.24 L) drip coffee: 115-175 mg

8 oz (0.24 L) brewed coffee: 80-135 mg

8 oz (0.24 L) instant coffee: 65-100 mg

2 oz (0.06 L) espresso: 100 mg

8 oz (0.24 L) energy drink: 80-300 mg

Caffeinated energy gels: 25-50 mg

Health concerns: Caffeine ingestion may increase urine formation within an hour after consumption; however, moderate levels (<300 mg) do not seem to have a detrimental impact on hydration status during exercise. In fact, in their meta-analysis, Zhang and colleagues (2015) stated that "concerns regarding unwanted fluid loss associated with caffeine consumption are unwarranted particularly when ingestion precedes exercise." This conclusion is strengthened when considering that brewed coffee, tea, and even energy drinks provide fluids to help offset any mild diuretic effect. The Food and Drug Administration (FDA) recommendation is to limit caffeine to less than 400 mg/day (FDA, 2023). Effects of caffeine toxicity (e.g., seizures) may occur with rapid consumption of around 1,200 mg or 0.15 tbsp of pure caffeine (FDA, 2023). A dose this high is unlikely to occur through consumption of coffee, tea, or even most energy drinks, but instead due to mismeasurement of highly concentrated liquids and powders. Individual tolerance, for genetic and other reasons, must be observed; according to a recent paper on caffeine misconceptions by Antonio and colleagues (2024) and others, caffeine itself has commonly described and dose-dependent side effects such as jitters, insomnia or reduced sleep quality, anxiety, tachycardia and/or heart palpitations, and usually small increases in blood pressure (Guest et al., 2021;, Haskell-Ramsay et al., 2018;, Lowery et al., 2023). The lethal dose of caffeine has been indicated at 70 to 90 mg/lb (31.8-40.9 mg/kg), or the equivalent of approximately 80 to 100 cups of coffee.

Calcidiol, Calcifediol, Calcitriol

(see *vitamin D*)

Calcium (Ca)

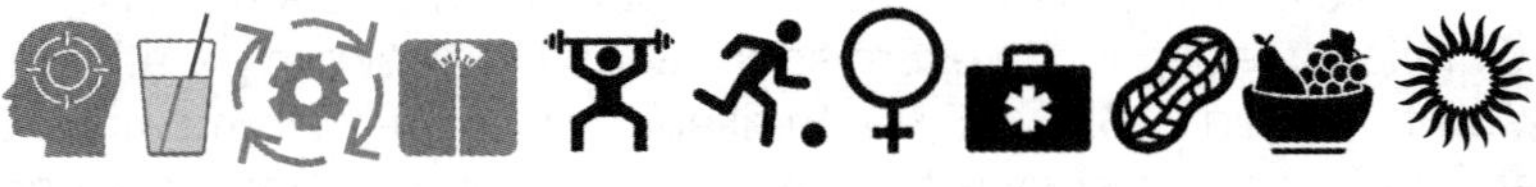

aka *calcium carbonate, calcium citrate, calcium gluconate, calcium lactate, calcium phosphate*

What it is: Although calcium has long been known to be an important mineral for the development and maintenance of strong bones, its other functions in muscle contraction, vasodilation, nerve transmission, and hormone secretion are also critical. These functions require a constant concentration of calcium be present in the blood (National Institutes of Health, 2012). With 99% of the body's calcium stores, bones represent a reservoir of stored calcium that can be called on to raise calcium levels when needed. The demand for calcium varies throughout life, depending on different growth needs in childhood and adolescence or during pregnancy and lactation (Fischer et al., 2018). The development of calcium deposits in bone or bone mineral density peaks around 17 to 23 years of age, with women peaking 2 to 3 years before men.

Function: Calcium intake determines skeletal calcium retention during bone growth, thus contributing to peak bone mass achieved in early adulthood (Zhu & Prince, 2012). Low calcium levels in the diet can contribute to a catabolic effect on the bone through the activation of parathyroid hormone. Aside from calcium intake, other diet and lifestyle choices such as inactivity, smoking, and excessive caffeine or alcohol intake can negatively affect development of bone mineral density (Patel et al., 2011). The aging process exacerbates calcium losses from bone, especially for women following menopause. Decreased calcium absorption can also occur as a result of many diseases, including malabsorption syndrome, primary cirrhosis, and celiac disease (Raszeja-Wyszomirska & Miazgowski, 2014; Theethira et al., 2014; Trotta et al., 2013). And although the calcium requirements to support the skeleton during growth and development and during aging are unlikely to be notably different between athletes and the general population, an additional consideration would be dermal calcium losses in athletes, particularly ultraendurance athletes (Sale & Elliot-Sale, 2019).

Performance benefit: Calcium supplementation for athletes could provide protection against bone loss and the development of stress fractures. It is also proposed that supplementing with calcium before or during prolonged exercise might compensate for dermal calcium losses and help maintain serum calcium levels, meaning that there would be no associated increase in parathyroid hormone release or bone resorption (Barry et al., 2011; Sale & Elliot-Sale, 2019).

Research: Studies on the effectiveness of calcium supplementation alone and in combination with vitamin D on losses in bone mineral density and risk of fracture have produced mixed results. In 2011 a meta-regression that reviewed results from 15 randomized, placebo-controlled trials involving calcium with or without vitamin D supplementation concluded that calcium does reduce the risk of fracture (Rabenda, Bruyere, & Reginster, 2011). However, a 2015 meta-analysis (Bolland et al, 2015) revealed that neither dietary calcium intake nor milk and dairy intake were associated with fracture in the bulk of studies reviewed; the authors also concluded that evidence of calcium supplementation preventing fractures is weak and inconsistent. Even so, it is well established that adequate calcium levels increase bone protection and protect against osteoporosis and fracture, though other nutritional habits, such as an energy availability of 45 kcal/kg of lean body mass/day (Papageorgiou et al., 2017, 2018), adequate carbohydrate availability (DeSousa et al., 2014; Sale et al., 2015), and optimal protein intake (Rizzoli et al., 2018), have been argued to be equally important to overall bone health, particularly for athletes (Sale & Elliot-Sale, 2019). In addition, supplementing with 1,000 mg of calcium 20 minutes prior to exercise, specifically a 35 km cycling time trial, also showed a significant reduction in exercise-induced increases in parathyroid hormone and bone resorption (Barry et al., 2011). Similarly, a pre-exercise meal containing ~1,350 mg of calcium has been shown to attenuate the subsequent response of both parathyroid hormone and bone resorption to a 90-minute cycling session in competitive female cyclists (Haakonssen et al., 2015). Additional research needs to evaluate the chronic impact this strategy has on bone mass and strength in athletes as well as quantify the amount of calcium lost in endurance and ultraendurance athletes as well as athletes who train in hot and humid climates.

Common usage: The RDA for calcium ranges from 1,000 mg/day to 1,300 mg/day for people ages 4 years and up. Peak absorption is achieved in doses under 500 mg; therefore, it is recommended that calcium be supplemented 3 times/day in 300 to 400 mg doses. Types of calcium supplements include carbonate, citrate, gluconate, lactate, and phosphate. Calcium carbonate is most effectively absorbed with food, whereas citrate forms can be absorbed with or without food. Food sources rich in calcium include milk, yogurt, cheese, fish such as salmon and sardines, and some vegetables including kale, bok choi, and broccoli. Calcium is also commonly fortified in fruit juices and cereals. The acidity in orange juice, for example, may help absorption of the calcium. Adding calcium, not typically present in the beverage, makes it an example of a functional food.

Health concerns: In some cases individuals may experience GI tract side effects, including constipation, bloating, or gas.

Calcium Ascorbate

(see *vitamin C*)

Calcium Pantothenate

(see *pantothenic acid*)

Calcium Pyruvate, Calcium Pyruvate Monohydrate

(see *pyruvate*)

Capric Acid, Caproic Acid, *Caprylic Acid*

(see *medium-chain triglycerides*)

Cannabidiol (CBD) 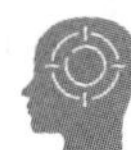 

aka *Epidiolex (brand name)*

What it is: Cannabidiol (CBD) is one of at least 80 cannabinoids in the *Cannabis sativa* plant. The plant in its entirety is also called marijuana or hemp. Unlike the delta-9-tetrahydrocannabinol (THC) found in marijuana, CBD is nonintoxicating, although it does produce some psychoactive effects.

Function: Preclinical (animal) studies suggest CBD has neuroprotective, anti-inflammatory, analgesic, and anxiolytic properties that may be of interest to hard-training, stressed athletes. It also appears to affect aspects of the sleep–wake cycle, although more research is needed.

Performance benefit: CBD could benefit neuromuscular recovery after exercise as well as ease competitive anxiety, although this is speculative. Its use immediately before competition needs to be studied, as most induced (anti-) anxiety research with CBD has involved public speaking.

Research: According to observational and retrospective investigations, CBD may provide modest benefits in conditions that are of common interest to athletes, including pain, anxiety, and sleep problems. However, there are very little clinical data on CBD directly related to exercise and athletes. Further, laws and regulations surrounding CBD can be difficult to navigate—as noted by Gamelin and colleagues (2020) noted that "cannabis is prohibited by the World Anti-Doping Agency (WADA) across all sports in competition since 2004 [but] the Agency has removed CBD itself from the list of prohibited substances—in or out of competition - since 2018."

Common usage: A broad range of CBD products (e.g., oils and capsules) at suggested doses of 5 to 50 mg/day have become readily available online and over the counter. According to McCartney and colleagues (2020), this includes products marketed specifically to recreational and elite athletes.

Health concerns: Impurities in some CBD products notwithstanding, the substance itself appears to be safe when taken orally or sprayed under the tongue by healthy persons free of liver disease. Research suggests doses up to 1,500 mg (very high) of CBD can be taken orally for up to 4 weeks and be relatively safe. Side effects do include mood changes, lightheadedness, and sleepiness, as well as dry mouth, diarrhea, and decreased appetite. Also, like certain other botanicals in this book, CBD may increase or decrease the metabolism or clearance of particular drugs—or have its own concentrations affected by them. For example, drugs used for opioid addiction, depression, epilepsy, and organ rejection may elevate CBD in the circulation.

Capsicum 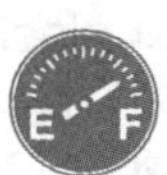 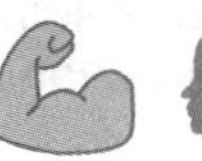 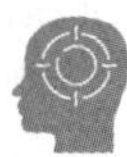 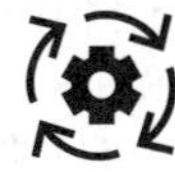

aka *capsaicin, capsiate, cayenne, chili pepper, green pepper, hot pepper, red pepper, sweet pepper*

What it is: A plant widely known for the hot, pungent properties of its fruits and seeds, capsicum (Greek, meaning *to bite)* is not only used for culinary purposes but also as a common ingredient in topical athletic balms because of its apparent ability to provide temporary relief from muscle and joint pain associated with arthritis, backache, strains, and sprains. Capsaicin and capsiate are active ingredients found within the capsicum plant; these have been the center of many recent studies evaluating the performance benefits of ingested capsicum.

Function: The fruit of the capsicum plant contains capsaicin at an estimated potency of 0.1% to 1.5%. Long-term exposure to capsaicin, generally via topical application, has been shown to decrease the activity of transient receptor potential vanilloid 1 (TRPV1), or capsaicin receptors. This effect helps desensitize nerve endings and ultimately provides a natural treatment for nerve-focused as well as inflammatory pain. Furthermore, activation of TRPV1 also can stimulate nitric oxygen synthesis, initiating vasodilation, which, in turn, may enhance exercise performance by increasing blood, nutrient, and oxygen delivery to the working muscles as well as aiding the clearance of metabolic byproducts. Reductions in rating of perceived exertion and pain have also been reported with consumption of capsaicin, as have improvements in force output.

Performance benefit: Athletes might benefit from reduced pain with topical application as well as improvements in both muscular and aerobic endurance with pre-exercise ingestion.

Research: Previous research on capsaicin and capsiate confirmed clinical benefits for a wide array of pain conditions, including those associated with athletic injury, when used topically or as a plaster following orthopedic surgery (Armstrong et al., 2011; Chrubasik et al., 2010; Kim et al., 2009). Over the past decade, there has also been a dramatic increase in research evaluating how capsaicin and capsiate can affect endurance performance and recovery, although findings are inconsistent. A 2022 random-effects meta-analysis of 14 studies ($n = 183$) looked at the effects of capsaicin and capsiate on aerobic endurance (e.g., time trials or time-to-exhaustion tests), muscular endurance (e.g., repetitions performed to muscular failure), and rating of perceived exertion (RPE) (Grgic et al., 2022). The most common dose provided was 12 mg of capsaicin or capsiate with instructions to consume 45 minutes prior to exercise. No significant differences were discovered between the placebo and capsaicin or capsiate when looking at aerobic performance or studies that used time trials or time-to-exhaustion tests. However, when evaluating muscular endurance, capsaicin or capsiate had a significant effect in improving total volume load in 3 sets of resistance exercise tests and reducing RPE. Though capsaicin and capsiate have shown promise as an ergogenic aid, additional research is warranted to further investigate their effects on chronic resistance training, aerobic exercise, and combination training as well as to establish a consistent mechanism of action before definite conclusions can be made (de Moura et al., 2021).

Common usage: The fruit and seeds of capsicum can be dried and ground into powder to provide a culinary kick to foods. For treatment of pain, application of a cream containing 0.025% to 0.075% capsaicin concentration 3 to 4 times/day over a period of 2 or more weeks is indicated. Additionally, the use of capsicum-containing patches at 8% concentration or plasters providing 11 mg of capsaicin per plaster can be applied once daily and left in place for 4 to 8 hours. Studies evaluating ingested forms have used doses of 1.2 mg to upwards of 12 mg taken 45 minutes prior to exercise.

Health concerns: Topical application of capsicum on skin is considered safe for most adults but may produce skin irritation, burning, and itching. Athletes with sensitive skin should test the product on a small patch of skin before using liberally. Capsicum should not be applied around the eyes, nose, or throat. Oral administration is also considered safe although acute symptoms may include stomach irritation, sweating, flushing, and runny nose. Athletes undergoing surgery should avoid oral use, as capsicum has been shown to increase bleeding.

Carbohydrate (CHO)

aka *saccharides (mono-, di-, poly-, oligo-), sugars*

What it is: Put simply, carbohydrate is sugar (saccharides) and starch found naturally in such foods as fruits, vegetables, dairy, legumes, and grains as well as in manufactured products such as sport drinks, energy bars, energy chews, and energy gels. Carbohydrate provides 4 kcal of energy/g. See descriptions of the common carbohydrate types in table 3.2.

TABLE 3.2 Types of Carbohydrates

Carbohydrate type	Carbohydrate description	Oxidation rate
Fructose	Fructose is a monosaccharide found naturally in fruits and honey.	Slow
Galactose	Galactose is a monosaccharide that, together with glucose, makes up lactose, the sugar found in milk.	Slow
Isomaltulose	Also known as palatinose, isomaltulose is a natural constituent of honey and sugar cane that is manufactured from sucrose.	Slow
Trehalose	Also known as mycose, trehalose is made up of a unique chemical bond of two glucose molecules.	Slow
Amylose	Amylose is an unbranched chain of glucose found in plants that, along with amylopectin, make up starch.	Slow
Glucose	Also known as dextrose or grape sugar, glucose is a monosaccharide produced commercially from several forms of starch, including corn, rice, and wheat.	Fast
Sucrose	Also known as table sugar, sucrose is a disaccharide made up of glucose plus fructose.	Fast
Maltose	Maltose is a disaccharide made up of two units of glucose.	Fast
Maltodextrin	Maltodextrin is a polymer of glucose that can enzymatically be derived from any starch, generally corn and wheat.	Fast
Amylopectin	Amylopectin is a highly branched chain of glucose molecules that are found in plants that, together with amylose, make up starch.	Fast
Waxy maize starch	Comprised primarily of amylopectin, waxy maize starch is a highly branched starch derived from corn.	Fast

Function: Upon digestion, carbohydrate is broken down into glucose and oxidized for immediate energy use or stored as glycogen in the liver and muscles for later energy use. Athletes who balance out their meals with 45% to 65% carbohydrate while meeting daily energy demands will store enough carbohydrate energy to fuel up to 3 hours of moderate-intensity exercise. Failure to consume adequate calories and carbohydrate to support training or inadequate supplementation with carbohydrate during moderate to high intensity exercise lasting more than 90 minutes increases the risk for glycogen depletion and low blood sugar levels. Consuming carbohydrate after a workout is essential for optimal immune function and recovery.

Performance benefit: Athletes who consume adequate carbohydrate will benefit from increased endurance during both high- and low-intensity training and competition as well as improved recovery times. Increasing the intake of carbohydrate (3.6-5.5 g/lb or 10-12 g/kg) for the final 72 hours leading up to endurance competition, a practice known as carbo-loading, can increase muscle glycogen stores by as much as 40%, especially when training volume is reduced in conjunction. This practice helps delay the onset of muscle fatigue (Sedlock, 2008). Using multiple sources of carbohydrates will produce better results compared to using a single source.

Research: Because it is well established that carbohydrate can enhance performance and recovery, modern-day research has focused on specifics, evaluating the best type, blend, and quantity of carbohydrate for the most efficient delivery of energy to an athlete's working muscles. Two categories of carbohydrate exist: those that are oxidized quickly (up to 1 g/minute) and those that are oxidized at slowly (up to 0.6 g/minute). Oxidation rates of the di- and polysaccharides sucrose, maltose, and maltodextrin, along with the monosaccharide glucose, fall on the fast side of the spectrum, whereas fructose and galactose are oxidized at slow rates. Additionally, a series of studies has shown carbohydrate oxidation rates can increase another 20% to 30%—to values of 1.7 g/minute—when a combination of carbohydrate that use different intestinal digestion and transport systems (such as glucose and fructose) are used (Currell & Jeukendrup, 2008; Jeukendrup, 2004, 2014). A 2011 meta-analysis of 73 well-designed studies, for example, confirmed these findings and also discovered a blend of maltodextrin plus fructose at a dose of approximately 0.32 and 0.09 g/lb (0.14 and 0.04 g/kg), respectively, taken each hour in an incremental fashion yields the most favorable effect on exercise time to exhaustion (Vandernbogaerde & Hopkins, 2011). It is important to note that although most studies have utilized a 2:1 glucose-to-fructose ratio, there is some evidence to suggest a ratio closer to unity (1 g of glucose/0.8 g of fructose) may be superior with respect to oxidation efficiency as well as gut comfort for the athlete (Rowlands et al., 2015). The recovery benefits of the maltodextrin plus fructose combination have also been shown to be significant, with a dose of 70 g taken in a 2:1 ratio within 1 hour post-workout doubling rates of liver glycogen compared to a calorie-matched maltodextrin plus glucose combination (Décombaz et al., 2011). Follow-up studies have supported this, strengthening the recommendations for athletes to consider postworkout ingestion of carbohydrates from a combination of glucose-based carbohydrates and fructose to optimally stimulate both liver and muscle glycogen synthesis and quick recovery of glycogen stores (Kerksick et al., 2017; Maunder et al., 2018; Podlogar & Wallis, 2020; Podlogar & Wallis, 2022).

Common usage: The most common carbohydrate supplements used by athletes include sport drinks (both liquid and powder form), energy gels, energy chews, and energy bars. For high-intensity training and competition lasting longer than 1 hour, merely rinsing the mouth with a carbohydrate solution can enhance endurance. For high-intensity events lasting 1 to 2.5 hours, ingestion of quickly oxidized carbohydrates (see table 3.2) at a rate of 30 to 60 g/hour is recommended. For prolonged training and competition over 2.5 hours, multiple carbohydrates should be used at a rate of 60 to 90 g/hour. Based on current research, the following combinations are recommended: glucose, maltodextrin, amylopectin, or waxy maize starch (60 g/hour) plus fructose (30 g/hour); glucose, maltodextrin, amylopectin, or waxy maize starch (60 g/hour) plus sucrose (15 g/hour) plus fructose (15 g/hour). When weather conditions on competition day are trending warm or when competing at higher elevations, particularly in the absence of acclimatation protocols, carbohydrate supplementation should be reduced by 10% to accommodate reduced rates of carbohydrate oxidation (Young et al., 2018). Ingestion of 0.6 to 1.0 g/kg of carbohydrate from a combination of glucose- and fructose-based carbohydrates within the first 30 minutes of completing glycogen-depleting exercise and again every 2 hours for the next 4 to 6 hours is recommended for quick recovery of glycogen stores (see table 3.3).

TABLE 3.3 Carbohydrate Intake Recommendations

	Dosing recommendations	Preferable carbohydrate sources
Daily intake	2.7-4.5 g/lb (1.2-2.0 g/kg) body mass	Whole grains, legumes, fruits, vegetables, yogurt, milk
Before competition	1-1.5 g/lb (0.45-0.68 g/kg) body mass in the 2-3 hours leading up to start	Easy-to-digest low-fiber carbohydrates: Plain bread, pretzels, potatoes, white rice, cream of rice cereal, pasta, pulp-free juices, sports drinks
During competition	<1 hour: Carbohydrate rinse 1-3 hours: 30-60 g/hour >3 hours: 60-90 g/hour	Glucose, sucrose, maltodextrin, maltose, amylopectin, waxy maize starch Glucose, sucrose, maltodextrin, maltose, amylopectin, waxy maize starch Multiple sources: Maltodextrin + sucrose, maltodextrin + fructose, maltodextrin + glucose + fructose
After competition	0.5-0.7 g/lb (0.2-0.3 g/kg) body mass within 30 minutes + every 2 hours for 4-6 hours or until calorie deficit is replenished	Immediate: Maltodextrin + sucrose, maltodextrin + fructose , maltodextrin + glucose + fructose Long-term: Whole grains, legumes, fruits, vegetables, yogurt, milk

Health concerns: Because the amount of carbohydrate transporters in the gastrointestinal tract is limited and oxygen availability for digestion and absorption is low during exercise, consuming too many carbohydrate calories, especially from one type of sugar, can overwhelm the metabolic pathway being used. Doing so delays emptying of fuel from the gut and increases the risk for such unpleasant gastrointestinal symptoms as bloating, nausea, cramping, and diarrhea. Athletes are encouraged to practice carbohydrate supplementation at target competition efforts as well as in general training to prepare the gut to optimally perform in competition (Vitale & Getsin, 2019).

Carnitine 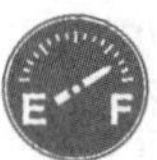 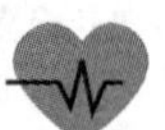 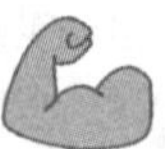 

aka *acetyl-L-carnitine (ALCAR), glycine propionyl L-carnitine (GPLC),*
L-carnitine, L-carnitine L-tartrate (LCLT)

What it is: Carnitine is a dipeptide synthesized in the liver, kidneys, and brain from the amino acids lysine and methionine and stored predominantly within heart and skeletal muscle. It is also naturally obtained from many foods, particularly those of animal origin. Carnitine plays an important role in energy production as well as the regulation of metabolic pathways involved in skeletal muscle protein balance. There are several compounds of carnitine, including L-carnitine (LC), acetyl-L-carnitine (ALCAR), L-carnitine L-tartrate (LCLT), and glycine propionyl L-carnitine (GPLC). ALCAR, or L-carnitine to which an acetyl group has been added, is thought to be the most bioavailable form of L-carnitine, whereas LCLT is one of the most common forms found in sports supplements due to its rapid absorption rate (Grivas, 2018; Scafidi, 2010).

Function: Carnitine serves as a key player in substrate utilization, helping transport long chain fatty acids into the mitochondria so that they can be oxidized to produce energy in the form of adenosine triphosphate (ATP). It also serves as a basin for excess production of acetyl-CoA, helping the flow of carbohydrate through the citric acid cycle (Stephens, 2018; Wall et al., 2011).

Performance benefit: Because of its multifaceted impact on different physiological and metabolic pathways, increasing and maintaining a high muscle carnitine level through supplementation is hypothesized to spare glycogen via increased fat oxidation at lower exercise intensities as well as promote a more effective oxidation of carbohydrate and reduced lactate accumulation at high intensities, thereby delaying the onset of fatigue and enhancing endurance performance. In addition, it is thought that carnitine may enhance recovery after exercise by increasing blood flow and oxygen supply to muscle tissue through improved endothelial function, increasing antioxidant enzyme activity and reducing hypoxia-induced cellular and biochemical disruptions that may otherwise interfere with optimal muscle recovery.

Research: Current data on carnitine supplementation has demonstrated equivocal outcomes. A systemic review of 11 studies, filtered based on methodological quality by the McMaster Critical Review Form, revealed that both acute and chronic LC supplementation could improve the performance of high-intensity exercise ($\geq$80% $\dot{V}O_2$max), yet do not seem to elicit the same benefit for more moderate-intensity exercise (50%-79% $\dot{V}O_2$max) (Mielgo-Ayuso et al., 2021). One study showed a dose of 3 to 4 g of LC or GPLC ingested 60 to 90 minutes before exercise to improve lactate threshold as well as lower levels of perceived exertion during incremental tests until exhaustion, as well as increasing peak and average power in the Wingate cycle ergometer test. Similarly, a slightly lower dose of 2 to 2.72 g/day of LC for longer periods of 9 to 24 weeks resulted in lower blood lactate accumulation and ratings of perceived exertion as well as increases in work capacity in "all out" tests, peak power in Wingate tests, and the quantity and weight load in leg press exercises. Similar dose patterns, 2.72 to 3 g/day of LC with or without carbohydrate intake over 4 to 24 weeks or 2 to 3 grams of LC taken 30 minutes to 3 hours before exercise, however, failed to demonstrate improvements in performance parameters during moderate-intensity exercise (50%-79% $\dot{V}O_2$max). A 2016 study discovered no effect on muscle function, energy metabolism, or $\dot{V}O_2$max during both submaximal or maximal exercise tests, and although plasma carnitine levels increased in both habitual meat eaters and vegetarians, the impact on muscle stores was minimal with a 12-week supplementation protocol consisting of 2 g/day of LC administered in a split-dose manner (Novakova et al., 2016). Because the bioavailability of LC supplements has been shown to be only 14% to 18% of dose, with the bulk being degraded by microorganisms in the large intestine (Rebouche, 2004), it is postulated that whole body carnitine retention and potential performance benefit can be increased when the supplement is co-ingested with an insulin stimulus like carbohydrate. Indeed, a chronic supplementation protocol consisting of 2 g of LC plus 80 g of carbohydrate taken twice daily over 24 weeks led to a 21% increase in muscle carnitine, which, in turn, decreased muscle glycogen utilization during submaximal cycling (30 minutes at 50% $\dot{V}O_2$max) by 55% and better matched the metabolic flux during high-intensity cycling (30 minutes at 80% $\dot{V}O_2$max), leading to an 11% boost in work output during a 30-minute time trial. On the recovery front, a double-blind, randomized, placebo-controlled trial including 80 healthy male and female participants aged 21 to 65 found that a supplementation protocol with 2 g/day of LCLT over 5 weeks, taken either 30 minutes prior to exercise or with the first meal of the day on nonexercise days, helped improve perceived recovery and soreness and lower serum creatine kinase as well as blunt declines in strength and power following an exercise challenge, independent of gender and age (Gnoni et al., 2020; Stefan et al., 2021). So, although data is not conclusive, there has been promising research supporting the use of carnitine, especially in conjunction with carbohydrate, to enhance the performance of high-intensity exercise as well as support recovery. Because differences in exercise intensity, amount and type of carnitine administered, and route and timing of administration relative to the exercise have led to conflicting experimental results, it is clear that additional research is warranted. This is also necessary to clarify the efficacy and safety of following prolonged supplement regimes before practical recommendations for use can be made.

Common usage: As a dietary supplement, carnitine is available as a solo entity or combined with other ingredients with amounts ranging from 3 mg to upwards of 5,000 mg. The most common dose demonstrated in the studies provided ranged from 2 to 4 g taken daily over 4 to 24 weeks (Office of Dietary Supplements & National Institutes of Health, 2022).

Health concerns: Because carnitine metabolism produces trimethylamine *N*-oxide (TMAO), a substance in the body linked to elevated cardiovascular disease risk, chronic use of carnitine as a dietary supplement must be carefully reviewed (Gatarek & Kaluzna-Czaplinska, 2021). Additional adverse reactions noted include agitation, nausea, and vomiting (Sawicka, Renzi, & Olek, 2020).

Casein 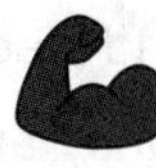  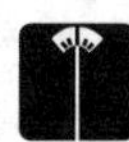    

aka *milk protein (see also whey protein)*

What it is: Milk contains two main proteins: casein and whey. Roughly 80% of protein found in milk is casein, which is considered a complete protein because it contains all the essential amino acids. The amino acid profile of casein is similar to whey, although not completely identical.

SUPPLEMENT FACT

Consuming milk, yogurt, and certain cheeses, like cottage cheese, either before or after training can provide a good natural source of casein and whey proteins because they are more isolated sources of slow-acting casein.

Function: Casein is much more slowly digested than whey and releases amino acids into the blood at a slower and more prolonged rate.

Performance benefit: Because of its ability to release amino acids into the blood more slowly, casein is thought to be especially beneficial at night before bed, as well as in combination with fast-digesting proteins either before or after exercise. Supplying the body with a slow and prolonged release of amino acids at night during sleep is thought to improve muscle recovery.

Research: Most research suggests that fast-acting proteins, such as whey, are most beneficial for stimulating protein synthesis and muscle recovery following exercise and are superior to casein or soy protein alone. However, it is unknown if whey protein in combination with casein provides additional benefits immediately following exercise or longer term, such as over the span of a 6- to 12-week training cycle. One study found that milk, which contains a combination of whey and casein protein, was superior to soy protein isolate in stimulating protein synthesis following exercise (Wilkinson et al., 2007). Another study of 16 resistance-trained men discovered supplementation with 40 g of casein taken 30 minutes before bed yielded a 22% boost in protein synthesis as well as extended amino acid availability throughout the night, which, in turn, led to an overall positive effect on protein balance (Res et al., 2012). More recently, a double-blind, crossover study (Martinez et al., 2021) evaluated the impact of 20 g of whey protein, casein protein, an 80:20 whey and casein combo, a 20:80 whey and casein combo, and a placebo on branched-chain amino acid (BCAA) blood profiles, markers of protein metabolism, and delayed onset muscle soreness (DOMS) after a single session of resistance exercise. The key takeaways from study investigators were the following:

1. BCAAs peaked at the same time, approximately 60 minutes after ingestion, for whey protein and both types of whey and casein combos. The casein treatment promoted the peak of BCAAs later, at 120 minutes post-treatment.

2. Both whey and casein blends promoted higher amino acid concentrations, which were similar to the whey protein treatment when compared to casein and placebo treatments.

3. The BCAAs leucine and isoleucine presented a longer period of permanence in the whey protein and the combination whey and casein treatments.

4. Although a single dose of whey protein and both whey and casein combos increased amino acid concentration, this did not influence performance; however, muscle soreness was minimized compared to casein and placebo.

Overall, the data suggest that the whey protein and the whey and casein combo treatments promoted a similar positive effect in skeletal muscle recovery. Additional studies with larger sample sizes are needed to evaluate the impact of whey protein and casein blend supplementation on exercise recovery and postexercise BCAA profiles in a long-term intervention before definite recommendations for use of casein over whey protein can be given.

Common usage: Typically, 20 to 40 g of casein proteins are used in combination with whey proteins either before or following exercise or at night before bed.

Health concerns: High-protein diets (less than 3 g/kg of body mass) do not appear to pose any health concerns; however, athletes must understand that excessive intakes of protein at the expense of other important nutrients such as carbohydrate, healthy fat, and those found in nutrient-dense fruits and vegetables can negatively affect performance.

Cat's Claw 

aka *Uncaria guianensis, Uncaria tomentosa*

What it is: Cat's claw, a thick woody vine native to the Amazon and tropical areas of South and Central America, has been used for thousands of years for medicinal and sacred purposes. The name is derived from the hook-like thorns that grow along the vine in a pattern that resembles the claws of a cat. Several species of the plant exist; however, *Uncaria tomentosa* is preferred for use in dietary supplements because of its higher alkaloid content. Cat's claw is believed to strengthen the immune system, inhibit inflammation, and suppress tumor growth and the replication of viruses (Erowele & Kalejaiye, 2009). In Germany and Austria cat's claw can only be dispensed with a prescription.

Function: Cat's claw contains a variety of components that are believed to be responsible for its positive impact on health. These include a variety of alkaloids, glycosides, triterpenes, and steroids. Specifically, quinovic acid, beta-sitosterol, and stigmasterol have been isolated in the plant. The exact mechanisms for all the beneficial effects of cat's claw are unclear, but recent research suggests its anti-inflammatory properties are related to the inhibition of nuclear factor kappa beta (NF-κβ) (Erowele & Kalejaiye, 2009).

Performance benefit: Cat's claw is most commonly marketed for its anti-inflammatory effects, especially for relief of osteoarthritic (OA) conditions. These effects could benefit athletes needing to treat inflamed tissues. It may also help prevent immune system suppression resulting from heavy training.

Research: There are still not a significant number of well-controlled research trials for cat's claw, although early in vitro studies and animal studies were positive (Carvalho et al., 2006). As of 2017, there were no known randomized control trials or published human outcome studies (DellaValle, 2017), although a number of inflammatory states have reportedly been improved by its use. One study did find that treatment of knee OA in 45 patients with 100 mg of cat's claw capsules improved pain associated with activity versus a placebo (Piscoya et al., 2001). This is the only known study using cat's claw alone for treatment. Other studies have used a combination of cat's claw and other herbal remedies, making it difficult to distinguish benefits exclusive to cat's claw (Miller et al., 2005, 2006). There are also no studies on athletic populations, nor research related to a beneficial impact on immune suppression during prolonged intense exercise; therefore, real-life evidence to support cat's claw's use in athletes is lacking.

Common usage: Unfortunately, the lack of scientific studies performed on human subjects makes it difficult to conclude a best-use strategy. Most dietary supplements are sold In 500 to 1,000 mg doses in either capsule or liquid form. Athletes should proceed with caution as the nutritional components of herbal dietary supplements can vary depending on growing and harvesting conditions as well as extraction methods and plant parts included.

Health concerns: The use of cat's claw appears to be safe, and few adverse events have been reported. According to the National Institute of Diabetes and Digestive and Kidney Diseases (2012), "Because cat's claw inhibits microsomal CYP 3A4 activity, it has a potential to cause herb-drug interactions and raise the levels of other drugs that are metabolized by CYP 3A4." Some possible adverse effects include GI tract distress, diarrhea, and increased risk of bleeding. Athletes with bleeding disorders or those taking drugs such as Warfarin should proceed with caution when using cat's claw.

Cayenne

(see *capsicum*)

Cevitamic Acid

(see *vitamin C*)

Chia Seeds 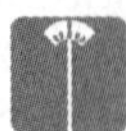  

aka *Salvia hispanica*

What it is: Naturally derived from the desert plant *Salvia hispanica,* chia seeds are a valuable source of omega-3 fatty acids, dietary fiber, protein, antioxidants, and minerals. Historically, they were used as a key fuel source by the Tarahumara people, whose traditions included ultraendurance running journeys across tough Mexican terrain. Claims that just a small amount can provide the energy to cover long distances have made the seed quite popular among endurance athletes.

Function: Chia seeds, which contain gummy fibers known as mucilage, form a gel-like substance when mixed with water. Scientists believe this also occurs in the gut, allowing a barrier to form between digestive enzymes and carbohydrate that works to slow the breakdown of carbohydrate and help maintain better blood sugar control, an attractive feature for athletes competing in ultraendurance events. It is also thought that the hydrophilic nature of chia seeds, which can absorb 10 times their weight in water, may allow an athlete to stay better hydrated during competition, another critical component to endurance and overall performance.

Performance benefit: Athletes may benefit from more stable blood sugars and extended endurance when using chia seeds before and during events lasting longer than 90 minutes. Because they are rich in omega-3 fatty acids, chia seeds may also help promote better recovery by reducing the chronic inflammation associated with high-intensity and high-volume sport training.

Research: There is limited scientific data regarding the efficacy of chia seed use beyond the scope of general health; however, increased interest and use by endurance athletes has led sport science researchers at a few universities to start collecting data. One crossover study failed to discover any added performance benefit in highly trained athletes who consumed a 50% chia and 50% sport drink (Gatorade) mix in preparation for a 1-hour aerobic treadmill run followed by a 10K time trial on a track, versus those who consumed 100% sport drink. A 2-week washout period separated each trial. Although the chia seeds provided no performance advantage, however, there were also no detriments, which led the scientists to conclude that chia seeds may provide a viable option for reducing dietary intake of sugar during a carbo-loading protocol (Illian, Casey, & Bishop, 2011).

Common usage: To form a gel for use leading up to as well as during athletic competition, mix 2 tbsp of seeds into 16 oz (0.47 L) of solution containing 50% sports drink and 50% water. For health benefits, chia seeds can also be eaten raw, ground, roasted, or baked; they are commonly served on top of cereal, yogurt, and salads and added to smoothies and baked goods.

Health concerns: The high dietary fiber content of chia seeds may cause digestive issues, including bloating and gas, especially when consumed before or during competition.

Chili Pepper

(see *capsicum*)

Chinese Caterpillar Fungus

(see *Cordyceps sinensis*)

Chinese Club Moss, *Huperzia serrata*

(see *Huperzine A*)

Chitosan 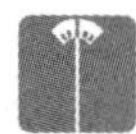

What it is: Chitosan is produced from chitin, which is a structural element in the shell of crustaceans such as crabs, shrimp, and lobster. It is commonly made into supplement form and sold as a weight-loss product.

Function: Chitosan can bind dietary fats and bile acids to itself, giving it potential as a weight-loss supplement as well as a treatment for high cholesterol. A meta-analysis found that 1.2 to 6.75 g of chitosan/day reduced the total cholesterol of hypercholestertolemic patients by approximately 11.5 mg/dL (Baker et al., 2009).

Performance benefit: Chitosan may assist with weight loss by binding fat consumed in the diet and limiting its absorption in the small intestine. As a result, calorie intake would be reduced, resulting in weight loss. It's important that athletes realize that dietary fat is essential for many functions of the body, and decreasing its absorption might have a negative impact on performance. Dietary fat provides essential fatty acids, aids in the absorption of fat-soluble vitamins, and is an important component of cell membranes.

Research: According to a meta-analysis by Moraru and colleagues (2018), "Erratic results have been published concerning the influence of the dietary supplement chitosan used as a complementary remedy to decrease the body weight of overweight and obese people." After reviewing 14 randomized control trials concerned with the effect of chitosan on body weight, serum lipids, and blood pressure, they reported that the use of chitosan as a dietary supplement for up to 52 weeks seems to only slightly reduce body weight (−1.01 kg). This finding is in line with earlier work suggesting chitosan is mildly effective at reducing body weight and body fat. A 2006 study of overweight adults found that 3 g of chitosan/day for 60 days reduced body weight by 2.8 lb (1.3 kg) compared to a 0.8 lb (0.4 kg) gain in body weight for a placebo group (Kaats, Michalek, & Preus, 2006). These results are similar to those of three other studies (Egras, 2011). Earlier reviews of chitosan concluded that effects were minimal and unlikely to be clinically significant (Jull et al., 2008; Mhurchu et al., 2005). Data are still limited, and conclusive recommendations cannot be made at this time. In addition, it is unknown if athletic performance or recovery is negatively affected as a result of binding essential fatty acids or limiting absorption of fat-soluble vitamins.

Common usage: Chitosan is typically supplemented in 1,500 to 3,000 mg dosages and should be taken in either two 1,500 mg doses before the two biggest meals of the day or in three separate 1,000 mg doses before meals.

Health concerns: Chitosan should be avoided by anyone with a shellfish allergy. Otherwise, chitosan appears to be safe and well tolerated. However, adverse effects such as constipation, flatulence, increased stool bulkiness, bloating, nausea, and heartburn have been reported.

Choline 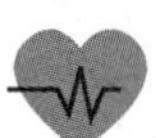 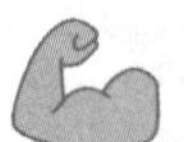 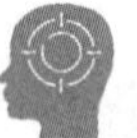 

aka *choline bitartrate, phosphatidylcholine, lecithin* (see also *citicoline, alpha-GPC*)

What it is: Choline, a member of the B-vitamin family, is derived from the Greek word *chole,* meaning "bile." Like bile acids, choline was identified when scientists discovered its ability to prevent fatty build up in the liver. Although choline was discovered in 1864, it was not classified as an essential nutrient by the Food and Nutrition Board of the Institute of Medicine until 1998. Humans can produce choline endogenously in the liver, mostly as phosphatidylcholine, but the amount that the body naturally synthesizes is not sufficient to meet human needs. This may be especially true when folate intake is low. The interest in choline and acetylcholine began in the 1990s when scientists discovered that levels of choline were significantly reduced in marathon runners after completion of the 26.2 mi (42.2 km) run and required 48 hours to return to normal (Conlay, Saboujian, & Wurtman, 1992).

Function: Choline serves as a methyl group donor, important for multiple aspects of metabolism. Choline has a number of significant roles in the body, including neurotransmitter synthesis, cell membrane signaling, lipid transport, and homocysteine metabolism (Sanders & Zeisel, 2007). Most important for athletes is choline's role as a precursor in acetylcholine (ACh) synthesis. The neurotransmitter ACh is released at the neuromuscular junction and binds to receptors on muscles to activate muscle contraction.

Performance benefit: As an essential micronutrient for energy production as well as muscle and cognitive function, choline is purported to help improve an athlete's strength, endurance, and mental focus during sport activity.

Research: Although true deficiency is very rare, most people in the United States consume less than the adequate intake (AI) for choline. According to NHANES data for adults, the average daily choline intake from foods and beverages is 278 mg in women and 402 mg in men. Researchers are studying whether this affects athletic gains. In a study by Lee and colleagues (2023), older participants (60-69 years old) underwent 12 weeks of resistance training (3 times/week, 3 sets of 8-12 reps at 75% of maximum strength [1RM], with 8 exercises) and had their diet records analyzed. The subjects' mean choline intakes were categorized into low (2.9-5.5 mg/kg lean mass/day), med-low (5.6-8.0 mg/kg lean mass/day), or adequate (8.1-10.6 mg/kg lean mass/day) groups— intakes corresponding to under 50%, ~63%, and ~85% of the AI for choline, respectively. Results indicated that gains in composite strength (leg press + chest press 1RM) were significantly lower in the low group compared with the other groups. Reduced gains in lean mass were also observed in the low group compared with higher choline intakes. From an acute standpoint, studies have provided evidence that only strenuous, prolonged exercise decreases choline levels significantly. Exercise must be longer than 2 hours in duration and at intensities greater than 70% to significantly decrease choline (Penry & Manore, 2008). Supplementation with choline has not been shown to be beneficial unless choline levels are significantly depleted or intakes are low, as noted. Sandage and colleagues (1992) have conducted one of the few studies examining the potential use of choline during prolonged, choline-depleting exercise. They found that 2.8 g of choline supplemented 1 hour before and halfway through a 20 mi (32.2 km) run improved finish times. A few studies have examined whether supplementation with choline above normal concentrations can improve physical performance; however, no benefits were found (Deuster & Cooper, 2002; Buchman, Jenden, & Roch, 1999; Burns, Costill, & Fink, 1988; Warber et al., 2000). More research is needed, especially in team sports such as football, basketball, and soccer. Currently, choline has potential benefit; however, this applies only during prolonged, high-intensity exercise.

Common usage: According to ODS.gov, the forms of choline in dietary supplements include choline bitartrate, phosphatidylcholine, and lecithin. Scientists have used fluids containing 2.43 to 2.8 g of choline consumed 1 hour before exercise and another 2.43 to 2.8 g dose provided during exercise as a means of preventing choline depletion. The AI for choline is 425 mg/day and 550 mg/day for adult women and men, respectively. Higher-fat meats such as beef liver and eggs are excellent sources of choline. One whole egg contains 113 mg of choline. Chicken, milk, and soybeans also contain relatively high amounts of choline, as do cauliflower and spinach.

Health concerns: The Office of Dietary Supplements at the National Institutes of Health note that high intakes of choline are associated with a fishy body odor, vomiting, excessive sweating and salivation, hypotension, and liver toxicity. The tolerable upper limit of choline as established by the National Academy of Sciences is 3 to 3.5 g for men and women.

Chondroitin  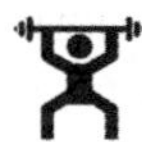

aka *chondroitin sulfate (see also glucosamine)*

What it is: Chondroitin is a large gel-forming molecule that is a constituent of hyaline cartilage, which covers the bones of synovial joints and absorbs shock and reduces friction during movement. Chondroitin is commonly supplemented orally in the form of chondroitin sulfate made from extracts of cartilaginous tissues in fish, birds, cows, or pigs (Black et al., 2009).

Function: In a healthy joint there should be minimal narrowing of the space between bones. As cartilage is lost, joint space narrows and increases the likelihood of developing osteoarthritis (OA), resulting in pain and loss of function. As a constituent of hyaline cartilage, chondroitin is beneficial in preventing the degeneration of joints such as the knee, hip, ankle, shoulder, and spine. It is hypothesized the availability of chondroitin is a limiting factor in the synthesis of different components of cartilage.

Performance benefit: Because the physical demands of sport and daily training place a significant amount of stress on joints, many athletes experience chronic joint pain. In addition, many athletes suffer injuries to joints that require surgery or joint reconstruction. Recovery from these types of surgeries can result in changes to the joint, and chondroitin could have a positive effect on recovery.

Research: The majority of research on chondroitin has focused on older populations suffering from OA of the knee or hip. Chondroitin's ability to improve joint pain and function is equivocal, with some but not all studies showing mild improvement. Long-term supplementation has shown to be most effective; in some cases chronic supplementation for over 1 year is required before structural changes in the joint are observed. Chondroitin is commonly supplemented in combination with glucosamine sulfate, another popular joint supplement. The effects of combining these supplements (versus using them alone) has shown mixed results. The Glucosamine/Chondroitin Arthritis Intervention Trial (GAIT), conducted by the National Institutes of Health, is one of the largest studies ever done related to chondroitin. The results of this study found neither chondroitin, glucosamine, nor the combination to significantly relieve pain compared to a placebo. However, patients suffering from higher levels of pain (moderate to severe) did show improvements in pain scores from a combination of chondroitin and glucosamine (Sawitzke, 2010). Another meta-analysis concluded that chondroitin was mildly effective in preventing joint space narrowing or degeneration over time; however, over 2 years of supplementation were required before effects were realized (Ho Lee et al., 2009). A more recent meta-analysis of eight randomized control trials concluded that the combination of glucosamine and chondroitin is effective and superior to other treatments as it relates to specifically to knee OA (Meng et al., 2023). Although there is some promising evidence of the benefits of chondroitin used in conjunction with glucosamine in mitigating the negative effects of OA, additional research is warranted, particularly in a healthy athletic population, before definite conclusions can be made.

Common usage: Typically, 800 to 1,200 mg of chondroitin sulfate are supplemented in either one large dose or two to three smaller doses throughout the day. There is no evidence to suggest that multiple doses consumed throughout the day are more effective than one large dose. Chondroitin is commonly supplemented in combination with glucosamine sulfate, SAMe (S-adenosyl methionine), or MSM (methylsulfonylmethane).

Health concerns: Chondroitin appears to be safe. It has been used in many short- and long-term research studies without any adverse health effects reported, although some preclinical concerns have appeared in the media suggesting chondroitin may encourage the development or recurrence of melanoma, a potentially deadly form of skin cancer. Concerned consumers should check with their physician.

Chromium (Cr) 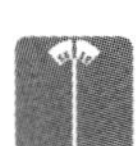 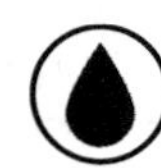

aka *chromium picolinate*

What it is: Only small amounts of chromium are needed for optimal health. Chromium can be found in a diverse selection of whole foods such as meats, whole grains, fruits, and vegetables. Broccoli, grape juice, whole wheat English muffins, and potatoes are among some of the higher chromium-containing foods. Chromium and picolinic acid are not naturally found together, but studies in animals have found that when supplemental sources of chromium are complexed with picolinic acid (forming chromium picolinate), absorption is improved.

Function: The exact mechanism of chromium is not known, but it is believed to improve insulin's ability to bind to cells and upregulate (or increase) receptors (Lukaski et al., 1996). It is hypothesized that this ability could enhance the anabolic properties of insulin, thus increasing lean body mass. In addition, chromium may stimulate metabolism and suppress appetite.

Performance benefit: If the proposed benefits of chromium are true, it would be of benefit for athletes wanting to gain lean muscle mass, improve body composition, and lose body fat and weight.

Research: Excitement about the potential fat-burning and muscle-building effects of chromium picolinate began in the late 1980s following a study in which males who supplemented with 200 mcg/day of chromium picolinate saw greater gains in strength and improvements in body composition than placebo (Lukaski et al., 1996). The results of this study were followed by several duplicate research trials that were unable to produce the same positive results. A meta-analysis of 10 studies by Pittler, Stevinson, and Ernst (2003) concluded that chromium picolinate provided a relatively small reduction in body weight, roughly 1.1 to 1.2 kg over 10 to 13 weeks in overweight and obese individuals. More recently, in 2010, a pilot study was conducted on overweight adults to assess the impact of 1,000 mcg of chromium picolinate over a 24-week supplementation period.

The results found no significant benefits from supplementation. The authors of this trial concluded that chromium picolinate does not appear to be beneficial for healthy over-weight populations (Yazaki et al., 2010). In conclusion, although there is evidence for the efficacy of chromium supplements in improving conditions in metabolic syndrome and in some patients with type 2 diabetes, there isn't data to support its use to initiate favorable body composition changes in a healthy athletic population (Maret, 2019).

Common usage: Typically, 200 to 1,000 mcg of chromium picolinate are supplemented daily, in either one or two smaller doses per day.

Health concerns: Few adverse events have been linked to high intakes of chromium; therefore, the Institute of Medicine of the National Academies has not established an upper tolerance limit. Certain medications may interact with chromium, especially when taken on a regular basis. It is advisable to check with a doctor or a qualified health care provider before supplementing with chromium.

Chrysin

aka *5,7-dihydroxyflavone*

What it is: Chrysin is a naturally occurring flavonoid present in plants. Significant amounts can be found in honey and honeycomb, and it can be chemically extracted from the blue passionflower or Indian trumpet flower. Flavonoids are natural antioxidants that exhibit a wide range of biological effects. Currently, more than 4,000 types of active flavonoids have been identified, including flavonols, flavones, flavanols, flavanones, anthocyanins, and isoflavonoids. The effects of flavonoids can include antibacterial, anti-inflammatory, antiallergic, antithrombotic, and vasodilatory results (Khoo, Chua, & Balaram, 2010).

Function: Chrysin is largely promoted as an antiestrogen and testosterone-boosting supplement. It is purported to inhibit aromatase, an important enzyme involved in the production of estrogen. Because aromatase is involved in the conversion of androgens into estrogens (Monterio, Azevedo, & Calhua, 2006), its inhibition would theoretically increase androgens, such as testosterone, and limit the concentrations of estrogens. Another potential mechanism is chrysin's ability to bind to estrogen receptors, limiting estrogen binding and estrogen's effects in the body.

Performance benefit: Athletes, mostly bodybuilders, have used chrysin supplements to promote anabolic hormones such as testosterone and limit estrogen. Anabolic hormones help build lean body mass and increase strength and power. Athletes' concerns with estrogens are that they might soften the physique, encourage growth of breast tissue if high enough, or cause other side effects.

Research: In recent years, chrysin has not seen much human research relative to sports nutrition. Early studies in vitro related to chrysin's ability to inhibit aromatase were positive (Campbell & Kurzer, 1993). Unfortunately, studies in animals and humans have not been effective, and though more research is needed, our current understanding is that chrysin does not inhibit aromatase activity (Monteiro, Azevedo, & Calhua, 2006; Saarinen et al., 2001). Gambelunghe and colleagues (2003) found no changes in levels of testosterone in males after 21 days of treatment with propolis and honey containing chrysin. Other studies have also failed to show a positive effect of chrysin on testosterone: In a 2001 study, the effects of a natural testosterone-boosting cocktail that included androstene-dione, dehydroepiandrosterone, saw palmetto, indole-3-carbinol, chrysin, and *Tribulus terrestris* were evaluated for 28 days. Total testosterone was unchanged, and though free testosterone levels were increased, so too were levels of estradiol, which can increase levels of estrogen and result in the development of female sex characteristics in males (Brown et al., 2001).

Common usage: Chrysin has been sold individually as a dietary supplement, often with a recommended daily dose of 1,000 to 2,000 mg. It is also commonly sold in combination with a variety of other so-called natural testosterone-boosting ingredients.

Health concerns: The use of chrysin appears safe. No known adverse effects have been noted in scientific research studies. However, many natural testosterone boosters are not typically effective and could contain other ingredients such as prohormones, which have been largely removed from the market since the early 2000s and can cause gynecomastia, lower HDL cholesterol, and negatively affect a person's psychological state. Athletes should use extreme caution when considering the use of these types of supplements.

Cinnamon

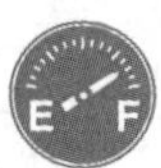  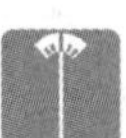  

aka *cinnamomum*

What it is: Cinnamon is a common spice used for cooking. It originates from the bark of two medicinal herbs, *C. zeylanicum* and *C. cassia*. Aside from its use in cooking, cinnamon has been used for many years as a medicinal herb to treat stomach complaints and other ailments. However, scientists recently have discovered that cinnamon has a plethora of other potential benefits, most significant of which is its ability to control blood sugar levels and improve insulin sensitivity. In addition, cinnamon is also believed to have anti-inflammatory, antimicrobial, antioxidant, and blood pressure–lowering effects (Gruenwald, Freder, & Armbruster, 2010).

Function: Cinnamon comprises a number of components that are speculated to be responsible for its beneficial effects, including volatile oils such as cinnamaldehyde, eugenol, linalool, and camphor are found in different quantities within the bark, leaf, and root bark of *C. zeylanicum and C. cassia* (Gruenwald, Freder, & Armbruster, 2010). The quantities of these volatile oils vary within the different species of cinnamon. In addition, cinnamon contains powerful polyphenols that can function as antioxidants and have anti-inflammatory effects.

Performance benefit: Cinnamon's ability to increase the effects of insulin could have strong implications for athletes, especially postworkout. Cinnamon could improve glycogen restoration and further stimulate protein synthesis through its insulin-augmenting effects. Improvement of glycogen restoration and protein synthesis could aid and speed muscle recovery. In addition, cinnamon could protect against chronically inflamed muscles and joints, reducing the severity of delayed-onset muscle soreness (DOMS) and tendonitis.

Research: The majority of research has focused on the impact of cinnamon on blood glucose and potential benefits in the treatment of diabetes. A 2024 meta-analysis of 24 randomized control trials concluded that cinnamon supplementation significantly improves fasting blood glucose as well as insulin sensitivity and hemoglobin A1c in type 2 diabetics or prediabetics (Moridpour et al., 2024). In another study, 22 subjects with prediabetes and metabolic syndrome consumed 500 mg of cinnamon extract/day for 12 weeks, resulting in significantly lower fasting blood glucose levels as well as increases in lean mass (Ziegenfuss et al., 2006). However, results showing improvements in body composition have failed to be replicated by other researchers (Vafa et al., 2012); therefore, clear conclusions are difficult to make at this time, and more research is needed, particularly in a healthy population. In vitro studies have shown cinnamon extract to increase glucose uptake and glycogen synthesis (Couturier et al., 2010). Yet, again, no specific studies have involved athletes or investigated cinnamon's impact on glucose uptake and glycogen restoration postexercise or its impact on protein synthesis. In vitro and animal studies also support cinnamon as an anti-inflammatory and inhibitor of cyclo-oxygenase-2 (COX-2) (Gruenwald et al., 2010)—a benefit shown to translate to reducing the duration and intensity of pain associated with menstrual cramping (Xu et al., 2020). Similarly, a randomized, placebo-controlled trial discovered a supplementation protocol consisting of 600 mg of cinnamon taken 3 times/day over 2 months significantly reduced serum levels of interleukin-6 and nitric oxide, two markers associated with inflammation and neurogenic pain, which, in this study, translated to a significant decrease in the frequency, severity, and duration of migraine attacks (Zareie et al., 2020). Although cinnamon shows promise for improving insulin sensitivity in type 2 diabetic patients as well as mitigating specific types of pain, the benefits as they relate specifically to athletes are currently unknown until more research is conducted on this population.

Common usage: Supplementation dosages of cinnamon between 3 to 6 g/day appear to be most effective, though higher doses (6 g taken 3x/day over 2 months) were used to elicit a positive benefit in migraine sufferers. In addition, the source of cinnamon (either *C. zeylanicum* or *C. cassia*) may have different effects, and further well-designed studies are needed to confirm the most effective sources.

Health concerns: Cinnamon appears to be safe, especially within recommended doses of 3 to 6 g/day. Preclinical and other human trials have not shown any significant toxic effects (Nuffer et al., 2023; Ranasinghe et al., 2012).

Cissus Quadrangularis 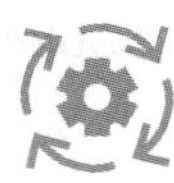 

aka *bone setter, devil's backbone, veldt grape*

What it is: *Cissus quadrangularis* is a perennial herb of the Vitaceae family, common to tropical and subtropical xeric wood. It is a beefy desert plant common in India and used in Ayurvedic medicine for a variety of disorders.

Function: The antioxidant effects of *Cissus quadrangularis* may affect specific tissues.

Performance benefit: *Cissus quadrangularis* may be useful for athletes suffering from joint pain or a recent fracture. More research is warranted, but a discussion with a health care provider may be helpful.

Research: According to Sundaran and colleagues (2020), methanol extract of *Cissus quadrangularis* exhibits strong antioxidant activity and methanol root extract comprises saponins that exhibit powerful sedative action, suppressing spontaneous motor action in mice. The antioxidant effects are at least in part due to high amounts of vitamin C, carotenoids, and polyphenols. Oxidative stress, which such antioxidants may decrease, is typically connected to inflammation, pain, or tissue damage. Perhaps related are the claims surrounding reduced joint pain, which do have limited data to support them, interestingly in exercising men (Bloomer et al., 2013). Further, some clinical data suggest hastened healing of bone fractures (Brahmkshatriya et al., 2015; Singh et al., 2013).

Common usage: 300 to 1,000 mg/day is common, but more data are needed; as with many supplements, doses can vary depending on age, weight, other supplements or medications, and individual tolerance.

Health concerns: Potential side effects include headaches, dry mouth, diarrhea, insomnia, and drowsiness. Others may be possible in sensitive individuals.

Citicoline 

aka *CDP-choline, Cognizin (brand name), cytidine-5-diphosphocholine (see also choline)*

What it is: Originally a prescription drug in Japan for stroke patients, citicoline is now sold as a dietary supplement for cognition enhancement.

Function: Citicoline appears to increase phosphatidylcholine in the brain.

Performance benefit: Citicoline has neuroprotective properties due to a greater availability of phosphatidylcholine, which may stimulate the repair and regeneration of damaged cell membranes of neurons. Athletes interested in sharpening psychomotor recovery should stay abreast of this body of literature.

Research: In addition to a mechanistic rationale, there are data to support the cognition-enhancing effects of citicoline. For example, in a randomized study of 100 individuals aged 50 to 85 with age-associated memory impairment, those supplemented with citicoline showed significantly greater improvements in secondary outcomes of episodic memory compared with placebo ($p = 0.0025$) (Nakazaki et al., 2021). Composite memory (a secondary outcome) was also significantly improved to a greater degree following citicoline supplementation ($p = 0.0052$). The effect is not just seen among the aging or impaired: McGlade and colleagues (2019) concluded that adolescent males receiving 28 days of Cognizin citicoline (250 or 500 mg) showed improved attention and psychomotor speed and reduced impulsivity compared to placebo.

Common usage: Citicoline has been used by adults in doses of 500 to 1,000 mg twice daily by mouth for up to 12 months.

Health concerns: Adverse effects could include hypotension, changes in heart rate, transient headaches, and restlessness.

Citrimax

(see *hydroxycitric acid*)

Citrulline Malate (CM) 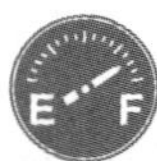 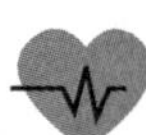 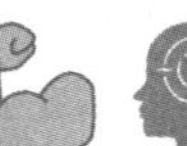 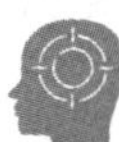 

What it is: A nonessential amino acid (L-citrulline) bound to an organic salt compound (malate), citrulline malate (CM) is a special nutrient combo marketed as an ergogenic aid for its purported role in reducing muscle fatigue, enhancing aerobic energy production, and facilitating optimal recovery.

Function: Individually, citrulline is synthesized within the intestines from the amino acid glutamine and plays a part in a series of biochemical reactions important for the removal of ammonia. Ammonia is a byproduct of both anaerobic and aerobic exercise that at high levels can negatively affect the production of energy, thereby leading to fatigue and reduced performance. Malate, also known as malic acid, is found naturally in fruits such as apples and plays a role in the Krebs cycle, which produces energy from carbohydrate, fats, and protein within the mitochondria. Furthermore, malate is able to recycle lactate for energy production, critical in protecting the muscles from fatigue and aiding recovery. Together, CM is thought to enhance aerobic performance or recovery by accelerating the clearance of fatigue-inducing ammonia, recycling lactate for improved energy production, or enhancing blood flow (Gough et al., 2021; Sureda & Pons, 2013). It may also play a role as a nitric oxide (NO) enhancer.

Performance benefit: Athletes may benefit from increased endurance during aerobic training and competition as well as faster recovery between high-intensity bursts of energy common in interval training as well as stop-and-go sports such as soccer. CM supplementation may also improve the use of amino acids, especially branched-chain amino acids, during exercise, which may further improve recovery from exertion (Sureda et al., 2010).

Research: According to Gough and colleagues (2021), "To date, a single acute 8 g dose of CM on either resistance exercise performance or cycling has been the most common approach, which has produced equivocal results." They also note that quality control issues have been reported among some manufacturers regarding citrulline-to-malate ratios and concluded that, until further studies are completed, the efficacy of CM supplementation to improve exercise performance remains ambiguous. Although limited in quantity, some earlier human studies evaluating the impact of CM did show some promise. One well-designed study found a single dose of 8 g of CM to increase the total number of repetitions completed by healthy men during 8 sets of flat barbell bench presses by nearly 53%, a significant improvement from the placebo trial. Furthermore, a 40% reduction in muscle soreness at 24 hours and 48 hours after training was reported as compared to the placebo trial. Study investigators concluded that CM demonstrated promise for athletes engaged in high-intensity anaerobic exercises with short rest times as well as for any athlete looking to reduce muscle soreness and improve recovery (Pérez-Guisado & Jakeman, 2010). A lower dose of 6 g/day taken over 15 days also yielded positive results with healthy men, demonstrating a significant reduction in the sensation of fatigue, a 34% increase in the rate of ATP production during exercise, and a 20% increase in the rate of phosphocreatine recovery after exercise, indicating a reduced energy cost of muscle contraction as compared to presupplementation trials (Bendahan et al., 2002). An animal study essentially replicated these data, demonstrating a significant decrease in both phosphocreatine (28%) and oxidative (32%) costs of contraction with CM supplementation, leading authors to conclude CM has an ergogenic effect associated with an improvement of muscle contraction efficiency (Giannesini et al., 2011).

Common usage: Research-supported dosages for CM range anywhere from 4 to 8 g/day. For use as a single dose, athletes may consume 8 g of CM 30 to 40 minutes before competition. For use as a daily supplement taken throughout a competitive season, athletes may consume 4 to 6 g split into two doses so that 2 to 3 g are taken 30 to 40 minutes before exercise and another 2 to 3 g are taken at bedtime, preferably on an empty stomach.

Health concerns: CM appears to be safe for use, though there are some reports of stomach upset at doses of 8 g/day.

Citrus Aurantium

(see *synephrine*)

Cobalamin

(see *vitamin B_{12}*)

Cochin Ginger

(see *ginger*)

Cocoa 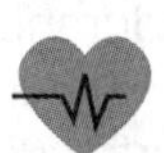 

aka *cacao, cocoa flavanols, dark chocolate, gallated flavan-3-ols, Theobroma cacao*

What it is: Foods and beverages that contain chocolate or cocoa are made from the beans of the *Theobroma cacao* tree. Cocoa liquor is a paste made from fermented cocoa beans that have been ground, roasted, and shelled. The percent cocoa referred to on food packaging is the percentage of cocoa liquor within the product. Cocoa powder, used in baking, is made by removing the cocoa butter from the liquor (Katz, Doughty, & Ali, 2011).

Function: Cocoa contains fatty acids; minerals such as magnesium, copper, potassium, and calcium; and polyphenols. Polyphenols include a variety of compounds, but cocoa is particularly rich in flavonoids, which include epicatechin, catechin, and procyanidins. Flavonoids can have cardioprotective effects through their antioxidant activity. In addition, flavonoids have immunoregulatory properties and beneficial effects on the vascular system. Flavonoids in cocoa can prevent the formation of atherosclerosis and lower blood pressure. Epicatechins appear to affect vascular function the most (Jalil & Ismail, 2008; Katz, Doughty, & Ali, 2011).

Performance benefit: Cocoa could benefit athletes through its impact on vascular function. Improved vascular function would result in increased blood flow and nutrients to muscles during training, resulting in improved performance. Improved postexercise blood flow would also benefit recovery. The antioxidant and immunoregulatory effects of cocoa provide additional benefits to athletes.

Research: The majority of research trials suggest that cocoa is capable of decreasing blood pressure and cholesterol and improving vascular function. No study to date has looked at the impact of cocoa on immune function in humans, although early animal studies are positive. Only recently have trials investigated the impact of cocoa on exercise. Studies investigating the impact of 40 g and 100 g of dark chocolate before prolonged cycling found dark chocolate to be beneficial in reducing oxidative stress and increasing mobilization of free fatty acids; however, no effect was seen on immune and endocrine response, nor on time trial performance (Allgrove et al., 2011; Davison et al., 2012). A systemic review of 13 randomized control trials demonstrated a positive impact of both acute (2 weeks) and chronic (3 months) intake of cocoa flavanols on vascular function, exercise-induced oxidative stress, and substrate utilization during exercise, demonstrating further promise for use to improve exercise performance and recovery (Decroix et al., 2018). However, the bulk of subjects evaluated were either untrained or obese, so additional research is needed to further clarify the impact of cocoa and its polyphenols on athletes and exercise performance.

Common usage: As little as 5 mg of the polyphenol epicatechin has been shown to provide health benefits. Typically, research trials have used 300 to 800 mg/day of cocoa polyphenols, which is the recommended supplementation level. Roughly 50 mg of polyphenols are present in 1 g of cocoa powder, 300 to 600 mg in a 40 g dark chocolate bar, and 100 to 200 mg in a 40 g milk chocolate bar.

Health concerns: The biggest concerns related to cocoa and dark chocolate are the high calorie and fat content and the risk of associated weight gain. No other health concerns are known at this time.

Coconut 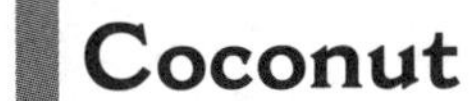 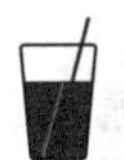  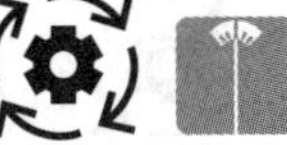

aka *coconut milk, coconut water, Cocos nucifera, virgin coconut oil*

What it is: Coconut is the fruit harvested from the *Cocos nucifera* tree. It is a dietary staple and common complementary medicine in Philippian, Polynesian, and Malaysian cultures. Coconut water, milk, and oils (found in the fleshy component of the fruit) are commonly used portions of the fruit and are becoming more popular as dietary supplements.

Function: Coconut's uses in medicine include its antibacterial, antifungal, and antiviral properties. In addition, coconut contains powerful antioxidants and is an immunostimulant. Coconut is unique in that it contains large amounts (roughly 70%-80%) of medium-chain triglycerides (MCTs), which can be absorbed directly into the blood, unlike longer chains, which must travel through the lymphatic system and the liver before being oxidized by the muscles as fuel.

Performance benefit: Coconut water is speculated to enhance fluid replacement and prevent dehydration, limiting the resulting drops in physical performance. Coconut milk, oil, and to some extent water provide powerful antioxidants and support healthy immune function. These properties could aid athletes in managing the stresses of training that can suppress the immune system, as well as limit the inflammation produced by muscle damage or injury. MCTs can also be quickly oxidized as a source of fuel during exercise, enabling endurance athletes to spare muscle glycogen and improve performance. Some evidence exists that MCTs can increase metabolic rate, assist in weight loss, and improve body composition.

Research: Kalman and colleagues (2012) examined coconut's hydrating abilities compared to water and a carbohydrate-electrolyte sport drink and found no significant differences in performance or markers of rehydration. Other studies have produced similar results. Although coconut water is equally effective in promoting rehydration, it is not superior to sport drinks and has also been noted to be less tolerable, causing GI tract distress (Kalman et al., 2012; Pérez-Idárraga & Aragón-Vargas, 2014; Saat et al., 2002). Information related to the immune-stimulating and anti-inflammatory properties of coconut is limited, though early work in animals is positive, showing coconut's anti-inflammatory effect at high doses. How this effect translates in humans or with specific inflammation-related conditions in athletes is currently unknown (Intahphuak, Khonsung, & Panthong, 2010). In weight-loss studies, data has been equivocal, with some studies showing coconut oil to aid abdominal body fat loss and others concluding that coconut oil failed to elicit any benefit as it relates to satiation, thermogenesis, and weight loss (Assuncao et al., 2009; Liau et al., 2011; Santos et al., 2019). It is evident that additional research specific to a healthy population is warranted before definite conclusions on the benefits of coconut and associated recommendations can be made.

Common usage: Weight-loss studies have used 30 mL (2 tbsp) of coconut oil per day. Recommendations for coconut water as a fluid replacement are similar to those for other fluids: 4 to 8 oz (0.12-0.24 L) every 15 minutes during exercise and 20 oz/lb (266 mL/kg) lost during exercise.

Health concerns: Although they are high in saturated fats, coconut milk and oils do not negatively affect blood cholesterol levels, and consumption is safe in the absence of allergy. However, it is still recommended that total intake of saturated fat not exceed 10% of daily calories.

Coenzyme Q10 (CoQ10) 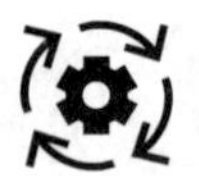 

aka *ubidecarenone, ubiquinone*

What it is: A vitamin-like, fat-soluble compound of the ubiquinone family, coenzyme Q10 (CoQ10) functions in all cells of the body, serving as a coenzyme for several of the key enzymatic steps that facilitate ATP production. CoQ10 also doubles as a potent antioxidant, helping destroy free radicals before they can cause damage to normal cells within the body. CoQ10 is naturally found in the highest concentration within organs and muscles that demand the most energy, such as the heart. It can also be found in such dietary sources as meat, poultry, and fish.

Function: The human body is on a continuous mission to generate enough energy to support the performance of every cell. Increased dietary intake of CoQ10, through whole food or supplementation, may help the body keep up the demand for mitochondrial ATP synthesis, especially when demand exceeds production, such as during the stress of physical exertion or recovery from injury. In addition, as a potent antioxidant in both the mitochondria and lipid membranes, CoQ10 helps to combat the 10- to 20-fold increase in reactive oxygen species (ROS) during physical exercise that can contribute to muscle injury and decreased performance.

Performance benefit: Purported performance-focused benefits of CoQ10 supplementation include improved oxygen usage in the heart and skeletal muscles, leading to increases in maximal aerobic capacity, anaerobic endurance, and overall work capacity. CoQ10 is also marketed as a recovery agent, helping to reduce exercise-induced muscle injury. Athletes with muscle-wasting diseases (e.g., muscular dystrophy) or diabetes as well as master-level athletes are thought to carry lower levels of CoQ10 and might benefit the most from supplementation.

Research: Although research has shown intense physical training to lower blood levels of CoQ10, there are mixed results on the validity of daily supplementation to produce enhancements in cardiovascular-focused performance variables. The majority of double-blind, placebo-controlled studies fail to demonstrate any significant enhancement with a daily supplementation protocol of 60 to 150 mg over 4 to 8 weeks regardless of fitness status (trained vs. untrained) (Bloomer et al., 2012; Ostman et al., 2012; Zhou et al., 2005). Some scientists believe this may be due to inefficient absorption of CoQ10 into the mitochondrial membrane, leaving open the possibility of better results with increased bioavailability (Liao et al., 2007). Nonetheless, although the current consensus on CoQ10's impact on cardiovascular performance remains primarily negative, the studies evaluating its impact on muscle recovery remain positive. A double-blind study on elite martial arts athletes, for example, discovered that a daily supplementation protocol of 300 mg of CoQ10 for 20 days during a period of intense training significantly lowered levels of the lipid peroxide (a free radical that contributes to oxidative stress in the body) and creatine kinase (an enzyme that signals muscle damage and injury), thereby helping protect against exercise-induced muscle injury and improving recovery (Kon et al., 2008).

Common usage: Per study protocols, recommended doses for adult athletes range from 60 to 300 mg/day taken continuously for at least 3 weeks. For doses higher than 100 mg/day, it is best to split the doses into two to three smaller doses and take them with meals containing some fat to facilitate more efficient absorption. Although CoQ10 is available in many forms, softgels tend to be better absorbed than capsules or other preparations.

Health concerns: CoQ10 is generally safe, with the exception of infrequent reports of nausea, loss of appetite, upset stomach, and diarrhea. Due to several drug–nutrient interactions, however, athletes taking any form of medication are advised to consult a physician before starting a supplementation protocol.

Colostrum 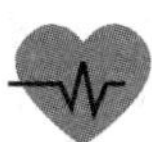 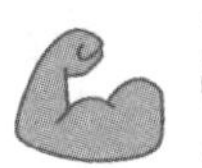  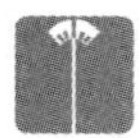

aka *bovine colostrum (BC), mother's milk*

What it is: Bovine colostrum (BC)—the milk secreted by a cow during the first few days after giving birth—contains a wide array of nutrients essential to the overall health of the athlete as well as growth-promoting and disease-fighting compounds that are thought to facilitate quicker recovery times during intense cycles of training and competition. BC contains 3 to 4 times more protein than regular cow's milk—an estimated 150 g/L—and is lactose free.

Function: A review of studies exploring the performance-focused attributes of BC and corresponding mechanisms of action concluded that supplementation seems to elicit a favorable impact on the recovery of athletes engaged in high-intensity or high-volume training (Shing, Hunter, & Stevenson, 2009). Several reasons were cited. First, BC seems to increase blood levels of a hormone called insulin-like growth factor 1 (IGF1), which enhances glucose and amino acid transport to cells, promotes protein synthesis, and protects against protein breakdown—all key factors to recovery. IGF1 may also help contribute to lean body mass gains. BC also appears to improve intramuscular buffering capacity, helping protect against muscle fatigue during high-intensity training as well as enhancing recovery between high-intensity exercise sessions. Finally, BC has been shown to increase levels of an antibody called immunoglobulin-A (IgA) within saliva that may help activate immune defenses, protecting the athlete from various sidelining bugs throughout training and competition.

Performance benefit: Athletes may benefit from quicker recovery times and enhanced immune function, especially when the body is exposed to increased stress levels at the peak of training and competition or when exercising in extreme environments (e.g., heat, altitude). BC taken in doses of 5 to 20 g/day over 14+ days before completing high-intensity exercise in heat may also help reduce the incidence of gastrointestinal symptoms (upset stomach or diarrhea) often seen as a result of endurance competition (Dziewiecka et al., 2022; Hałasa et al., 2017; March et al., 2018; Marchbank et al., 2011).

Research: The bulk of current research evaluating the performance impact of BC has produced mixed results. One double-blind study failed to demonstrate an impact on blood or saliva immunoglobulin levels after a 4-week daily supplementation protocol incorporating 25 g of a low-protein colostrum; however, the incidence of upper respiratory symptoms reported by elite swimmers decreased by 36% as compared to a calorie-matched placebo (Crooks et al., 2010). In contrast, an earlier double-blind, placebo-controlled study of adult male and female athletes found a BC dose of 20 g taken during 2 weeks of training produced significant increases in serum IGF1 and saliva IgA (Mero et al., 2002). Additionally, a lower dose (10 g/day) of BC taken over 10 weeks not only reduced the incidence of upper respiratory symptoms but also yielded significant improvements in highly trained cyclists compared to a placebo group in a 40 km time trial performance after completing a high-intensity training session (Shing et al., 2006). Researchers attributed these results in part to a significant level of favorable changes in the concentration of several antibodies. However, results from a recent meta-analysis of 10 randomized control trials with a total of 239 subjects concluded BC supplementation has no or a fairly low impact on improving the concentration of serum immunoglobulins (IgA, IgG), lymphocytes and neutrophils, and saliva immunoglobulin (IgA) in athletes and physically active participants, signaling a gap in scientific knowledge on the mechanisms underlying its immunological effects (Główka et al., 2020). Of worthy note to athletes competing in stop-and-go sports, supplementation with just 3.2 g of bovine colostrum over 6 weeks following an intermittent task designed to simulate the physiological demands of soccer attenuated inflammatory and muscle-damage-related markers induced by their protocol and speeded the recovery of explosive power (assessed by squat jump performance) (Kotsis et al., 2017). It is evident that the performance impact of BC supplementation is likely multifaceted, meaning small improvements across several variables rather than a single variable contribute to the potential benefits. Future studies should focus on the impact of a standardized supplement protocol (e.g., dose, length of time) on the proposed mechanisms of actions and the performance of athletes in a variety of exercise protocols.

Common usage: BC is available in a variety of forms, including tablets, powders, bars, and liquids. Research-supported doses are variable but, on average, a dose of 5 to 50 g/day has been used.

Health concerns: Although BC is generally well tolerated, there have been some reports of gastrointestinal distress, including such symptoms as bloating, nausea, vomiting, and diarrhea, as well as diminishing performance returns at high doses (>50 g/day). Of special note, while colostrum is not a substance specifically banned by the US and World Anti-Doping Agencies, IGF-1 is. Thus, athletes are advised to exercise caution using supplements containing colostrum for fear of causing increased concentration of plasma insulin-like growth factor 1 and impacting the outcome of anti-doping tests (IGF1).

Coneflower

(see *echinacea*)

Conjugated Linoleic Acid (CLA) 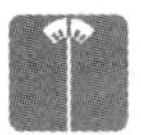

What it is: Conjugated linoleic acid (CLA) is an isomer of common linoleic acid but unlike it metabolically. Linoleic acid is an omega-6 fatty acid, one of two essential fatty acids that must be consumed in the diet; such as through milk, butter, and meat fats. The chemical formula of CLA is the same as linoleic acid; however, its chemical structure is different. CLA is commonly found in two shapes, known as 10-CLA and 9-CLA. Roughly 75% to 90% of the CLA found in milk is of the 9-CLA variety.

Function: CLA is believed to improve body composition by lowering fat mass and increasing fat-free mass. There are a variety of proposed mechanisms, which include decreased enzyme activity leading to a decreased uptake of triglycerides by fat cells. CLA is also believed to influence transcription factors that regulate production of new fat cells. Lastly, CLA is thought to increase beta-oxidation, the metabolic pathway used to burn fat.

Performance benefit: CLA is a popular supplement among bodybuilders and fitness competitors interested in reducing body fat and establishing a lean appearance. It is also used by athletes to help reduce unwanted body fat and increase lean body mass.

Research: A significant amount of research has been done on CLA, producing a wide variety of results. Early studies in animals were positive: CLA use led to losses in body fat and increases in lean body mass, especially in mice. However, studies in humans were not nearly as conclusive or effective. A meta-analysis of 18 scientific studies related to CLA and its impact on body composition concluded that a 50:50 mixture of 10-CLA and 9-CLA did produce a slow decrease in fat mass (0.05 kg/week) over the course of 6 months to 2 years. Fat loss peaked between 1 and 2 years (Whigham et al., 2007). A similar meta-analysis on the same 18 studies, completed to determine if fat-free mass or muscle mass was affected, concluded that CLA was not effective in increasing muscle mass (Schoeller, Watras, & Whigham, 2009). More recently, in a 2011 study of the effects of CLA on body composition in overweight men, 8 weeks of CLA did not affect body weight, composition, or beta-oxidation, which is a marker of fat use (Joseph et al., 2011).

Common usage: Research suggests that 10-CLA is most effective in producing changes in body fat; however, when supplemented alone, it produces insulin resistance. This negative affect is counteracted when 10-CLA is supplemented with 9-CLA. A dosage of 3.2 g/day of a 50:50 ratio of 10-CLA and 9-CLA is suggested; higher doses are not recommended.

Health concerns: Higher intakes of CLA increase liver and spleen size and can result in insulin resistance. In addition, some studies have found CLA to increase markers of inflammation, such as C-reactive protein.

Copper (Cu)   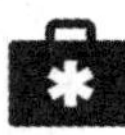

What it is: An essential trace mineral that is not synthesized by the body and thus must be consumed in the diet, copper plays a role in a wide range of biochemical processes key to optimal health and performance. It can be obtained naturally from such foods as organ meats, seafood (especially shellfish), nuts, seeds, whole grains, legumes, and chocolate as well as in dietary supplement form.

Function: Because copper is lost in small amounts via sweat during exercise, athletes may be more vulnerable to deficiencies if intake from whole foods or supplementation does not offset these losses. Deficiencies in copper can lead to a number of symptoms detrimental to health and performance. For one, the body requires copper to produce ATP; without it, energy wavers. Copper is also critical for optimal use of iron. If iron is hindered, oxygen delivery to red blood cells becomes impaired, leading to diminished respiratory function as well as muscle fatigue and weakness. Furthermore, copper is important for the function of a variety of enzymes essential to an athlete's health. One of these enzymes, superoxide dismutase (SOD), is considered one of the most powerful antioxidants, helping to scavenge damaging free radicals and counteract some of the damage the body's own defense mechanisms cannot offset during particularly hard training cycles. Copper's antioxidant defenses may support an athlete's immunity as well as aid recovery. Another enzyme, lysyl oxidase (LOX), aids in the formation of collagen and elastin, two proteins necessary for bone and connective tissue health.

Performance benefit: Athletes may benefit from enhanced energy and endurance as well as better immune support and quicker recovery times. Integration of copper at a dose of 2.5 to 3 mg/day may also slow down bone mineral loss and reduce resorption markers, thereby supporting bone metabolism and aiding maintenance of bone health (Rondanelli et al, 2021).

Research: Most available research has evaluated the impact of strenuous exercise on copper status and the ramifications for a variety of body functions important to health and performance; however, many studies are animal based and merely draw conclusions based on purported benefits of increased copper intake through diet or supplementa-tion. One study evaluated the correlation between neutropenia (abnormally low numbers of white blood cells called neutrophils), a marker of immune status, and serum copper levels in an Olympic sailing crew during training for the Beijing Olympic Games. As suspected, the serum copper concentration of sailors with neutropenia was significantly lower than those with normal neutrophil content, leading authors to conclude that low serum copper may be a cause of impaired immune function in elite athletes and that supplementation may be helpful for this population (Lewis et al., 2010). Another study of race dogs determined prolonged run training over 3 days and a 12- to 15-day sled race depressed the blood activities of three copper enzymes with antioxidant qualities: plasma ceruloplasmin, plasma diamine oxidase, and erythrocyte superoxide dismutase. Study investigators concluded this effect could have been prevented by increased copper intake (DiSilvestro, Hinchcliff, & Blostein-Fujii, 2004). Future research needs to focus on the actual impact of copper supplementation on the variables important to human athletic performance in both deficient and nondeficient populations.

Common usage: The current RDA for copper is 0.9 mg, though up to 3 mg may be consumed through whole food or dietary supplementation, generally in multimineral form, to support health. Copper should be taken separately from vitamin C and zinc for optimal absorption. Although the recommended daily intake for copper is met by most North American diets, athletes, especially those who follow a vegetarian diet or who have undergone gastric bypass surgery, are at greater risk for deficiency due to special circumstances that increase daily requirements.

Health concerns: Excessive copper intake, generally defined by levels above the upper safe and adequate daily dietary intake of 1.5 to 3 mg/day for adults, can trigger severe stomach pain, nausea, vomiting, and diarrhea. Copper can be toxic to the body at levels above 10 mg/day.

Cordyceps Sinensis 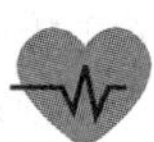 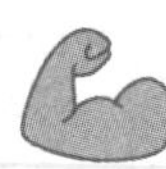  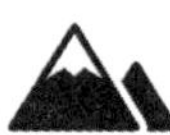

aka *Chinese caterpillar fungus, Dong Chong Xia Cao* (see also *medicinal mushrooms*)

What it is: A wild fungus discovered at high altitude in China, *Cordyceps sinensis* (CS) has long been used in Chinese medicine to protect the lungs from a variety of ailments. Nicknamed "summer plant, winter worm" due to its growth on the larvae of a Lepidoptera moth, a cycle that takes approximately 6 years, CS is an extremely rare find in nature and expensive in its wild form. As a result, CS is generally cultivated. The popularity of the supplement in sports boomed in the early 1990s after a series of records set by Chinese elite distance runners were attributed by their coach to a dietary protocol that included CS during training.

Function: Animal studies have shown CS to increase the ratio of ATP to inorganic phosphate in the liver, allowing for more efficient use of oxygen and a higher tolerance to acidosis, thereby showing potential performance applications for sports that require both aerobic and anaerobic endurance.

Performance benefit: As exertion level increases, so does the demand for oxygen. By improving oxygen usage, CS may help an athlete better respond to these demands, enhancing anaerobic threshold, reducing lactate, and extending time to exhaustion. Animal studies have also shown CS to improve stress-induced physiological changes within the adrenal gland, thymus, and thyroid, thus presenting promise for immune function, resistance to fatigue, and recovery. CS may further help enhance the body's defense against infections and inflammation by stimulating the activity and numbers of several immune markers, including T-helper cells and natural killer cells.

Research: Although animal studies have demonstrated several potential positive applications for athletes, especially those competing in endurance events, the translation to sport performance in human studies has not been consistent. For example, a 2004 double-blind study found no significant differences in $\dot{V}O_2$max, peak power output, blood lactate levels, time to exhaustion, and overall time trial performance between a placebo-fed and a CS-fed group of trained cyclists after 5 weeks of supplementation. Similar results were documented just a year later in a smaller double-blind, placebo-controlled study on trained cyclists (Parcell et al., 2004). However, a 2010 double-blind, placebo-controlled, prospective trial yielded significant improvements in the metabolic and ventilatory performance of active older subjects (ages 50-75) completing a symptom-limited incremental exercise protocol on a cycle ergometer after a supplementation protocol of 333 mg of CS taken 3 times/day for 12 weeks (Chen et al., 2010). Such results are consistent with animal studies demonstrating a higher tolerance to acidosis and resistance to fatigue (Kumar et al., 2011). Some research suggests that potential positive effects of CS may be enhanced when supplemented in conjunction with other plant extracts like *Rhodiola crenulata*, with supplementation of 2,000 mg/day demonstrating a positive effect on physiological stress induced by high-altitude training as well as aerobic performance (Chen et al., 2014). However, the data have been inconsistent, making recommendations for supplemental use as it relates to athletic performance inconclusive.

Common usage: Research-supported doses of CS range from 4.5 to 10 g/day, often split into two to three doses.

Health concerns: Although CS is generally considered safe, there is little known about the safety of long-term use. In the short term, reported side effects include diarrhea, dry mouth, and nausea. Athletes with immune system disorders such as multiple sclerosis, lupus, and rheumatoid arthritis or who are pregnant or breastfeeding are advised against using CS.

Creatine 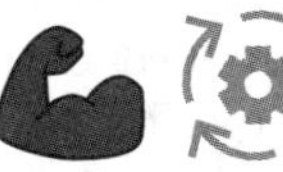  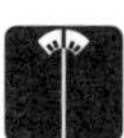 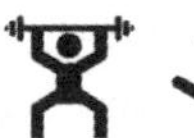 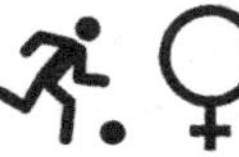 

aka *creatine citrate, creatine ethyl ester, creatine monohydrate, N-(aminoiminomethyl)-N-methylglycine, phosphocreatine*

What it is: Creatine is a naturally occurring nutrient that can be obtained in the diet from meat and fish. It can also be synthesized in the liver and pancreas from the amino acids arginine, glycine, and methionine. Approximately 95% of the body's creatine is stored in muscle, mostly in the form of phosphocreatine. Phosphocreatine and creatine provide a vital reservoir of energy that is used to replenish ATP during high-intensity exercise. In 1992 the London *Times* revealed that Linford Christie, a British sprinter and gold medalist in the Barcelona Olympic Games, used creatine (Rawson & Venezia, 2011); since then creatine has become increasingly popular and to date is among the best-selling dietary supplements on the market.

Function: During high-intensity anaerobic exercise lasting 5 to 15 seconds, muscles rely on stores of phosphocreatine to resynthesize ATP. Once these stores become depleted, the body is forced to rely on other forms of metabolism for ATP, and performance begins to decline. Supplementation with creatine increases stores of phosphocreatine, allowing muscles to work at higher intensities for a longer time. This is extremely beneficial for performance in high-intensity, strength, and power sports that rely heavily on phosphocreatine stores for energy. Interestingly, recent evidence suggests that creatine might have additional health benefits in the treatment of a broad range of diseases, including neurodegenerative disorders, cancer, rheumatic diseases, and type 2 diabetes, in addition to improving cognitive function in older adults (Buford et al., 2007).

Performance benefit: Creatine offers a number of performance benefits. It can produce small but immediate effects on maximum strength and power. This allows athletes to perform more high-intensity work in competition and training, resulting in improved performance and an enhanced training effect.

Research: Scientific research has proven that supplementation with creatine results in 10% to 40% increases in phosphocreatine stores within muscles. Athletes who consume diets low in meat and fish or who are vegetarian typically see the highest increases in phosphocreatine stores. Short-term supplementation has been shown to improve maximal strength and power by 5% to 15%, single-effort sprint performance 1% to 5%, and work performed during multiple sets of maximal strength training or sprinting 5% to 15%. In addition, long-term creatine supplementation can improve the training effect by 5% to 15%, improving gains in strength, power, and lean body mass (Kreider, 2003). A number of forms of creatine exist, including creatine salts (creatine citrate, maleate, fumarate, tartrate, pyruvate), creatine ethyl ester, and Kre-alkalyn. No forms of creatine have been scientifically proven to be more effective than creatine monohydrate. D-pinitol and Russian tarragon (*Artemisia dracunculus*) have been added to creatine supplements to improve effectiveness; however, evidence to support this is inconclusive (Jager et al., 2011). One of two research studies on D-pinitol found low doses to be effective and enhance creatine uptake; however, results from another research trial found no benefits (Greenwood et al., 2001; Kerksick et al., 2009).

Common usage: It is advised that athletes use a loading protocol for the most immediate effect on phosphocreatine stores. This involves consuming 0.3 g/kg of body mass or 0.25 g/kg of fat-free mass for 3 to 5 days followed by a dose of 3 to 5 g/day thereafter. The uptake of creatine within the muscle is best when creatine is consumed in combination with protein and carbohydrate. During the 3- to 5-day loading phase, the total daily dose should be separated into four or five smaller servings consumed throughout the day. Following loading, a 3 to 5 g maintenance dose can be consumed before or after workout. A longer-term strategy of consuming 4 to 6 g/day without a loading phase can also be used; however, the effect is not as immediate (Buford et al., 2007). Typically, phosphocreatine stores remain elevated for 4 to 6 weeks after supplementation stops.

Health concerns: Creatine is considered safe despite early speculation that it negatively affects renal function. This concern was the result of a misunderstanding surrounding creatine's irreversible breakdown product, creatinine, commonly used to assess renal clearance of bloodborne waste. Creatine has also been scrutinized because of a lack of long-term research; however, long-term use has been studied up to 5 years. Despite inducing fluid retention within muscle tissue (not unlike glycogen), creatine does not increase the risk of cramping nor cause dehydration.

Creatine Pyruvate

(see *pyruvate*)

Curcumin  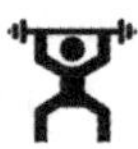  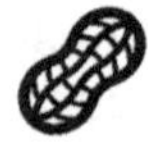

aka *Curcuma longa, turmeric*

What it is: Curcumin is a constituent of *Curcuma longa,* also known as turmeric. Turmeric is cultivated in India and other parts of Southeast Asia, where it is a commonly used spice in Indian dishes such as curry. In addition to its use as a spice, turmeric has been used in Ayurvedic medicine for a wide variety of conditions, most commonly those related to inflammation. Curcumin polyphenols are the active constituents in turmeric.

Turmeric is what gives many dishes their strong yellow color. Note that potentially dangerous yellow chemicals, added to boost the coloration, have been a problem in recent years because the vividness of the color was attractive to consumers.

Function: Curcumin exerts a postexercise anti-inflammatory effect by modulating the proinflammatory cytokines TNF-α, IL-6, and IL-8, and it may also have a slight antioxidant effect. Likewise, curcumin is able to decrease muscle damage through the reduction of muscle creatine kinase (CK) activity (Fernández-Lázaro et al., 2020).

Performance benefit: Athletes commonly use anti-inflammatories to limit inflammation and pain from muscle injury, arthritic joints, or DOMS (delayed-onset muscle soreness) resulting from heavy, intensified training. Curcumin is a promising supplement for athletes looking for an alternative to nonsteroidal anti-inflammatories such as ibuprofen. Curcumin could also be used to lessen muscle soreness and speed recovery following training, thus improving and speeding athletic gains.

Research: Numerous studies related to the use of curcumins as a therapy for cancer, rheumatoid arthritis, and osteoarthritis have been positive (Jurenka, 2009). Animal and human trials have confirmed the anti-inflammatory and antioxidant effects of curcumin. In addition, clinical trials are uncovering the various mechanisms by which curcumin works. Davis and colleagues (2007) were the first to test the impact of curcumin on DOMS produced in rats via a downhill running protocol. Results indicated that curcumin blunts various inflammatory markers, improves muscle recovery, and improves performance in a time trial 48 to 72 hours after induction of DOMS. A double-blind, placebo-controlled trial on a human population discovered that daily supplementation with 1.5 g of curcumin over 4 weeks significantly blunted markers of inflammation, namely CK, and also resulted in decreased muscle soreness following a muscle-damaging exercise protocol (Basham et al., 2020). In 2021 Suhett and colleagues reviewed the available human evidence regarding curcumin supplementation on sport and physical exercise and concluded that most of the existing studies displayed positive effects. Specifically, curcumin is helpful in reducing exercise-induced muscle damage (EIMD) and perceived muscle soreness without negatively affecting the body's natural inflammatory response following exercise. Indeed, a recent systemic review and meta-analysis of randomized control trials concluded that curcumin supplementation, through its role in reducing serum CK levels, shows promise in improving some aspects of DOMS, including muscle damage, muscle soreness, inflammation, muscle strength, and joint flexibility (Fang & Nasir, 2021). However, it is important to note that, though recent studies have shown promise—especially for curcumin's potential effect on EIMD and muscle performance, recovery, better psychological responses, and DOMS—there have been inconsistencies in study protocols and outcomes. This highlights the need for more human trials that replicate supplementation procedures (i.e., doses, type of curcumin) before absolute guidelines for supplement use are set (Oxley & Peart, 2024).

Common usage: Curcumin's acceptable daily intake, as supported by the European Food Safety Authority database, is currently listed at 3 mg/kg. Supplementation doses of clinical trials evaluating curcumin have ranged from a total of 500 to 3,000 mg/day, either taken as a single dose or split into two doses. Timing postexercise curcumin supplementation seems to elicit a more beneficial effect in attenuating muscle soreness (Tanabe et al., 2019). Because the bioavailability of curcumin is poor and variable between subjects, scientists are working to develop strategies to improve bioavailability.

Health concerns: Curcumin is on the FDA's Generally Recognized as Safe (GRAS) list (Sharifi-Rad et al., 2020). However, there is some concern that turmeric or curcumin can cause urinary oxalate levels to rise, resulting in an increased risk of kidney stones. For this reason, keeping turmeric intake below 3 g (1 tsp) daily is advised (Tang et al., 2008).

Cyanocobalamin

(see *vitamin B$_{12}$*)

Dark Chocolate

(see *cocoa*)

Deer Antler (DA)

aka *deer antler extract, deer velvet, elk velvet antler*

What it is: Deer antler (DA) has been used for over 2,000 years in Chinese medicine. It is purported to provide a range of benefits, including enhancement of musculoskeletal and immune function, rapid healing of tissues and bones, and improved vitality (Allen, 2002). Supplement companies claim that DA is a natural source of insulin-like growth factor 1 (IGF1), which is a substance banned by the NFL. DA received extensive media attention in 2013 when Baltimore Ravens All-Pro linebacker Ray Lewis was accused of using DA spray to speed recovery of a torn biceps tendon he suffered early in the season.

Function: DA contains an array of nutritional compounds, including proteins, peptides, and minerals as well as omega-3 fatty acids, glycosaminoglycans, and prostaglandins, which could be responsible for its beneficial effects. More significantly, DA is purported to be a natural source of IGF-1, a powerful anabolic hormone that can promote the building and recovery of muscles and connective tissues. Aside from its impact on muscle and connective tissue, DA has been used in clinical studies to improve treatment of arthritic conditions.

Performance benefit: If DA does contain bioavailable IGF-1 and can increase levels of IGF-1 in the body, it could assist athletes in muscle recovery and regeneration, allowing faster recovery from intense workouts and promoting gains in lean body mass. In addition, DA could benefit athletes with arthritic joints and tendinitis.

Research: More data are needed despite some positive statements found in articles published in journals related to integrative medicine or ethnopharmacology. In a 2003 study by Sleivert and colleagues, no effects on circulating levels of testosterone, IGF-1, or erythropoietin were noted with DA supplementation during 10 weeks of a strength program. Furthermore, no differences in six-repetition maximum strength or $\dot{V}O_2$max were observed. A similar study by Syrotuik and colleagues (2005) that used 10 weeks of DA supplementation also found no significant effects on rowing performance and showed no altered hormonal responses at rest or during exercise. A review of the health benefits of DA concluded that claims for DA are not based on research from human trials (Gilbey & Perezgonzalez, 2012). Currently, there is no evidence to suggest that DA can naturally increase levels of IGF-1, nor does it affect muscular strength, recovery, and growth.

Common usage: DA is sold in spray form as well as in capsules and powder. Doses used in clinical trials range from 430 to 1,300 mg in capsule form (Allen, 2002). Similar doses are suggested when used in spray form.

Health concerns: The safety of DA has been suggested by some clinical human trials as well as animal studies. However, Angers and colleagues (2009) caution that humans who consume DA are at risk for exposure to prion diseases, a set of lethal disorders caused by protease-resistant abnormally shaped proteins. Further, athletes should use caution with supplements that claim to naturally affect anabolic hormones, which could be adulterated with pharmaceutical drugs not listed on product labels.

Dehydroepiandrosterone (DHEA) 

What it is: Dehydroepiandrosterone (DHEA) is an anabolic prohormone or precursor to testosterone. Prohormones became very popular in 1998 when baseball player Mark McGwire admitted to using a supplement called *andro*—an over-the-counter supplement that contained the hormone androstenedione—to help gain muscle mass, strength, and power and subsequently improve his hitting abilities. DHEA is not the same as andro, but is part of a similar biosynthetic pathway.

Function: In men over the age of 30, serum-free testosterone concentrations decline 1.2% each year. Oral supplementation with DHEA is believed to increase the availability of precursors to testosterone and prevent this decline. It is also speculated that young athletes would also experience increases in testosterone. However, there are two significant problems with this thought. First, oral intake and absorption of DHEA must bypass uptake and degradation by the liver. Secondly, DHEA must be converted into either androstenediol or androstenedione, both of which must then be converted into testosterone. In reality, both androstenediol and androstenedione can take a variety of paths that end in the production of testosterone or female sex hormones like estrogen.

Performance benefit: Athletes may benefit through increased testosterone or other androgen production; higher testosterone levels could result in increases in lean body mass, strength, and power.

Research: Oral supplementation of 50 to 100 mg of DHEA raises serum levels of DHEA and DHEA-S (DHEA sulfate) 7-fold and increases androstenedione 4-fold. Chronic supplementation of 50 to 1,600 mg of DHEA appears to affect these weaker androgens, with doses greater than 1,600 mg resulting in greater effects. Unfortunately, acute and chronic supplementation have no impact on testosterone (Brown, Vukovich, & King, 2006). However, estradiol and female sex hormones do increase. This effect is most clear in young adolescent and adult athletes. Research in older individuals and those with abnormally low testosterone levels is less clear, with some studies showing DHEA capable of increasing testosterone and others showing no effect. Brown, Vukovich, and King (2006) studied the effects of 50 mg of DHEA taken 3 times/day on young, untrained weightlifters and concluded DHEA did not improve strength or lean muscle mass. A more recent study found similar results in 19- to 22-year-old soccer players consuming 100 mg/day for 28 days; there were no significant changes in body fat or muscle mass (Ostojic, Calleja, & Jourkesh, 2010).

Common usage: Research studies have used a variety of doses ranging from 50 to 100 mg up to 1,600 mg/day.

Health concerns: Extreme caution should be used when using DHEA and other prohormone supplements. The side effects of supplementing with DHEA are less severe than those of other prohormones like androstenedione, which can cause gynecomastia (enlarged breasts in men), lower HDL cholesterol levels, and negatively affect a person's psychological state. Dietary supplements marketed as natural testosterone boosters often contain prohormones, which are not listed on labels, and purity is a concern.

Delta-Tocopherol, Delta-Tocotrienol

(see *vitamin E*)

Dendrobium

aka *dendrobine, Dendrobium nobile*

What it is: Plants in the orchid family (a large genus containing more than 1,800 species) are common to temperate and tropical parts of Asia. These plants have been used in traditional Chinese medicine for a wide range of effects, including astringent, analgesic, antipyretic, neuroprotectant, and anti-inflammatory, as well as to nourish the stomach and enhance production of body fluids. Today dendrobium, in particular *Dendrobium nobile*, is a component of some preworkout supplements.

Function: According to Cakova and colleagues (2017), the most active constituents are polysaccharides, phenanthrene derivatives, and alkaloids. Dietary supplement purveyors claim stimulant effects.

Performance benefit: As a preworkout stimulant, dendrobium supplements are purported to increase a sense of energy, alertness, and motivation, potentially combined with caffeine or other known stimulants. Benefits are difficult to speculate on, as little human research exists and lawsuits surrounding contamination with known stimulants have occurred.

Research: Human data are sorely lacking.

Common usage: There is no recommended dosage for dendrobium, and proprietary supplement blends can mask any knowledge of a specific dose.

Health concerns: Few data exist in humans, let alone in athletes. According to the Consortium for Health and Military Performance (CHAMP, 2018), "dendrobine taken in sufficient amounts can slow breathing and heart rate and cause an unsafe drop in blood pressure. If dendrobium nobile is part of a proprietary blend, there is no way to tell how much dendrobine is present without laboratory testing. Therefore, dendrobium as a dietary supplement ingredient may pose health risks, including convulsions, seizures, or low blood pressure."

Devil's Claw

aka *grapple plant, Harpagophytum procumbens, wood spider*

What it is: Devil's claw is the common name of *Harpagophytum procumbens,* an herb native to regions in South Africa, Botswana, Zambia, and Zimbabwe. The name *devil's claw* was given to the plant because of its hook-shaped fruit. The roots of the plant are used for medicinal purposes to treat pain, inflammation, and degenerative disorders. Devil's claw contains a variety of phytochemicals and nutrients. Harpagoside and glycoside beta-sitosterol are the major constituents believed to provide the greatest anti-inflammatory effects ("Harpagophytum procumbens [Devil's Claw]," 2008).

Function: Devil's claw inhibits two major inflammatory mechanisms known as lipopolysaccharide-induced nitric oxide and cyclooxygenase-2 (COX-2). Many popular pharmaceutical drugs prescribed as anti-inflammatories and pain relievers inhibit COX-2. In addition, devil's claw is chondroprotective, meaning it protects against the degradation of cartilage (Sanders & Grundmann, 2011).

Performance benefit: Devil's claw is one of a variety of supplements for athletes looking for an alternative to nonsteroidal anti-inflammatories (NSAIDs) such as ibuprofen in the treatment of pain and loss of function in degenerative and arthritic joints. Devil's claw may also aid in protecting joints from the degenerative stresses of sports and training.

Research: Data in the National Library of Medicine regarding devil's claw and sport are very limited. Additionally, many trials are problematic because of smaller sample sizes, short treatment periods, and insufficient quality control. Although more research is needed, early results were somewhat promising. Research trials have examined the effectiveness of devil's claw in relieving symptoms of pain and improving joint function in a variety of conditions such as osteoarthritis, fibromyalgia, and rheumatoid and degenerative joint disorders. Few studies to date have looked at long-term supplementation over 1 year, making the safety of long-term use questionable. A 2004 meta-analysis of 14 studies involving devil's claw determined there was strong evidence for the use of harpagophytum extract at a daily dose of 50 mg of harpagoside (the glucoside constituent responsible for the beneficial effects of devil's claw) for acute, nonspecific, lower back pain (Gagnier et al., 2004). This is somewhat in contrast to a 2006 review of the efficacy of devil's claw, which concluded that "the methodological quality of the existing clinical trials is generally poor, and although they provide some support, there is a considerable number of methodologic caveats that make further clinical investigations warranted" (Brien, Lewith, & McGregor, 2006). Further, Crawford and colleagues (2019) recommended against the use of devil's claw to treat musculoskeletal pain. Additional better-controlled, long-term research trials should be undertaken before definitive conclusions are made.

Common usage: The quality of extract found in many dietary supplements can be a concern and affect usage. Typically, 1,000 to 3,000 mg of devil's claw extract is recommended; however, the harpagoside content is most important, with 50 to 100 mg of harpagoside recommended. A dose of 1,800 to 2,400 mg dried devil's claw root powder contains 50 to 100 mg of harpagoside ("Harpagophytum procumbens [Devil's Claw]," 2008).

Health concerns: Devil's claw should not be used in combination with NSAIDS, anticoagulants such as warfarin, hypoglycemic medications, or antacids. Adverse events involve gastrointestinal complaints. Effects on heart rhythm and force of contraction have also been noted (Sanders & Grundmann, 2011).

Dihydrolipoic Acid

(see *alpha-lipoic acid*)

Dimethylamylamine (DMAA) 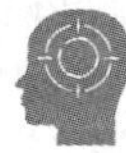

aka *Geranamine (brand name), geranium oil extract, geranium stem, methylhexanamine, 1,3-dimethylamylamine, 1,3-dimethylpentylamine*

What it is: Dimethylamylamine (DMAA) is a pharmaceutical amphetamine derivative originally introduced by Eli Lilly in 1948 as a nasal inhaler. Although it was withdrawn from the pharmaceutical market in the 1980s, it remained commonly recommended as a preworkout enhancer or a so-called fat burner, with sales topping $100 million in 2010, until it was banned by the FDA in 2014. According to current FDA rules and regulations, for DMAA to be sold as a dietary supplement, it must be naturally occurring and have a documented history of use before 1994. Currently, significant controversy exists because a scientific study found that geranium oil contains a small amount of DMAA (0.07%), thereby allowing supplement companies to meet the FDA's criteria with claims that their products contain this ingredient (Cohen, 2012). However, since this study, several others have been unsuccessful in confirming this finding, leading the FDA to conclude that DMAA is not found naturally in geranium oil and thereby disqualifying it as a natural ingredient.

Function: DMAA has strong stimulatory effects on the body. Its exact mechanisms are unknown. Some speculate that DMAA works in a fashion similar to ephedrine and other amphetamines by binding to sympathetic nervous system or adrenal receptors and initiating a strong sympathetic response, thus increasing heart rate, heightening alertness, and increasing force production within the muscles.

Performance benefit: DMAA is believed to improve exercise performance by delaying fatigue and potentially increasing force production. In addition, it may increase resting metabolic rate and lipolysis at rest and during exercise, resulting in improvements in body composition.

Research: Limited scientific data are available related to the effectiveness of DMAA. A 2011 study found DMAA increased systolic and diastolic blood pressure; meanwhile, plasma norepinephrine and epinephrine were relatively unaffected (Bloomer et al., 2011). Use of DMAA has been found to result in serious and life-threatening adverse events (Gee, Jackson, & Easton, 2010).

Common usage: Most supplements list, or listed, DMAA as an ingredient included in a proprietary blend; therefore, the amount of DMAA found in most dietary supplements is unknown.

Health concerns: DMAA has been implicated in a number of serious adverse events, including panic attacks, seizures, and two deaths. It has been described as having toxic effects on animals that were "greater than that of ephedrine and less than that of amphetamine" (Cohen, 2012).

⚠ SUPPLEMENT WARNING

Athletes should avoid using products containing DMAA, which has many health risks and can result in positive drug tests for amphetamines (Vorce et al., 2011). The U.S. military has removed DMAA-containing supplements from all its military exchanges worldwide, and Health Canada has banned DMAA from all supplements (Cohen, 2012). However, it may be listed in the nutrition facts panel under a variety of names, making it difficult to identify in many dietary supplements in the United States. In addition, the FDA has stated that, "There are inadequate safety data and general recognition of safety cannot be established" regarding DMAA as an additive to foods. "Indeed, the available data indicate that the use of DMAA in food is a cause for concern. As such, the use of DMAA in food constitutes use of an unapproved food additive, rendering the product unsafe" (2016).

Dimethylethanolamine (DMAE) 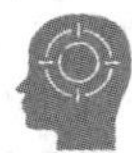

aka *Deanol (brand name), DMAE bitartrate*

What it is: Once a pediatric drug for behavioral and motor issues, dimethylethanolamine (DMAE) is now a dietary supplement. It is a colorless viscous liquid used in skin care products and also taken orally as a potential nootropic (cognition enhancer).

Function: One mechanism by which it purportedly exerts effects is by increasing production of the neurotransmitter acetylcholine (ACh). It also has antioxidant effects.

Performance benefit: Based on anecdotal reports among nonathletes, DMAE may enhance mood and memory, which could play a role in cognitive aspects of sport; however, data are lacking.

Research: Data collection that was underway during the time DMAE was sold as the drug Deanol was ultimately discontinued. Additionally, little research has been done with athletes.

Common usage: Dietary supplements are sold with a wide range of doses from 50 mg to perhaps 600 mg. 250 mg is probably most common.

Health concerns: Because DMAE may affect ACh in the brain, persons taking acetylcholinesterase inhibitors or anticholinergics should avoid it and discuss their interest with their physician. There are also lay reports of drowsiness, muscle tension or twitching, and confusion (which seems contrary to the hope for nootropic effects). Clinical research is needed to clarify.

Dimethyl Sulfone

(see *methylsulfonylmethane*)

D-Leucine

(see *leucine*)

Docosahexaenoic Acid (DHA)

(see *omega-3 fatty acids*)

Dong Chong Xia Cao

(see *Cordyceps sinensis*)

D-Ribose

(see *ribose*)

Ecdisten, Ecdysone

(see *ecdysteroids*)

Ecdysteroids 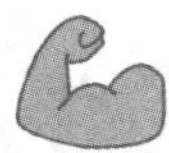 

aka *beta-ecdysterone, β-ecdysterone, Ecdisten (brand name), ecdysone, ecdysterone, isoinokosterone, 20-beta-hydroxyecdysterone, 20-hydroxyecdysone (20-HE)*

What it is: There are three classes of steroid hormones: The vertebrate steroid hormones (androgens, estrogens, progestogens, etc.); brassinolides, growth-promoting hormones found in plants; and ecdysteroids, found in insects and plants (Bathori et al., 2008).

Thus far nearly 300 ecdysteroids have been discovered; 20-hydroxyecdysone (20-HE) is the main biologically significant ecdysteroid found in insects and is also one of the most common plant-derived ecdysteroids (Bathori et al., 2008). Spinach, quinoa, and chestnuts are noted to contain considerable amounts of ecdysteroids such as 20-HE (Bathori et al., 2008; Gorelick-Feldman et al., 2008).

Function: Ecdysteroids are believed by some to produce anabolic and cholesterol-lowering effects. In addition, they may stimulate and strengthen the immune system and allow individuals to better adapt to various stresses placed on the body. Within this proposed framework, ecdysteroids promote vitality and increase resistance to stress. The mechanisms are somewhat unknown. Unlike androgens, which act on androgen receptors and initiate a response, ecdysteroids behave differently because specific receptors do not exist. However, various nonreceptor-induced signaling pathways have been implicated as potential mechanisms (Bathori et al., 2008), and more recently, there is some suggestion in the literature that effects may be mediated by estrogen receptor binding (Isenmann et al., 2019).

Performance benefit: If the claims about ecdysteroids are true, athletes would benefit from the anabolic and adaptogenic effects. Similar to anabolic steroids, ecdysteroids could promote gains in lean body mass, increasing muscle size, strength, power, and performance. The adaptogenic effects of ecdysteroids would allow athletes to adapt to the stresses of training and potentially handle higher volumes and intensities, inducing adaptation and improved performance over time.

Research: Early studies on mice in the 1960s and 1970s found that ecdysteroids promoted protein synthesis (Otaka, Okui, & Uchiyama, 1976), and more recent studies have produced similar results (Gorelick-Feldman et al., 2008; Gorelick-Feldman, Cohick, & Raskin, 2010; Toth et al., 2008). A 2009 study found 20-HE is capable of improving insulin resistance and decreasing weight and body fat gain in diet-induced obese mice (Kizelsztein et al.). From a very broad perspective, Eastern European, Russian and Asian researchers appear to have greater interest than U.S. researchers in this area of study. Historically, research conducted on humans is relatively weak. Wilborn and colleagues conducted a study in 2006 looking into the effects of three supplements often marketed as natural alternatives to steroids including 20-HE, on 45 resistance-trained men who supplemented for 8 weeks while lifting 4 days/week. No beneficial effects on changes in lean body mass, levels of anabolic hormones, or improvements in strength and power were observed. Other proposed benefits of ecdysteroids, such as promoting adaptogenic effects during training, are unstudied and speculative at this time.

Common usage: One of the few human trials used 200 mg/day of 20-HE (Wilborn et al., 2006). Mice models typically use 5 to 10 mg/kg of ecdysteroids or 20-HE (Bathori et al., 2008).

Health concerns: Ecdysteroids have low acute toxicity at doses of 6 to 9 g/kg in mice; 2 g/kg in rabbits resulted in no toxic symptoms (Kizelsztein et al., 2009). The common consumption of vegetables with high ecdysteroid content is further evidence of safety.

⚠ SUPPLEMENT WARNING

Maral root, a perennial herb originating in the mountains of southern Siberia (also known as *Leuzea carthamoides, Rhaponticum carthamoides, Russian leuzea)*, was first observed as a medicinal plant when native hunters noticed that maral deer appeared to renew their strength after eating its roots. The plant is now grown in

Ecdysteroids

central and eastern Europe. In traditional Siberian medicine it is used to restore strength after illness and prevent overtraining; Soviet and Russian athletes have also used maral root as an ergogenic aid to assist in handling the physical and psychological stress of intense training (Kokoska & Janovska, 2009). Maral root contains a variety of potentially beneficial compounds, such as 20-hydroxyecdysone (20-HE), believed by some to have anabolic properties. In addition to ecdysteroids, various sterols such as beta-sitosterol, flavonoids or anthocyanins, and triterpenoid glycosides can provide potential health benefits, such as stimulating and supporting the immune system, preventing free radical damage, increasing protein synthesis, improving work capacity, and supporting cognitive function. Maral root is also believed to enhance performance during aerobic endurance events and prolonged, intermittent, high-intensity team sports

Some animal studies have found ecdysteroids derived from maral root can promote growth, increase fat-free mass, and in some cases decrease fat mass (Slama et al., 1996; Stopka, Stancl, & Slama, 1999). Other animal trials in mice have shown an increase in work capacity running on treadmills and in swimming endurance protocols (Azizov & Seifulla, 1998). Scientists note that significant differences are small in these studies, and small sample sizes limit the quality of results (Kokoska & Janovska, 2009).

Although some early studies were promising, there is a lack of current scientific evidence to conclude that maral root or its ecdysteroid components are beneficial for athletic performance. It should be noted that one modern Bulgarian study suggested a potential for antiadipogenic effects, which the authors (Todorova et al., 2024) suggested warrant further research. Whether this would result in clinically meaningful fat reductions over time in athletes remains unknown.

Echinacea 

aka *coneflower, Echinacea angustifolia, Echinacea pallida, Echinacea purpurea*

What it is: Also known as coneflower, echinacea is an herbal remedy prepared from both the stems and leaves of the plant and often used to ward off the common cold, flu, and other infections. Although several species of echinacea exist, the three types commercially available include *Echinacea angustifolia* (narrow-leaved coneflower), *Echinacea pallida* (pale coneflower), and *Echinacea purpurea* (purple coneflower).

Function: The physical stress associated with training and competition can suppress an athlete's immune function, increasing risk for infection. Antibodies known as immunoglobulins are critical to an athlete's immune defense against bacterial and viral infection; however, following periods of intense training, decreases in these antibodies have been reported along with increased incidence of upper respiratory infection. Echinacea contains several bioactive compounds—including alkamides, caffeic acid, and polysaccharides—that may help bolster an athlete's immune function by increasing the number and activity of antibodies as well as white blood cells and natural killer cells (Veldman et al., 2023). A new compound found within echinacea, echinalkamide, has been shown to improve bone regeneration, which has generated some interest for the purpose of osteoporosis prevention and treatment (Li et al., 2013). This may be of particular interest to postmenopausal women, who are at greater risk for bone loss.

Performance benefit: Athletes may benefit from less frequent and less severe upper respiratory infections throughout their competitive season.

Research: Although animal trials have demonstrated favorable immune responses through exposure to echinacea, applications to humans are less conclusive, with mixed results reported in healthy populations. For example, one large study of 755 healthy subjects found supplementation of an alcohol extract from freshly harvested *E. purpurea* (95% herb, 5% root) over a period of 4 months to reduce the total number and duration of cold episodes and protect against viral infections with maximal effects occurring on recurrent infections compared to the placebo (Jawad et al., 2012). Yet, according to a second large-scale study (713 subjects), a placebo effect may contribute to results. Study investigators evaluated whether the severity and duration of illness caused by the common cold are influenced by randomized assignment to open-label echinacea pills (root extracts of *Echinacea purpurea* and *angustifolia*) compared to conventional double-blind allocation to active and placebo pills and compared to no pills at all during a 5-day span. Although participants randomized to the no-pill group tended to have longer and more severe illnesses than those who received pills, the differences were not significant. There were also no significant differences between groups in a couple of key markers of immune function. For the subgroup that received pills and believed in the purported role of echinacea in immune function, illnesses were substantively shorter and less severe. This was the case regardless of whether the pills contained echinacea, confirming a placebo effect was indeed present (Barrett et al., 2011). Two systematic reviews also found limited to no evidence for echinacea preparations reducing cough as a symptom of upper respiratory infection or for treating and preventing the common cold compared to a placebo (Karsch-Völk et al., 2014; Wagner et al., 2015), making additional research on a healthy human population, including athletes, warranted before conclusive recommendations for use can be made.

Common usage: The stems and leaves of the echinacea plant are used fresh or dried to make teas, juices, extracts, tablets, and capsules. Research-supported doses are based on the type of preparation used: capsule 300 mg, dried root (or tea) 1,000 to 2,000 mg, freeze-dried plant 325 to 650 mg, juice 2 to 3 mL, tincture 3 to 5 mL, fluid extract 1 to 2 mL. Prescribed doses can be taken 3 times/day over a heavy training block or every 2 hours for 24 hours with the onset of cold-like symptoms.

SUPPLEMENT FACT

Echinacea loses its effectiveness with long-term use and thus should only be used cyclically throughout a season. For example, an athlete may use echinacea during a particularly hard 3-week training block and then cycle off during a recovery period or merely use echinacea throughout the duration of an infection.

Health concerns: Echinacea seems to be well tolerated by most people, though clinical trials have demonstrated gastrointestinal symptoms at doses above 2 g/day. Allergic reactions have been reported in those with allergies to plants within the daisy family, such as ragweed and marigold.

Egg Protein 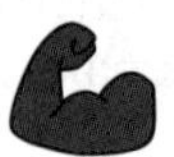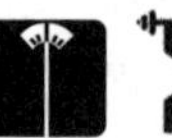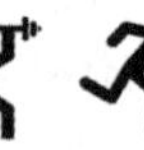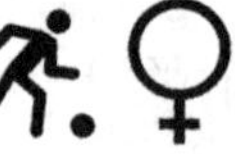

aka *albumin*

What it is: Eggs have long been known as a high-quality source of protein. Eggs are considered a complete protein, meaning they contain all of the essential amino acids.

Because of its high biological value, PDCAAS, and DIAAS (Protein Digestibility-Corrected Amino Acid Score and Digestible Indispensable Amino Acid Score, respectively), eggs are commonly used as the source of protein in powders and supplements.

Function: Egg proteins provide important amino acids that are used by the body as building blocks for the synthesis of new proteins, including muscle. These amino acids can also signal or turn on protein-building pathways in the body. Exercise and training push muscles to their performance limits, inducing damage and the breakdown of proteins within muscle. Supplying dietary protein throughout the day and in relation to workouts and training can help prevent damage during training and stimulate restoration of muscle. All protein sources are unique in the various combinations and amounts of amino acids they contain. Eggs could contain a superior combination of these amino acids, making them more effective for athletes than other protein sources.

Performance benefit: Eggs provide a valuable, high-quality protein source for athletes that assists in preventing muscle breakdown, maintaining lean body mass, stimulating the recovery of damaged muscle, and building new muscle.

Research: Egg protein is recognized as highly digestible and an excellent source of essential amino acids, with the highest attainable PDCAAS (Puglisi and Fernandez, 2022). In their review, Puglisi and Fernandez state that

> Research specifically assessing the effects of eggs on muscle protein synthesis is limited, but evidence from the field pointing to the importance of protein quality and data from Moore, et al. (2009) assessing muscle protein synthesis with egg consumption is promising. These authors provided 0, 5, 10, 20, and 40 g of whole egg protein to healthy young men after leg resistance exercise training on five separate occasions. Researchers found that 20 g of egg protein was sufficient for maximizing muscle protein synthesis, in line with the findings from Witard et al. (2014) that 20 g of whey protein also optimally stimulated muscle protein synthesis (*ibid*).

Studies comparing the consumption of protein sources before and after exercise tend to conclude that the fast-digesting properties of whey protein make it the best and quickest source of high-quality amino acids before, during, and after exercise. However, egg proteins tend to rank a close second. It should also be noted that although egg protein powders and supplements can provide an excellent source of amino acids, they lack many natural vitamins, minerals, phospholipids, and lipids found in whole eggs.

Common usage: Protein needs are based on body weight. A common recommendation is that 1.2 to 2 g of protein/kg is sufficient for nearly all athletes. Although many athletes exceed these recommendations, excessive protein consumption could interfere with the intake of other nutrients as they are crowded out by satiating protein foods or supplements, as noted below. Timing the consumption of protein before, during, and after exercise is also beneficial. The amount of per-dose protein needed for maximal benefits is roughly 20 to 40 g (Jager et al., 2017).

Health concerns: According to the ISSN position stand on dietary protein (Jager et al., 2017), the consumption of whole eggs has been criticized due to their cholesterol content. However, a growing body of evidence demonstrates the lack of a relationship between egg consumption and coronary heart disease, which is linked to high levels of LDL cholesterol in the blood. Further, this position paper points out that eggs are an example of a functional food, supplying physiologically active components and thereby providing a health benefit beyond basic nutrition. High-protein diets do not appear to pose any health concerns; however, athletes must understand that excessive intakes of protein could result in underconsumption of other important nutrients such as carbohydrate, healthy fat, and nutrient-dense fruits and vegetables.

Eicosapentaenoic Acid (EPA)

(see *omega-3 fatty acids*)

Elderberry  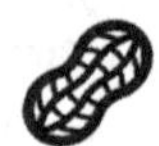

aka *elder, elder flower, Sambucus nigra*

What it is: A large shrub native to Europe, Africa, and parts of Asia, elderberry's bark, leaves, flowers, and berries have long been used for medicinal purposes in many European and Middle Eastern cultures and have more recently garnered attention in athletics for its immune-strengthening and antioxidant properties. Though several species of elder exist, European elder, also known as black elder or *Sambucus nigra*, is the most commonly used.

Function: The fruit, or more specifically the berry, of the elderberry plant is an excellent source of vitamins A and C as well as several plant compounds, including phenolic acids, flavonoids, catechins, anthocyanins, and proanthocyanidins that are thought to contribute to its therapeutic properties (Barros et al., 2012). Dietary flavonoids, in particular, carry antioxidant properties that may help offset some of the oxidative damage to cells, including those important to immune function, that occur during heavy training cycles. Additionally, animal models have shown elderberry to increase the number and activity of several key immune compounds as well as help initiate phagocytosis, which helps rid the body of harmful foreign particles, bacteria, and dead or dying cells that could otherwise sideline an athlete with infections such as the flu.

Performance benefit: Athletes may benefit from enhanced immune function, allowing them to rebound faster from illness during training and competition. There is also emerging evidence that the high polyphenol content and antioxidant capacity of black elderberry may enhance exercise performance as a result of lower oxidative stress and augmented nitric oxide production, with subsequent improvements in vascular function and skeletal muscle perfusion and metabolism (Kashi et al., 2019).

Research: Few human studies have been conducted to be able to confirm the efficacy of supplemental use in athletes. However, two double-blind, randomized, placebo-controlled studies demonstrate some promise. In the first study, elderberry extract (Sambucol) was given to adult patients in a daily dose of 60 mL (4 tbsp) within the first 48 hours after the onset of flu-like symptoms. These patients were able to recover significantly faster than the control group receiving the placebo. Over 93% of patients receiving the elderberry reported cessation of symptoms after only 2 days of treatment; the placebo group failed to report improvement until day 6. Furthermore, although serum samples analyzing various antibodies did not reveal a significant difference, the trend was in favor of the treatment group. The second study revealed similar results with a treatment protocol that incorporated 15 mL (1 tbsp) of elderberry extract (Sambucol) taken 4 times/day over 5 days; following this protocol essentially cut the duration of flu-like symptoms in half compared to a placebo (Zakay-Rones et al., 1995, 2004). Conclusions from a systemic review of five randomized control human trials revealed that while elderberry failed to prevent the onset of the common cold or flu, it did seem to reduce the severity and duration as well as adverse outcomes associated with infection (Wieland et al., 2021). Though these results suggest elderberry may be helpful in enhancing recovery from the flu—extremely helpful for an athlete who can't afford to be sidelined in the midst of a busy training and competition schedule—additional studies are warranted before definite guidelines for use can be implemented.

Common usage: Elderberry is available dried (tea); as a liquid, syrup, wine, extract, and tincture; and in capsule and lozenge forms. In the limited human research available, elderberry extract at a dose of 15 mL (1 tbsp) taken 4 times/day upon first onset of flu-like symptoms may be effective in reducing the duration of the flu. As an alternative, 3 to 5 g of dried elderflower, standardized to at least 0.8% flavonoids, can be prepared as a tea and consumed 3 times/day.

Health concerns: Although elderberry appears to be safe when used in recommended doses short term (up to 5 days), certain species such as *Sambucus ebulus* consumed uncooked can cause symptoms that resemble cyanide poisoning, including diarrhea, vomiting, vertigo, numbness, and stupor.

Elemental Iron

(see *iron*)

Elk Velvet Antler

(see *deer antler*)

Enterococcus

(see *probiotics*)

Epimedium, *Epimedium Grandiflorum*

(see *horny goat weed*)

Escherichia

(see *probiotics*)

Euterpe Oleracea

(see *acai berry*)

Evening Primrose Oil

(see *gamma-linolenic acid*)

Evodia Fruit, Evodiamine, *Evodia Rutaecarpa*

(see *rutaecarpine*)

Fenugreek 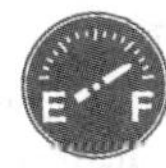 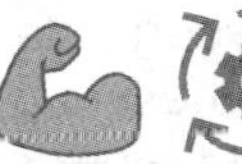 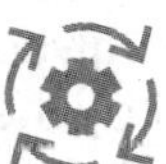 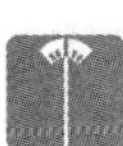 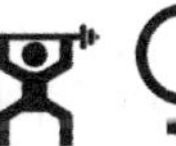  

aka *goat's horn, Trigonella foenum-graecum*

What it is: A white-flowered herbal plant from the pea family, fenugreek leaves and seeds are commonly used to flavor dishes, especially Indian curry dishes. Nearly 175 potentially health-promoting compounds have been identified in fenugreek seeds alone, including such active constituents as alkaloids, flavonoids, steroids and saponins (Shashikumar et al., 2018).

Function: Evidence from animal studies suggests that fenugreek may lead to a favorable metabolic response during exercise: Reliance on fatty acids, rather than glucose, to fuel activity is enhanced, helping to spare limited muscle glycogen stores and delay the onset of fatigue associated with depletion (hitting the wall). Additionally, fenugreek seems to help promote glycogen repletion, which is essential for optimal postworkout recovery. Of further ergogenic benefit, fenugreek is rich in antioxidant compounds known as flavonoids and polyphenols. Fenugreek has also been shown to display pharmacological effects, namely increases in free estrogen and testosterone levels in females and testosterone levels in males, which may have benefits related to muscle strength and body composition (Rao et al., 2016; Steels et al., 2017).

Performance benefit: Endurance-trained athletes may benefit from delayed onset of fatigue during training and competition as well as enhanced recovery. Strength-trained athletes may benefit from body composition alteration and increases in muscle strength and endurance. Of special note to master athletes, there is some evidence that supplementation with an extract of fenugreek may help improve pre- and postmenopausal symptoms and improve sexual function of healthy aging women (Steels et al., 2017). In addition, there is some evidence that it also reduces age-related symptoms of androgen decrease, increases testosterone levels, and improves sexual function in healthy aging males (Rao et al., 2016).

SUPPLEMENT FACT

Fenugreek seeds contain an amino acid called 4-hydroxyisoleucine that is commonly extracted and used to lower blood sugar in people with diabetes. In addition, some studies suggest it may help lower body fat through its role in insulin promotion and blood sugar regulation.

Research: Studies evaluating the impact of fenugreek on performance parameters in a trained population are limited. One human trial with trained cyclists found administration of 1.8 g/kg of dextrose in combination with 2.0 mg/kg of 4-hydroxyisoleucine from fenugreek seeds immediately and 2 hours after completion of a 90-minute exhaustive cycling exercise protocol enhanced the rate of glycogen repletion by 63% as compared to the placebo group, supporting the potential benefit of fenugreek for recovery (Ruby et al., 2005). However, another human study of similar double-blind design failed to replicate these results. In that study, the same dose of dextrose and 4-hydroxyisoleucine was administered immediately and 2 hours after cycling 5 hours at 50% peak cycling power. In addition, a standardized meal with or without fenugreek was consumed 4 hours after cycling for 5 hours at 50% peak cycling power and before concluding with a 40 km cycling time trial (Slivka et al., 2008). Contrary to previous studies, there was no difference between groups in muscle glycogen levels at any point during the study, nor was performance gain experienced by the fenugreek group during the 40 km time trial. It is evident more research is needed before conclusions can be drawn on the performance attributes of fenugreek related to fuel usage, endurance capacity, and recovery in endurance-trained athletes. However, there is emerging evidence demonstrating fenugreek's potential for body composition alterations as well as improved muscle strength and endurance in resistance-trained athletes. A recent meta-analysis of four randomized control trials found fenugreek supplementation to significantly improve muscle strength, repetitions to failure (muscle endurance), and submaximal performance index as well as lead to improvements in body composition parameters (Albaker et al., 2023). One trial reported that a fenugreek extract at a dose of 500 mg taken over 8 weeks of resistance training not only had a positive impact on upper and lower body strength but also showed a significant improvement in lean body mass and body fat reduction compared to the placebo group without any reported side effects (Poole et al., 2010).

Another trial evaluated found a dose of 900 mg of fenugreek extract in combination with 3.5 g of creatine taken over 8 weeks along with a structured resistance-training program significantly improved muscle strength (repetition maximum) for bench press and leg press and demonstrated similar results to supplementation with creatine (5 g) plus dextrose (70 g) in a group of resistance-trained males. Similarly, 300 mg of fenugreek seeds (*Trigonella foenum-graecum*) taken 2 times/day over 8 weeks of resistance training (4 sessions/week) yielded more substantial anabolic and androgenic activity as well as significantly more repetitions to failure (muscle endurance) and favorable body composition changes without negative impacts on muscle strength and without reported side effects compared to the placebo group (Wankhede et al., 2016). All the trials reported in Albaker and colleagues' (2023) meta-analysis were specific to resistance-trained male subjects, but Rao and colleagues (2023) discovered that females aged 25 to 45 following a supplementation protocol consisting of 600 mg of a fenugreek extract over 8 weeks of resistance training experienced significant improvements in lean body mass as well as decreases in body fat and increased repetition max (leg press) compared to the placebo group, indicating that benefits seem to span genders.

Common usage: The seeds and leaves of fenugreek are commonly formulated in powder and extract when used for medicinal and supplemental purposes (Poole et al., 2010). Fenugreek is available as seed powder capsules, teas, and pulverized seeds that can be mixed in water. The appropriate dose of fenugreek for athletes is still unclear, although dose recommendations appear to be weight dependent. A dose of 2 mg/kg of 4-hydroxyisoleucine (an active ingredient isolated from fenugreek seeds) has been administered to endurance-trained athletes to yield a performance benefit (Ruby et al., 2005). In strength-trained athletes, the doses of fenugreek extract used in favorable trials ranged from 500 to 900 mg/day taken over 8 weeks of resistance training.

Health concerns: Fenugreek is considered safe and well tolerated by most, although athletes sensitive to curry should be cautious as allergic symptoms (e.g., bronchospasm, wheezing, and diarrhea) have been reported. Additionally, because the leaves and seeds of fenugreek are rich in dietary fiber, consumption may initiate gastrointestinal disturbances such as diarrhea and gas. Thus, precompetition use is not recommended. Fenugreek may alter the color and smell of urine, a side effect that is not considered harmful to health.

Ferrous Bisglycinate, Ferrous Carbonate Anhydrous, *Ferrous Fumarate,* Ferrous Gluconate, Ferrous Pyrophosphate, Ferrous Sulfate

(see *iron*)

Fiber 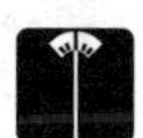 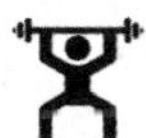 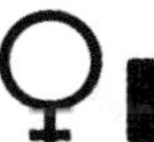 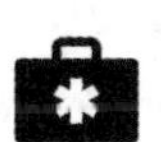 

What it is: Fiber is a type of carbohydrate commonly found in plants that resist digestion and absorption in the small intestine. Many types of fiber exist; however, they have historically been classified into two categories: soluble and insoluble. Soluble fiber is soluble in water and includes pectin, gum, beta-glucan, psyllium, inulin, and mucilage. Insoluble fiber is not soluble in water and includes cellulose, hemicellulose, and lignin. However, due to the complexities of other functional qualities such as fermentation, viscosity, bulking, and the ability to affect the adsorption of other compounds, the FDA has now largely moved beyond this simple classification. Although soluble and insoluble fiber share many physical properties, including water-binding capacity and capacity to bind mineral cations, their fermentability can vary according to the physicochemical properties of each compound (Williams et al., 2019).

The FDA's definition for dietary fiber that can be declared on the Nutrition and Supplement Facts label includes "non-digestible soluble and insoluble carbohydrates (with 3 or more monomeric units), and lignin that are intrinsic and intact in plants; isolated or synthetic non-digestible carbohydrates (with 3 or more monomeric units) determined by FDA to have physiological effects that are beneficial to human health" (FDA, updated 2024). The term "beneficial to human health" includes the following effects:

- Lowering blood glucose
- Lowering cholesterol levels
- Lowering blood pressure
- Increasing frequency of bowel movements (improved laxation)
- Increasing mineral absorption in the intestinal tract
- Reducing energy intake (e.g., due to the fiber promoting a feeling of fullness).

In addition to intact and intrinsic fiber, the FDA has identified the following synthetic and isolated nondigestible carbohydrates as meeting the dietary fiber definition:

- Beta-glucan soluble fiber
- Psyllium husk
- Cellulose
- Guar gum
- Pectin
- Locust bean gum
- Hydroxypropyl methylcellulose (HPMC)

For practical purposes, these additional nondigestible fibers have been added:

- Mixed plant cell wall fibers (a broad category that includes fibers like sugar cane fiber and apple fiber, among many others)
- Arabinoxylan
- Alginate
- Inulin and inulin-type fructans
- High amylose starch (resistant starch 2)
- Galactooligosaccharide
- Polydextrose
- Resistant maltodextrin/dextrin
- Cross linked phosphorylated RS4
- Glucomannan
- Acacia (gum arabic)

For more common questions on the most recent dietary fiber definitions and benefits, see: https://www.fda.gov/food/food-labeling-nutrition/questions-and-answers-dietary-fiber; updated 2021.

Current recommendations suggest 14 g of fiber/1,000 kcal be consumed daily. For the average women consuming 2,000 kcal/day, this is equivalent to 28 g of fiber; for the average male consuming 2,600 kcal/day, this is equivalent to 36 g of fiber/day (Anderson et al., 2009). These recommendations will be even higher for athletes whose caloric demands are much higher.

Unfortunately, the average American intake for fiber is less than half the recommended amount. Fruits, vegetables, and whole grain foods are all excellent natural sources of fiber (Papathanasopoulos & Camilleri, 2010), and fiber supplements have recently become popular as a means to meet recommendations for those whose diets are low in fiber.

Although there are a variety of types of fiber supplements available on the market, soluble fiber supplements are generally suggested. Psyllium and beta-glucans are the only two types of fiber with FDA approval as cholesterol-lowering agents (Anderson et al., 2009), with psyllium the most common type of fiber used in research trials. Inulin is another fiber found in foods and supplements; it is a better prebiotic fiber for promoting the growth of bacteria in the GI tract, but less specific research has been done on inulin relative to blood cholesterol and weight-loss effects. More research is needed on fiber and the advantages of specific fiber for targeted health benefits.

Function: Fiber is proven to provide a number of health benefits. Fiber reduces the risk of coronary heart disease, stroke, hypertension, diabetes, obesity, and certain gastrointestinal diseases (Anderson et al., 2009). Increasing fiber intake will lower cholesterol and blood pressure. Soluble fiber has been shown to improve glycemic control and insulin sensitivity in both nondiabetics and diabetics, and fiber supplementation in obese individuals significantly enhances weight loss. The prevention of weight gain and assistance in weight loss is often attributed to fiber's ability to increase satiety and stabilize blood glucose levels. Finally, fiber is a prebiotic and provides nutrients to support the growth of healthy bacteria in the GI tract. Creating a beneficial environment for growth of these bacteria will strengthen and bolster the immune system.

Performance benefit: Athletes might benefit from the potential weight-loss and weight-management benefits of fiber, especially those needing to maintain a lower body weight and leaner body composition. In addition, athletes could benefit from the immune-enhancing benefits of soluble fiber.

Research: Animal experiments, epidemiological studies (those identifying trends within population groups), and clinical trials provide support for high-fiber diets to help prevent weight gain (Papathanasopoulos & Camilleri, 2010). A recent assessment of five clinical research trials found high-fiber diets to improve weight loss by approximately 2.2 lbs (1 kg) over an 8-week period (Anderson et al., 2009). Fiber improves insulin sensitivity and satiety and supports the growth of healthy bacteria in the GI tract. It is clear that adequate intake of fiber is essential for optimal health of both athletes and nonathletes.

Common usage: The amount of fiber needed is relative to fiber intake from food. Typically, 5 to 20 g of fiber is supplemented at smaller doses before meals. Again, a total fiber intake of 14 g/1,000 kcal consumed is recommended. For an athlete burning 3,500 kcal/day, this is equivalent to 49 g of fiber/day. Diets high in fruits, vegetables, and whole grains naturally provide sufficient amounts of fiber.

Health concerns: It is recommended that fiber intake not exceed 60 to 70 g/day.

5-Diamino-5-Oxopentanoic Acid
(see *glutamine*)

5-Hydroxytryptophan (5-HTP)  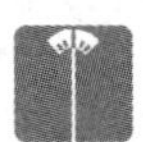

What it is: 5-hydroxytryptophan (5-HTP) is an aromatic amino acid naturally produced in the body from tryptophan. It is extracted from the seeds of the African plant *Griffonia simplicifolia*.

Function: The amino acid tryptophan is converted to 5-HTP before being converted to serotonin, an important neurotransmitter produced in the body that contributes to the regulation of mood, appetite, sleep, memory, and learning. This is why foods such as turkey that contain high amounts of tryptophan may induce sleepiness.

Performance benefit: For athletes, supplementation with 5-HTP may increase levels of serotonin, thereby improving sleep and recovery.

Research: Animal studies and human trials suggest that 5-HTP supplementation can increase serotonin levels (Birdsall, 1998), although no studies have looked specifically into the effects of 5-HTP on recovery in athletes. Most research has focused on the impact that increasing serotonin levels might have on depression. A review article by Turner, Loftis, and Blackwell (2006) noted that of 11 double-blind, placebo-controlled studies, 7 showed 5-HTP to be more effective than a placebo in treating depression. Research studies related to sleep have found 5-HTP supplementation to significantly increase the amount of non-REM sleep (Morrow et al., 2008); however, no known studies have evaluated whether this impact on sleep improves recovery for athletes. Interestingly, Evans and colleagues (2023) concluded that daily supplementation with 100 mg of 5-HTP over 8 weeks ($n = 48$) may affect some aspects of body composition (less fat mass) in exercise-trained men and women.

Common usage: When used for insomnia or to enhance sleep, a dose of 100 to 300 mg of 5-HTP before bedtime is recommended. When used to treat depression, 50 mg of 5-HTP taken 3 times/day has been suggested. If an effective response is not produced after 2 weeks, an increased dosage of 100 mg 3 times/day can be taken. Such self-treatment should be discussed with a health care professional such as a physician or behavioral therapist.

Health concerns: Caution is necessary when taking 5-HTP in combination with selective serotonin reuptake inhibitor (SSRI) antidepressants such as fluoxetine (Prozac), paroxetine (Paxil), sertraline (Zoloft), or fluvoxamine (Luvox) or monoamine oxidase inhibitor (MAOI) antidepressants such as phenelzine (Nardil) or tranylcypromine (Parnate). 5-HTP in combination with these drugs may lead to serotonin syndrome, characterized by agitation, confusion, delirium, and tachycardia. There are no adequate studies related to use of 5-HTP during pregnancy (Birdsall, 1998).

5,7-Dihydroxyflavone
(see *chrysin*)

Flaxseed 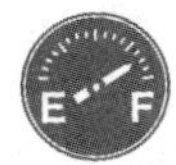

aka *flax oil, Linum usitatissimum, linseed oil*

What it is: Consisting of one-third oil and two-thirds fiber, flaxseed, whose scientific name *Linum usitatissimum* appropriately means "most useful," packs quite the nutritional punch. Its oil is a rich source of essential fatty acids (EFAs), especially alpha-linolenic (ALA) omega-3 fatty acid, and the fibrous byproduct of the seed is chock-full of vitamins and minerals as well as a group of chemical compounds called lignans. Flaxseed mucilage, found on the outermost layer of the seed's hull, consists mainly of water-soluble polysaccharide and makes up about 3% to 8% of the seed weight. These compounds are thought to have health benefits through their anti-inflammatory action, antioxidative capacity, and lipid-modulating properties (Parikh et al., 2019).

Function: EFAs, especially the omega-3s found in flaxseed oil, are needed for the synthesis of powerful hormones called prostaglandins, which help regulate several aspects of metabolism. EFAs appear to enhance the burning of excess fat to produce heat, a process known as thermogenesis, which may help produce fat loss and favorable changes in body composition. Soluble fibers from flaxseed mucilage increase the viscosity of intestinal contents, prolong absorption rate of nutrients (e.g., glucose), delay gastric emptying, decrease fat digestibility, and lower blood glucose level.

Performance benefit: For athletes, flaxseeds are most recognized for their apparent ability to enhance fat metabolism and promote favorable body composition changes. Of special interest to athletes who suffer from constipation or irritable bowel syndrome (IBS), flax mucilage, one of the key components of flaxseed, has prebiotic qualities that help bulk up the stools and regulate the beneficial composition of microbes in the gut that alleviate the symptoms of constipation and IBS (Dzuvor et al., 2018).

Research: Flaxseed is a promising candidate for the management of metabolic syndrome to control blood lipid levels, fasting blood sugar, insulin resistance, body weight, waist circumference, body mass, and blood pressure (Shayan et al., 2020). Results from a 2022 double-blind, randomized study concluded that flaxseed mucilage is an effective supplement for weight and body fat loss. In this study, both a high daily intake (5,120 mg) and low daily intake (2,560 mg) of flaxseed mucilage led to significantly greater body weight reduction after 12 weeks compared to the placebo group (Bongartz et al., 2022). In the high-dose group, nearly 70% of participants lost at least of their 5% baseline weight over 3 months. This study was conducted on a moderate to severely overweight population; however, it is of interest to athletes that the weight loss was primarily fat mass, with preservation of lean body mass noted. Similar results have been discovered with administration of 100 g/day of flaxseed meal (a byproduct of flaxseed after oil processing) over 60 days (Kuang et al., 2020). Follow-up research should evaluate the effect of flaxseed intake on the metabolic profile and body composition of a healthy, fit population; however, the current proven benefits make administration of flaxseed as part of an athlete's daily diet something that should be considered for general health.

Common usage: Flaxseed can be consumed in whole or crushed form as well as in powder form as meal or flour. Flaxseed oil is available in liquid and capsule form. For general health, 1 to 3 tbsp of whole or ground flaxseed and 1 tsp to 1 tbsp of flaxseed oil is recommended. Ground flaxseed can be sprinkled on yogurt and cereals and added to baked goods; its oil form can be mixed with vinegar to form a dressing for salads. Essential fatty acids in flaxseed can become rancid with exposure to heat, light, and oxygen, so storage in a cool, dark, dry place is essential. The oil should not be used in cooking.

Health concerns: Because flaxseed, specifically in whole or ground form, is high in dietary fiber, it is best introduced gradually and in small amounts with water to avoid stomach cramping and diarrhea. It is best taken after competition to avoid such digestive issues.

Folic Acid 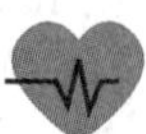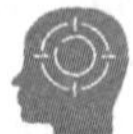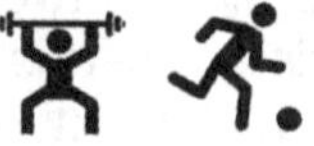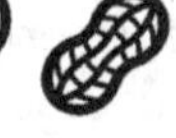

aka *folacin, folate, pteroyl-L-glutamic acid, pteroyl-L-glutamate, pteroylmonoglutamic acid, vitamin B$_9$*

What it is: Folic acid, which is a member of the B-vitamin family, is a synthetic and stable form of its naturally occurring sister, folate. It is a water-soluble vitamin and commonly used in vitamin supplements as well as fortified foods such as cereals and grains. Folate (derived from the Latin word *folium*, meaning "leaf") is found in dietary sources such as dark green leafy vegetables, liver, legumes, wheat germ, egg yolk, yeast, and sunflower seeds. Because only 50% of dietary folate is available for use in the body, deficiencies are common, making intake of fortified foods or vitamin supplements necessary.

Function: Folic acid plays a key role in several actions in the body that may benefit performance, especially as it relates to oxygen delivery. In conjunction with vitamin B$_{12}$, folic acid aids the production and maintenance of new cells, including red blood cells (also known as erythrocytes), which are vital to oxygen transport. A boost in red blood cell count may help facilitate more efficient oxygen delivery to muscles during exercise. Furthermore, by decreasing levels of homocysteine (an amino acid that has been shown to contribute to atherosclerosis or thickening of the arteries), folic acid is thought to enhance vascular function, thereby improving the delivery of oxygen and other nutrients essential to cardiovascular health and performance. This is especially relevant in light of the fact that intense, long-duration exercise has been correlated with increases in blood homocysteine levels, possibly heightening risk for heart attack and stroke in athletes, especially when folic acid intake is insufficient.

SUPPLEMENT FACT

Deficiencies in folate or vitamin B$_{12}$ can lead to megaloblastic anemia, which causes the production of abnormally large red blood cells that cannot effectively transport oxygen or remove carbon dioxide. Symptoms tend to manifest as neurological problems. Athletes who have undergone gastric bypass surgery or who are sensitive to gluten may be at greater risk for developing these symptoms.

Performance benefit: Folic acid may help increase oxygen delivery to and uptake by muscles, thereby enhancing aerobic performance.

Research: When energy intake is sufficient, athletes seem to consume adequate amounts of folic acid (Woolf et al., 2017). However, calorie-restricted diets, which are common among athletes looking to lose weight, often contain insufficient amounts of folic acid. Such dietary habits can lead to compromised vascular function and altered sex hormone levels in both males and females (Lanser et al., 2011). Fortunately, researchers discovered that a supplementation protocol incorporating 10 mg (10,000 mcg)/day of folic acid taken over 4 to 6 weeks provides a boost in the vascular function of female runners, regardless of baseline hormonal or serum folate status (Hoch et al., 2010). In addition, there is evidence that increased dietary intake and resulting plasma levels of folic acid are correlated with decreased homocysteine levels (Di Santolo et al., 2009). It is currently unknown whether this will aid performance, but based on data from clinical trials, it may help reduce risk factors related to cardiovascular disease in athletes (Asbaghi et al., 2023; Hankey et al., 2012). Findings from a 2017 clinical trial also demonstrate that folic acid ingestion, at a dose of 5 mg (5,000 mcg)/day over 6 weeks, may help improve blood flow in the exercising skeletal muscle of recreationally active adults aged 60 to 80 (Romero et al., 2017). This demonstrates the potential for the therapeutic use of folic acid to improve skeletal muscle blood flow, and perhaps exercise and functional capacity, in older adults.

Common usage: The current RDA for folic acid stands at 400 mcg for men and women over the age of 14 years, and recommendations increase to 600 and 500 mcg accordingly for pregnant and lactating women, respectively. Research-supported doses for improvements in vascular function range from 5,000 mcg to 10,000 mcg per day over 4-6 weeks.

Health concerns: As a water-soluble vitamin that is regularly removed from the body through urine, toxicity symptoms are rare, even with doses of 10,000 mcg/day. Some reports of stomach upset, sleep disturbances, and skin problems have been reported with doses above 15,000 mcg/day. Even so, the current tolerable upper intake level (UL) for folic acid remains at 1,000 mcg/day for adult men and women.

Frankincense

(see *Boswellia serrata*)

Fucoxanthin  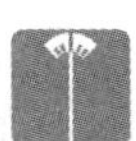 

aka *brown seaweed extract*

What it is: Fucoxanthin is a carotenoid isolated from edible brown seaweed.

Function: Aside from antioxidant effects, there is speculation that it may increase the expression of uncoupling proteins—mitochondrial transporters that increase energy expenditure and potentially fat loss. Further, some investigators, such as Zaharudin and colleagues (2019), have demonstrated inhibition of alpha-glucosidase, an enzyme important to intestinal carbohydrate digestion and glucose uptake.

Performance benefit: Reduced body fat can be important for athletes in weight class and physique sports such as bodybuilding or fitness competitions. If more human data reveal a consensus that fucoxanthin is biologically significant for weight-loss effects, this would be the most likely benefit.

Research: There is little data available relative to athletes. Hitoe and Shimoda (2017) reported reduced body weight and abdominal fat, with effects present in both visceral and subcutaneous fat, in mildly overweight adults using 1 to 3 mg fucoxanthin over 4 weeks. It is worth noting this is a short time frame to be measuring valid body composition changes. Also, very recent and novel data (Yang et al., 2022) suggest fucoxanthin has potential for therapeutic efficacy in neurodegenerative disorders.

Common usage: An indication of 2 to 8 mg/day is common in dietary supplement materials; this amount roughly coincides with research.

Health concerns: Hitoe and Shimoda (2017) reported no abnormalities of blood pressure, pulse rate, blood parameters, and urinalysis parameters. If inhibition of carbohydrate digestion is clinically meaningful, it would be problematic for athletes intentionally ingesting carbohydrate solutions before, during, and after exercise for performance benefits.

Gallated Flavan-3-Ols
(see *cocoa*)

Gamma-Aminobutyric Acid (GABA) 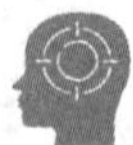

aka γ-*aminobutyric acid*

What it is: Gamma-aminobutyric acid (GABA) is an amino acid neurotransmitter found in the brain. The body synthesizes GABA from glutamic acid; GABA intake from dietary sources like tomatoes and fermented foods can also be considerable (de Bie et al., 2023). GABA acts as a major inhibitor of the central nervous system (Abdou et al., 2006). As a neural inhibitor, GABA is believed to have a beneficial role as an antistress agent. It is this ability that is commonly marketed to dietary supplement consumers.

Function: GABA can bind to receptors in the brain and induce neural inhibition, which has the potential to alleviate stress, induce relaxation, and improve the quality of sleep, concentration, and cognitive performance. In addition, GABA is believed to improve the ability to handle acute stress and reduce cortisol response. Interestingly, the levels of GABA synthesized in the brain decrease with age.

Performance benefit: If conflicting literature can be explained and refined, GABA could assist athletes in handling the daily physical and emotional stresses of training, improve an athlete's mood, support attention-related tasks, and lower the cortisol response to training. GABA could also benefit athletes by improving the quality of sleep and muscle recovery during sleep.

Research: One problem associated with GABA is that oral supplements are not believed to be able to cross the blood-brain barrier. A significant number of GABA receptors are located in the brain, and GABA's apparent inability to reach these receptors makes it less likely GABA will have any significant physiological effects on the body. However, conflicting evidence suggests other mechanisms could be at work, such as effects via enteric nervous system GABA receptors. As stated by Leonte and colleagues (2018): "Although there is controversy about whether oral GABA can cross the blood-brain barrier, our results offer preliminary evidence that GABA intake might help to distribute limited attentional resources more efficiently." Either way, most research has focused on drugs and other substances that can reach GABA receptors in the brain and induce the central nervous system inhibitory effects described previously (Goldberg, 2010). Relatively few well-controlled scientific studies have been carried out on oral GABA supplementation. These studies have found GABA to be beneficial in reducing nerve strain and psychological fatigue, but only in chronically fatigued populations (Kanehira et al., 2011; Nakamura et al., 2009); however, these studies are not considered to be of high quality, used small numbers of subjects, or came from the same group of researchers. Another trial found GABA capable of increasing alpha brain waves, which are associated with relaxation and reduced stress (Abdou, 2006); unfortunately, only 13 subjects were used for this trial. In 2015 Yamatsu and colleagues studied the effects of "two food materials, γ-aminobutyric acid (GABA) produced by natural fermentation and Apocynum venetum leaf extract, on the improvement of sleep." Their reported electroencephalogram (EEG) results suggested that oral administration of GABA (100 mg) and *Apocynum venetum* leaf extract (50 mg) had beneficial effects on sleep—specifically, it shortened sleep latency by 5.3 minutes. More recently, and perhaps due to challenges regarding control issues and population specificity, Imafuku and colleagues (2023) sought to identify new criteria for estimating the effects of dietary supplements for sleep. They examined the relationships among four dietary supplements, including GABA, as well as the life habits and sleep problems and conditions of subjects before supplementation. They concluded that, along with the other sleep aids, GABA (111.1 mg/day) was found to ameliorate sleep problems significantly. Further, preconditions specific to improved subjects were found to differ depending on the dietary supplements and sleep problems. Interestingly, subjects who consumed dairy products often showed improvement in their sleep problems with all the tested supplements. Taken together, this supplement remains controversial; more research is needed before definitive conclusions can be made.

Common usage: Research trials have varied in the amount of GABA provided, but typically 50 to 100 mg is recommended.

Health concerns: The use of GABA in 50 to 100 mg doses appears safe; however, no long-term studies are known at this time. In addition, little is known about drug–supplement interactions.

Gamma-Glutamylcysteinylglycine, Gamma-L-Glutamyl-L-Cysteinylglycine

(see *glutathione*)

Gamma-Linolenic Acid (GLA) 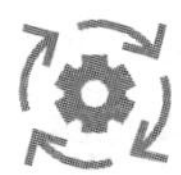 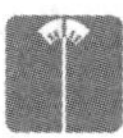

aka *black currant seed oil, borage oil, evening primrose oil*

What it is: Gamma-linolenic acid (GLA) can be found in a variety of oils in nature and is also produced in the body from the common omega-6 fatty acid linoleic acid. Linoleic acid can be found in vegetable oils such as soybean, safflower, corn, and rapeseed, all of which can be converted into GLA. Unfortunately, the rate of conversion of linoleic acid to GLA is very low, below 5% (Czernichow, 2010). GLA is commonly found in oils sold as supplements, including borage (18-26 g/100 g), evening primrose (7-10 g/100 g), black currant (15-20 g/100 g), and fungal oils (23-26 g/100 g). It can also be found in organ meats such as eggs and liver, as well as in human milk.

Function: Fatty acid metabolism is complex. It typically starts with a parent omega-6 or omega-3 fatty acid "parent molecule" and through multiple steps continues to elongate and otherwise modify it to make it more physiologically impactful. In the body, the common omega-6 fatty acid linoleic acid is inefficiently converted into GLA. GLA is then converted into dihomo-GLA (DGLA), which is finally converted into arachidonic acid (Wang, Lin, & Gu, 2012). Arachidonic acid is capable of exerting a variety of physiological effects in the body, and can be seen as a building block for pro-inflammatory molecules. It may seem contradictory to supplement an omega-6 like GLA; omega-6 fatty acids are typically seen as pro-inflammatory compared to omega-3s. As explained by Sergeant and colleagues (2016), "The anti-inflammatory effects of DGLA have been attributed to both 1) the anti-inflammatory properties of DGLA-derived metabolites and 2) the ability of DGLA to compete with AA in the synthesis of pro-inflammatory arachidonic acid products." Even this, however, is not the entire story. Some actions of arachidonic acid are anti-inflammatory, such as its ability to increase prostaglandin E1 (PGE1), which inhibits proinflammatory cytokines as well as inflammatory leukotrienes. As was noted in the entry for arachidonic acid, more research is needed given the complex nature of fatty acid–eicosanoid metabolism.

Performance benefit: GLA is most commonly used in the treatment of chronic inflammation for conditions such as dermatitis, eczema, and rheumatoid arthritis. It is also believed to help alleviate symptoms of menopause and premenstrual syndrome. The exact benefits of GLA supplementation for athletes are speculative; however, it is sometimes added to weight-loss supplements as a source of fatty acids believed to improve weight loss and body composition.

Research: Existing research is not promising since GLA is ineffective as an agent in the treatment of dermatitis and eczema, and insufficient evidence exists related to its effects on rheumatoid arthritis (Bayles & Usatine, 2009). According to Sergeant and colleagues (2016), "While there have been numerous *in vitro* and *in vivo* animal models which illustrate that GLA-supplemented diets attenuate inflammatory responses, clinical studies utilizing GLA or GLA in combination with omega-3 (n-3) PUFAs have been much less conclusive." One research trial has investigated potential benefits related to weight loss. The study examined the effects of GLA on weight regain. Formerly obese subjects consumed 5 g of borage oil or 5 g of olive oil for 1 year following initial weight loss. The results found the amount of weight regain to be significantly less for the borage oil group; however, only 13 of 17 subjects completed the trial (Schirmer & Phinney, 2007). More research is required before clear conclusions can be made relative to weight loss. Currently, there is little evidence to support the use of GLA.

Common usage: A range of 0.16 g to 0.64 g of GLA (160-640 mg) is commonly used in research trials. Because a standard 1 g capsule of evening primrose oil contains roughly 0.08 g of GLA, a 5 g dose would contain roughly 0.45 g of GLA.

Health concerns: Minor side effects have been reported, including abdominal pain, nausea, increased bowel movements, diarrhea, and headaches. GLA is safe when used in recommended doses (Bayles & Usatine, 2009). Insufficient research is available to know if any drug-supplement interactions exist.

Gamma-Tocopherol, Gamma-Tocotrienol

(see *vitamin E*)

Ganoderma Lucidum (Reishi)

(see *medicinal mushrooms*)

Garcinia Cambogia

(see *hydroxycitric acid*)

Garden Beet

(see *beetroot*)

Garlic 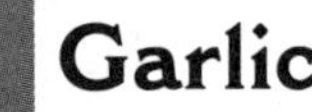  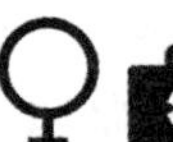  

aka *Allium sativum*

What it is: Garlic has been cultivated and used for over 6,000 years and is considered one of the first recorded performance-enhancing agents: It was used by the Olympic athletes of ancient Greece to increase strength and endurance during sporting competition and war. Though garlic is currently more widely used as a seasoning, scientists have started to evaluate whether the performance-enhancing claims made by early Olympians hold any merit. In particular, research has focused on the 30+ sulfur-based compounds within the plant that may provide antioxidant and anti-inflammatory benefits for athletes.

Function: The inflammatory process is an important component of the body's immune defense system. When kept temporary and local, it helps protect tissues and organs from damage; however, when inflammation spreads and becomes chronic—common among athletes walking the tightrope between training and overtraining—an array of problems from muscle damage and injury to illness can occur and hinder performance. Laboratory studies have demonstrated that sulfur compounds within garlic help regulate inflammation by inhibiting the activity of inflammatory enzymes. Preliminary evidence, primarily from animal studies using aged garlic extract, suggests that this may benefit the health of the musculoskeletal system during training.

Performance benefit: Athletes may benefit from enhanced recovery from exercise.

Research: Though the early Olympians may have believed garlic consumption enhanced strength and endurance during competition, there is no scientific evidence to support such claims, and thus a placebo effect was likely operating. For example, a small, single-blind, crossover study of 11 trained cyclists discovered no improvement in 40 km time trial performance with a supplement protocol including garlic extracts of 1,000 mg/day over 4 weeks compared to a placebo (Tsao et al., 2023). However, there was a significant increase in whole body antioxidant capacity, which attenuated blood indicators of systemic oxidative stress and inflammation and significantly reduced markers of muscle damage during the 40 km cycling exercise period ($p < 0.05$). Though it is prudent to hypothesize such positive adaptations could yield improvements in recovery and exercise performance, additional research with a larger subject size is warranted. A recent single-blind, cross-over, counterbalanced study, for instance, found that an acute oral supplemental dose of 2,000 mg of garlic extract taken immediately after exercise enhanced muscle glycogen replenishment—interestingly, without improvements in whole body insulin sensitivity (Cheng et al., 2024). Again, subject size ($n = 12$) was too small to draw definite conclusions. So, although the health benefits of garlic have strong evidence, additional research is needed before practical recommendations for use as it relates to sport performance can be made.

Common usage: Garlic can be consumed in whole or supplement form. The amount of active ingredients (sulfur compounds) in each supplement will vary based on how the supplement was processed. Further studies on the effectiveness of garlic from a performance standpoint need to be conducted before conclusive dosing recommendations are appropriate for an athletic population. For general purposes, consuming 1 chopped clove daily or using a standardized extract at a dose of 600 to 1,200 mg split into three doses/day is currently recommended.

ATHLETES' TIP

A compound in garlic called *ajoene* has been shown to carry strong antimicrobial properties, and topical application seems to be effective in fighting the fungus that causes athlete's foot. An at-home remedy can be made by mixing a few finely crushed garlic cloves with olive oil and rubbing small amounts on the affected area 2 to 3 times/day.

Health concerns: The most common adverse effects reported with oral ingestion of garlic and garlic supplements include bad breath and body odor, although such gastrointestinal issues as heartburn, abdominal pain, gas, nausea, and diarrhea have been reported. Rare occurrences include allergic reaction and uncontrolled bleeding. Topical application may cause skin irritation and blisters in a small number of users and are considered grounds for discontinuing use.

Geranamine, Geranium Oil Extract, Geranium Stem

(see *dimethylamylamine*)

Ginger

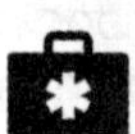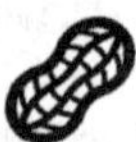

aka *African ginger, black ginger, cochin ginger, ginger essential oil, ginger root, Indian ginger, Jamaica ginger*

What it is: Derived from the horizontal stem of the plant *Zingiber officinale,* ginger is an herb commonly eaten raw or cooked. It is used to add spice to a wide spectrum of cultural cuisines, including such Western favorites as ginger ale and ginger snaps. Containing more than 50 types of antioxidants, ginger has been used in Chinese medicine for several thousand years and is recognized in athletics as a natural alternative to nonsteroidal anti-inflammatory drugs (NSAIDs).

Function: Ginger contains antioxidant compounds called gingerols that, like NSAIDs, block the enzymatic action of cyclooxygenase-1 (COX-1) and cyclooxygenase-2 (COX-2), which are responsible for the production of inflammation-inducing prostaglandins. Ginger also reduces the body's production of proinflammatory chemicals called cytokines while desensitizing TRPV1, a type of pain receptor found in peripheral nerves.

Performance benefit: Athletes may benefit from reduced levels of postworkout inflammation and muscle pain, thereby facilitating faster recovery from intense training.

Research: A pair of double-blind, placebo-controlled studies conducted by researchers from the University of Georgia determined that a 2 g/day dose of ginger, taken either in raw or in heat-treated form, over 11 days reduced exercise-induced muscle pain associated with weightlifting exercise by 25% compared to a placebo (Black et al., 2010). Furthermore, a systematic review of clinical trials concluded that there is preliminary support for the anti-inflammatory benefits of ginger or specific constituents found within ginger, thereby presenting promising applications for pain associated with arthritic conditions common among athletes, especially osteoarthritis (OA) (Terry et al., 2011). Follow-up studies have confirmed that oral supplementation with ginger shows promise in reducing inflammatory markers (C-reactive protein and concentration of nitric oxide) as well as proinflammatory cytokines (Mozaffari-Khosravi et al., 2016; Naderi et al., 2016); these clinical trials found a supplementation protocol that entailed 1 g/day of ginger in capsule form over 3 months to yield favorable results. Interestingly, a 2020 systemic review and meta-analysis—albeit of only four studies—failed to find sufficient evidence to support the use of oral ginger compared with placebo in pain relief and functional improvement in patients with knee OA (Araya-Quintanilla F, Gutierrez-Espinoza H, Munoz-Yanez MJ, Sanchez-Montoya U, Lopez-Jeldes, 2020). It is evident more research needs to be conducted, particularly exploring different supplemental doses and protocols in athletes, before conclusions can be drawn on the effectiveness of ginger supplementation in this population.

Common usage: Prepared from fresh and dried ginger root or from steam distillation of the oil in the root, ginger supplements are available as extracts, tinctures, capsules, and oils. In addition, ginger can be consumed in raw form or added as a spice in cooking. For treatment of muscle pain and inflammation, the research-supported dose ranges from 0.5 to 2 g/day, preferably split into two doses (e.g., pre- and postworkout). If ginger is consumed in capsule form, the recommended approach is a standardized extract with a gingerol content of 5%.

ATHLETES' TIP

A 2 g dose of raw ginger in capsule form is roughly equivalent to 1 tsp of powdered ginger, 0.5 tsp of ginger extract, or 1 tbsp finely chopped fresh ginger.

Health concerns: Although ill effects associated with use of ginger supplements are rare, there have been some reported cases of mild heartburn, stomach upset, and diarrhea with larger doses.

Ginkgo Biloba  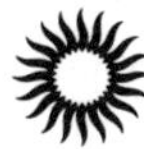 

aka *ginkgo leaf extract, ginkgo seed, Japanese silver apricot*

What it is: *Ginkgo biloba* is an herbal supplement prescribed to preserve memory, improve brain function, and prevent the decline in cognitive function associated with aging. Sales of ginkgo exceed $249 million annually in the United States, making it a popular nutritional supplement.

Function: A number of mechanisms are hypothesized to be responsible for ginkgo's ability to improve cognitive function and prevent cognitive decline. First, ginkgo acts as an antioxidant, preventing free radical damage. Secondly, ginkgo may have a neural protective effect on the central nervous system. Third, ginkgo potentially modulates neurotransmitter systems and improves blood circulation. Finally, ginkgo's antidepressant and adaptogenic effects are associated with a beneficial effect on mood.

Performance benefit: Ginkgo could provide a performance benefit for athletes involved in sports that require fast decision making and cognitive performance. In addition, ginkgo could reduce the stress of training, particularly in extreme environments like heat.

Research: Studies evaluating the cognitive benefits of ginkgo on a healthy, fit population are lacking, and even among disease states, such as dementia and Alzheimer's disease, positive results generally have not been shown (Birks, Grimley, & Van Dongen, 2009; Canter & Ernst, 2007). Ginkgo's antidepressant and adaptogenic attributes are less researched. In 2002 a group of scientists from the Institute of Experimental Endocrinology found administration of 120 mg/day of ginkgo reduced the rise in blood pressure and cortisol during experimentally induced stress compared to the placebo group (Jezova et al., 2002). However, these results have not been confirmed by additional research. Evolving research has shown the potential neuroprotective benefit of nanodelivery of traditional Chinese *Ginkgo biloba* extract and bilobalide (a derivative of ginkgo) on the pathophysiology of heat stroke. Study investigators found the extracts of *Gingko biloba* to attenuate more than 80% of the reduction in brain pathology in heat stroke compared to conventional drug delivery as well as improve functional outcomes after heat stroke (Sahib et al., 2021). This has favorable applications to athletes training and competing in heat as well as soldiers exposed to extreme temperatures in combat. Additional research exploring the potential benefits of administration of ginkgo as it relates to mitigating the detriments of stress situations in a healthy, fit population is warranted before conclusions on use can be made.

Common usage: Most research trials assessing the effects of a single dose of ginkgo on cognitive performance have used 120 mg, 240 mg, or 360 mg doses before performing cognitive tasks. Long-term studies typically have used 120 to 240 mg/day in either one dose or two smaller doses.

Health concerns: Ginkgo can interfere with a number of medications such as antidepressants, blood thinners, antiepileptics, diabetes medications, diuretics, and nonsteroidal anti-inflammatories (NSAIDs). Those taking any of these medications should check with a doctor before beginning supplementation.

Ginseng 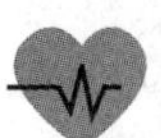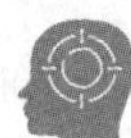

aka *American ginseng, Korean ginseng, Panax ginseng, Siberian ginseng*

What it is: A slow-growing herb native to East Asia with a light-colored root, single stalk, and long oval green leaves, ginseng is often called *man root* due to its resemblance to a human body. Ginseng is thought to have adaptogenic qualities that may help an athlete better cope with the mental and physical stresses associated with sporting competition, thereby providing a boost to performance.

TYPES OF GINSENG

American: Also known as *Panax quinquefolius* and belonging to the Araliaceae family of plants, American ginseng contains active compounds called ginsenosides and saponins that are thought to help fight fatigue and stress by supporting the adrenal glands and the use of oxygen by exercising muscles.

Panax: Derived from the Greek word *panacea* meaning "cure all," Panax ginseng, also known as Korean, Chinese, or Asian Ginseng, also contains ginsenosides and saponins as well as B-vitamins and dietary flavonoids. These are thought to strengthen the immune system by enhancing the number of immune cells in the blood, helping protect an athlete from a wide variety of ailments that can hinder performance.

Siberian: Also known as *eleuthero*, *ci wu jia*, or Russian ginseng, Siberian ginseng contains active compounds called eleutherosides that are thought to help enhance mental acuity and improve the use of oxygen by the muscles, thereby aiding endurance as well as enhancing recovery.

Function: The different varieties of ginseng all contain ginsenosides within the root of the plant. These compounds act on the central nervous system and have antioxidant and anti-inflammatory properties, as well as effects on cortisol modulation that are thought to improve overall energy and immune functionality, particularly during times of fatigue or stress.

Performance benefit: Athletes may benefit from increased ability to counter the potential detriments of physical and mental stress, including immune breakdown and compromised performance, thereby promoting recovery and allowing more training to be absorbed for increased performance.

Research: Studies evaluating the capacity of ginseng as a protective element in the physiological response to exercise have found consumption to reduce variables associated with catabolism, including muscle damage and fatigue, thereby aiding the recovery process (Zha et al., 2022). Flanagan and colleagues (2018) found a supplementation protocol that included 960 mg/day of Panax ginseng attenuated the cortisol and creatine kinase (CK) response to strength training exercise (5 series of 12 repetitions of leg press at 70% RM). Additionally, increased levels of glutathione, improved response of superoxide dismutase (SOD), and enhanced total antioxidant potency in plasma (TAP), were reported, leading study investigators to conclude that Panax ginseng may improve the acute antioxidant response to strength training and decrease muscle catabolism induced by exercise. This same supplementation protocol was shown to also improve subjective measures of effort and pain following an acute session of resistance-based exercise (Caldwell et al., 2018). In another study, both subjective perception of effort as well as muscle excitability (electrical activity of the vastus lateralis muscle) following completion of a series of half-squat exercises to concentric failure were shown to improve in trained track and field athletes with a supplementation protocol including 100 mg/kg/day of Panax ginseng. However, there was no difference compared to the placebo group when evaluating markers of muscle damage, nor did the supplementation protocol affect any delayed onset of muscle soreness (Cristina-Souza et al., 2022). Hsu (2010) found intake of 400 mg/day of American ginseng (AG) over 4 weeks to significantly decrease blood markers of oxidative stress and muscle soreness in active men both immediately and 72 hours after a 60-minute downhill treadmill run compared to a placebo. Similarly, Lin and colleagues (2021) evaluated the impact of a higher dose (1.6 g/day) of AG over 30 days on muscle damage parameters induced by downhill running and found improvements in the CK response as well as a decrease in lipid peroxidation. However, more robust studies are needed to explore different types of ginseng, dose and durations, and type of subjects—especially athletes—before definite guidelines for use in this population can be provided.

Common usage: Ginseng can be made into a powder, capsule, or liquid tincture with important data on supplement labels including the type of ginseng, the plant part used (root), the amount and form of ginseng (powder or extract), and the concentration of ginsenosides. The recommended dose of ginseng in dry ginseng root is 0.5 to 2 g for short-term dosing and 1 g for long-term dosing, equivalent to 200 to 600 mg of extract (Bostock et al., 2018).

Health concerns: Reported side effects include headaches, heart palpitations, high blood pressure, dizziness, nausea, vomiting, diarrhea, and flushing of the face. Consuming ginseng with caffeine can cause overstimulation and insomnia in some people. Ginseng directly increases the clearance of Warfarin; therefore, it is a contraindication for those taking this blood thinner.

Glucosamine 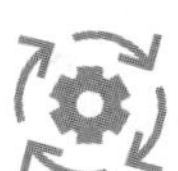 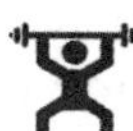 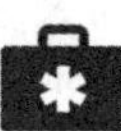

aka *glucosamine hydrochloride (HCL), glucosamine sulfate (see also chondroitin)*

What it is: Glucosamine is a naturally occurring amino sugar that is a building block for proteins of the connective tissue known as glycosaminoglycans. Roughly 50% of hyaline cartilage, which covers the bones of synovial joints such as the knee, hip, and shoulder, is composed of glycosaminoglycans. Cartilage functions to absorb shock and reduce friction during movement. Two supplemental forms of glucosamine exist: glucosamine sulfate and glucosamine hydrochloride (HCL).

Function: The availability of glucosamine is believed to be a limiting factor in the synthesis of glycosaminoglycan. Therefore, supplementation may prevent the degeneration and loss of cartilage in joints such as the knee, hip, ankle, shoulder, and spine. Glucosamine might also act by suppressing the expression of several mediators of cartilage degradation.

Performance benefit: Because the physical demands of sport and daily training place a significant amount of stress on joints, many athletes experience chronic joint pain. In addition, many athletes suffer injuries to joints that require surgery or joint reconstruction. Recovery from these types of surgeries can result in changes to the joint, and glucosamine could have a positive effect on recovery.

Research: A significant amount of research related to glucosamine has been conducted in combination with chondroitin, often with mixed results, making it difficult to come to clear conclusions. For example, a systematic review and meta-analysis specific to knee osteoarthritis (OA) by Meng and colleagues (2023) found that "the combination of glucosamine and chondroitin is effective and superior to other treatments in knee osteoarthritis to a certain extent." These researchers noted the limited number of studies and uneven trial quality, however, and called for more high-quality trials. An earlier, larger meta-analysis by Zhu and colleagues (2018) that included hip as well as knee OA found that, compared with placebo, chondroitin alone could help reduce pain symptoms and improve function, whereas glucosamine alone elicited significant effects only on stiffness improvement. Interestingly, the combination therapy did not have enough evidence to be superior to placebo. In any case, many scientists have tended to agree that glucosamine can improve symptoms of pain associated with OA and delay its progression. It appears that long-term supplementation over at least 1 year may be required before significant improvements take place. In 2005 Poolsup and colleagues reviewed a variety of research studies and concluded there was evidence to support improvement of symptoms with glucosamine sulphate; however, another group of researchers was more cautious, stating that overall, glucosamine was shown to have a moderately significant effect (Black et al., 2009). Early research work suggested that glucosamine sulfate was superior to glucosamine HCL in providing benefit, but some experts believe both are equally effective. Only one known research study has used postinjury glucosamine (Ostojic, 2007). This trial, involving athletes who had just suffered knee injuries, supplemented glucosamine for 4 weeks. No differences in pain, swelling, or passive knee flexion and extension were noted at 7, 14, or 21 days. However, after 28 days of supplementation, the glucosamine group demonstrated significant improvement in passive knee flexion and extension.

Common usage: Current recommendations are 1,500 mg/day of glucosamine sulfate or glucosamine HCL in three doses of 500 mg each. Recently, scientists have suggested that a 1,500 mg dose is relatively small compared to higher amounts used in successful animal studies (Aghazadeh-Habashi & Jamali, 2011). Some believe this is one of the reasons for mixed results in previous research trials. In some European countries and the United Kingdom, glucosamine is prescribed as a pharmaceutical drug to treat OA. However, not all countries are as convinced of its effectiveness.

Health concerns: Glucosamine is safe. Recently concerns have been raised related to glucosamine's impact on blood glucose levels, glucose metabolism, and insulin sensitivity. However, this concern is probably unwarranted (Simon et al., 2011).

Glucuronolactone

aka *d-glucuronolactone, glucurono-γ-lactone*

What it is: Often an ingredient in preworkout formulas and energy drinks, glucuronolactone is a metabolite of glucose. It's also a component of connective tissue in the body.

Function: Glucuronolactone's relationship to glucuronidation, part of the natural process of metabolizing drugs and other compounds for elimination, is sometimes seen in marketing materials. However, there is little research to suggest that it is important to the energizing effects of energy drinks.

Performance benefit: As part of a cocktail typically consisting of caffeine and taurine (among other ingredients), glucuronolactone may help effect a sense of energy and alertness.

Research: Modern data specific to glucuronolactone is lacking—a fact noted by various researchers.

Common usage: As part of a typical energy drink, 600 mg per serving is a common dose.

Health concerns: The opinion from the European Safety Authority (EFSA) Panel on Food Additives and Nutrient Sources Added to Food (ANS) was that exposure to d-glucuronolactone through regular consumption of energy drinks was not of safety concern (EFSA, 2009). There is little evidence in a sensory (stimulant) regard.

Glutamine 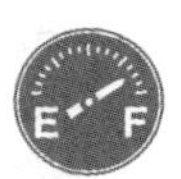  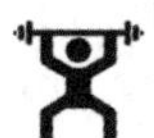 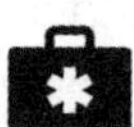 

aka aminoglutaramic acid, 5-diamino-5-oxopentanoic acid, gln, glutamic acid 5-amide, levoglutamide, L-glutamine, (S)-2, 2-aminoglutaramic acid

What it is: The most abundant amino acid found in the body, predominantly synthesized and stored in the muscles, glutamine participates in a number of reactions important to health and recovery. Glutamine is classified as conditionally essential, meaning that under normal circumstances the body can synthesize adequate amounts to support physiological demands. However, although the average Western diet has been reported to supply 5 to 10 g of glutamine, generally in the form of both animal- and plant-based protein sources, it is thought that athletes may require additional amounts to offset the heightened stress associated with heavy physical training.

Function: Prolonged periods of heavy training as well as ultraendurance competition (e.g., adventure racing, triathlon, marathon) are associated with significant drops in plasma (blood) glutamine levels, which is a postulated cause of exercise-induced immune impairment and increased susceptibility to infection, especially upper respiratory infection. Supplementation with glutamine is thought to provide athletes with immune support, thereby helping to offset these drops. Glutamine also promotes protein synthesis and thus may help protect athletes against muscle breakdown. As an important connector to an intermediate metabolite in the Krebs cycle, glutamine is also thought to help spare phosphocreatine and glycogen in muscle fibers, particularly type I (slow-twitch) fibers, which may extend endurance.

Performance benefit: Athletes may benefit from improved immune response and recovery times during heavy training cycles as well as enhanced ability to rebound from sport-oriented trauma or injury. Glutamine may be of particular benefit to athletes experiencing symptoms of burnout or overtraining, such as fatigue, frequent illness, and poor performance.

Research: It is thought that the drop in glutamine levels during exercise by itself may not be significant enough to compromise the immune function of healthy, well-nourished athletes. A 2012 study of ultraendurance athletes reported a 19% drop in plasma glutamine levels in trained men completing a 24-hour endurance trial consisting of kayaking, running, and cycling; however, intramuscular glutamine levels remained unchanged up to and during the immediate postexercise recovery period (Borgenvik et al., 2012). Furthermore, several studies have found no effect of supplementation with glutamine on postexercise alterations in several aspects of immune function (Gleeson, 2008). Even so, during extreme catabolic stress, such as that seen with traumatic injury, intracellular glutamine levels can drop by more than 50%, and plasma concentration can drop by 30%. At that point, supplemental glutamine certainly becomes an integral nutritional component to all aspects of recovery, including immune functionality and tissue repair (Askanazi et al., 1980). Additionally, a small study of competitive soccer players found that preworkout consumption of a carbohydrate-glutamine solution containing 50 g of maltodextrin and 3.5 g of glutamine was more effective in increasing the athletes' distance and duration of tolerance to intermittent exercise and lowering subjective feelings of fatigue than a calorie-matched carbohydrate-only solution (Favano et al., 2008).

Common usage: Glutamine is available in tablet, capsule, and powder form and is often added to recovery-focused sport drinks as well as infused into energy chews and gels. Research-supported doses for added immune and recovery support during intense training cycles range from 1.5 to 4.5 g, generally split into doses taken before, during, and after workouts or between meals. In addition, similar doses have been taken 30 minutes before exercise to enhance endurance performance.

Health concerns: Acute intake of glutamine by athletes in daily doses of 20 to 30 g over 2 weeks seems to be well tolerated, though a small number have reported symptoms such as constipation and bloating.

Glutathione 

aka *gamma-glutamylcysteinylglycine, gamma-L-glutamyl-L-cysteinylglycine, L-glutathione, reduced glutathione (GSH)* (see also *superoxide dismutase*)

What it is: is an antioxidant molecule that is generally considered endogenous (i.e., originating from within); however, its status can be affected by other nutrients. Exercise stress has been shown to lower glutathione levels in the body and negatively affect endurance performance, immunity, and recovery, making corrective measures to optimize glutathione levels of potential benefit to the athlete.

Function: As an antioxidant, glutathione is purported to aid performance by protecting against cellular damage incurred from the production of free radicals during exercise, especially when levels exceed the body's own natural defenses. This can occur when an athlete returns to training after a long layoff, enters a particular tough training cycle, or is exposed to other stressors such as altitude, smog, or extreme heat or cold. Research has shown exposure to such stressors can significantly decrease glutathione levels in the body (Gomes, Stone, & Florida-James, 2011; Pinho et al., 2010). Additionally, maintaining glutathione levels is thought to protect athletes from infection and reoccurring illness by enhancing nutrient and amino acid absorption in cells that are important to immune function, namely lymphocytes and phagocytes.

Performance benefit: Although sold as a supplement itself, it is more likely that athletes could benefit from other nutrients that increase glutathione tissue concentrations. Added antioxidant protection through supplementation of various glutathione-encouraging nutrients may enhance endurance, help speed recovery, and better maintain the health of an athlete throughout a competitive season.

Research: Exercise training itself enhances glutathione status. Further, research is still not particularly supportive of direct supplementation. Because glutathione is not well absorbed across the gastrointestinal tract, it is virtually impossible to raise circulating levels through direct oral use. Even an acute, high-dose (3 g) oral administration of glutathione failed to affect circulating levels in one study (Witschi et al., 1992). Research focusing on supplemental oral intake of glutathione alone is virtually nonexistent. Instead, research has focused on intravenous administration of glutathione or oral intake of glutathione precursors and derivatives such as N-acetylcysteine, L-cysteine, and L-glutamic acid. In a case study involving a 61-year-old trained endurance athlete, for example, four separate intravenous doses of 1,000 mg of glutathione over 36 days led to progressive and significant time improvements in an established 18.4 mi (29.6 km) time trial; the end result was a more than a 5-minute improvement, or 7.2% performance gain (Misner, 2003). In the case of oral supplementation, two separate double-blind, placebo-controlled studies found that 700 mg/day of cystine (a dipeptide of cysteine) and 280 mg/day of theanine (a precursor of glutamate) over 10 to 14 days provided a significant protective effect on natural killer cell activity, helping reduce incidence of infection in highly trained athletes during high-intensity resistance exercise and run training compared to a placebo (Kawada et al., 2010; Murakami et al., 2009). Both cysteine and glutamate play key roles in the formation of glutathione. Although it is evident that maintaining optimal levels of glutathione is important to an athlete's health and performance, there is not adequate evidence for its oral supplementation use, specifically when taken alone.

Common usage: Glutathione is available in capsule, tablet, and powder form. A combined amino acid cocktail that includes glutathione along with L-cysteine, N-acetylcysteine, L-glutamic acid, or glycine is thought to have a greater impact on body glutathione levels and consequent antioxidant benefit than taking glutathione alone. Doses generally range from 600 to 1,200 mg/day split into two doses. Hemolytic anemia, also known as hemolysis, which often occurs in runners, can lower circulating levels of glutathione; consequently, affected athletes may benefit from intravenous or oral supplement intervention.

Health concerns: Glutathione, taken either orally or by injection given by a qualified health care professional, appears to be safe; no adverse symptoms have been reported.

Glycerol  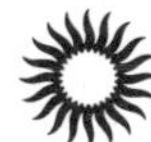

aka *1,2,3-propanetriol*

What it is: Glycerol, also known as a plasma expander, is a natural metabolite that is rapidly absorbed into the body and carries osmotic properties that enables greater fluid retention than water alone. It previously was on the World Anti-Doping Agency (WADA) banned substance list for use by competitive athletes, but in January 2018, it was officially removed, making it an accessible option for hyperhydration and postexercise rehydration strategies.

Function: As a water-attracting three-carbon compound, typically part of the "backbone" of a triacylglycerol (fat) molecule, glycerol temporarily increases plasma (blood) volume—an effect used for hyperhydration.

Performance benefit: Increasing plasma volume (about 5%-10%) is a phenomenon that naturally occurs when a training regimen starts and typically lasts for about 3 days upon cessation of exercise. Consuming glycerol in a large volume of water amplifies this fluid expansion, which can be advantageous for buffering the 5% to 10% plasma loss typically seen during exercise-induced sweating. The degree to which glycerol supplementation leads to improvements in thermoregulation or hemodynamics above baseline is not clear in the literature. What seems more plausible is a buffer against the ergolytic effects of dehydration.

Research: Research confirms the hyperhydrating effect of glycerol when consumed with water. For example, van Rosendal and colleagues (2010) stated that many studies have shown an increase in body water of about 1 L. The scientific literature regarding performance enhancement is equivocal, but the osmotic gradient and plasma volume expansion itself is not. An additional fluid retention of ~1,300 mL for a 70 kg athlete upward of 4 hours after exertion has been reported with the combination of glycerol (1.4 g/kg FFM) and sodium (3.0 g/L) in 25 mL of water/kg FFM, suggesting that combining osmolytes may be more effective than just using one (Goulet et al., 2018; Montner et al., 1996; Wingo et al., 2004).

Common usage: Athletes intending to hyperhydrate with glycerol typically ingest about 1.0 to 1.2 g/kg in about 1.5 to 1.8 L of fluid over a period of 60 minutes, 30 minutes prior to exercise. For endurance athletes, current data supports the consumption of 1.2 to 1.4 g of glycerol/kg fat-free mass (FFM) paired with ~25 mL of fluid/kg FFM 90 to 180 minutes before exertion (Goulet et al., 2018; van Rosendal et al., 2010). The translation into a performance benefit is unlikely to be significant unless effort is high and conditions, such as heat, warrant increased uptake of fluid to maintain hydration (Goulet et al., 2007).

Health concerns: Although not a health concern by itself, Koehler and colleagues (2013) noted that glycerol hyperhydration may be misused to mask the effects of blood doping by diluting the very high level of hemoglobin and hematocrit induced by such practices. Nonetheless, its effects are modest on these variables. Side effects from glycerol ingestion are rare, but include nausea and gastrointestinal discomfort, likely from the fluid shifts.

Glycine Betaine

(see *betaine*)

Goat's Horn

(see *fenugreek*)

Golden Root

(see *Rhodiola rosea*)

Grape Seed 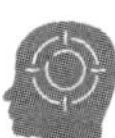  

aka *grapeseed, grape seed oil, muskat, Vinis vinifera*

What it is: According to Elejalde and colleagues (2021), grapes are an important source of natural antioxidants due to their high polyphenol content, which has potential benefits for the reduction of the effects of intense exercise. Indeed grapes, a member of the berry fruit family, have long been considered a nutrition powerhouse with medicinal use dating back to ancient Greece. Their seeds contain a unique class of plant compounds called oligomeric proanthocyanidin complexes (OPCs), which contain strong antioxidant qualities of potential benefit to a highly trained athlete.

Function: As an athlete hits the peak of training, where total volume and intensity often reach uncharted levels, the production of free radicals and oxidative stress may exceed the body's natural defenses, causing damage to muscle tissue and inhibiting optimal recovery from training. Grape seed, whose antioxidant abilities have been shown to be 20 to 50 times more potent than such popular antioxidants as beta-carotene, vitamin C, and vitamin E, helps strengthen and protect cell membranes, including that of muscle tissue, from oxidative damage caused by elevated levels of circulating free radicals during times of exercise stress. Grape seed also helps inhibit the release of chemicals called prostaglandins, which can generate inflammation during an allergic or asthmatic response, making supplementation potentially beneficial for athletes who suffer from allergies or asthma.

Performance benefit: Athletes may experience less muscle damage and inflammation during heavy training, thereby facilitating faster recovery times.

In a double-blind, randomized, placebo-controlled study, a group of elite sportsmen in the midst of training and competition saw nearly a 10% increase in antioxidant capacity, resulting in reduced biomarkers of skeletal muscle damage, when supplementing with 400 mg of grape seed extract for 1 month; this result equated to significant increases in performance, including a 6.4% boost in explosive power, during a structured jumping exercise protocol (Lafay et al., 2009). There is also some evidence that OPC in grape seed offsets some of the swelling triggered by athletic injury and surgery (Constantini, De Bernardi, & Gotti, 1999; Fine, 2000; Teixeira, 2002; Xu et al., 2012). A 2021 review by Elejalde and colleagues concluded that there is "promising evidence, although still limited" and that "more pilot studies on the effect of grape polyphenols on the oxidative stress produced by sport should be conducted to determine the optimal concentration, dosage and effect on the oxidative stress for target athletes."

Common usage: Grape seed is available as a liquid extract or as a capsule. Research-supported treatment doses for antioxidant protection in athletes range from 25 to 50 mg taken up to 3 times/day. The highest quality grape seed products are standardized for purity and control of the substance to 40% to 80% proanthocyanidins or have an OPC content of at least 95%.

Health concerns: Grape seed seems to be well tolerated, although there have been reports of headache; dry, itchy scalp; dizziness; and nausea in a small population. Animal studies have shown doses up to 100 mg/kg/day to be safe for use; however, safety trials on humans are limited, so it is advisable to consult with a physician before supplementation, especially if taking any medications.

Grapple Plant

(see *devil's claw*)

Green Pepper

(see *capsicum*)

Green Tea Extract  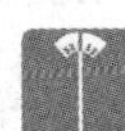 

aka *epigallocatechin-3-gallate (EGCG) (see also caffeine and theanine)*

What it is: Green tea is made from the dried leaves of *Camellia sinensis*. Unlike black tea, which undergoes fermentation, green tea leaves are steamed and unfermented. Extracts of green tea may be caffeinated or decaffeinated. Although there are small amounts of caffeine in green tea, the unique properties are partly a result of the catechin polyphenol epigallocatechin-3-gallate (EGCG). Potential benefits to athletes probably involve both. Green tea as a whole also contains theanine, an unusual amino acid known to interact with caffeine in different ways.

Function: EGCG and related green tea polyphenols possess antioxidant and anti-inflammatory properties. Further, increased metabolic rate and fat oxidation are a principal interest and have some support in the literature.

Performance benefit: The purported benefit of green tea extract for the athlete is an increase in fatty acid oxidation (as a substrate for exercise performance), or, harder to achieve, modestly decreased body fat over time.

Research: A systematic review by Vázquez Cisneros and colleagues in 2017 reported that 100 to 460 mg of EGCG/day has shown effectiveness for body fat and body weight reduction when consumed over 12 weeks or more. Co-consumption of 80 to 300 mg caffeine was a contributing factor.

Common usage: A typical dose of green tea extract is 250 to 500 mg/day.

Health concerns: Published meta-analyses indicate that green tea is safe for moderate and regular consumption. There is some indication in the literature that elevated liver enzymes may occur in susceptible individuals. Hu and colleagues (2018) suggested a safe intake level of 338 mg EGCG/day for adults when ingested as a concentrated solid bolus dose.

Grifola Frondosa (Maitake)

(see *medicinal mushrooms*)

Gymnema Sylvestre (GS)  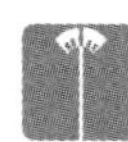 

aka *gurmar*

What it is: *Gymnema sylvestre* (GS) is a large woody herb grown in central and southern India as well as tropical regions of Africa and Australia. For centuries it has been used as a medicinal plant in traditional Ayurvedic medicine. Its leaves, which are typically the active part of the plant, are believed to assist in reducing blood sugar, resulting in its use as a treatment for diabetes. In addition, the plant is believed to affect taste sensations, benefit digestion, promote circulation, protect against viral infection, and prevent obesity. GS is sold by itself as a dietary supplement to promote health and is also an ingredient in so-called fat-burning supplements.

Function: According to Turner and colleagues (2022), one application of *Gymnema sylvestre* is to block lingual sweet taste receptors, thereby reducing pleasantness and intake of sweet food. However, there remains a lack of quality research studies on GS; as a result, how it works is relatively unknown. Because GS's mechanisms are speculated to involve insulin production and sensitivity, the majority of research has focused on its applications to diabetes. GS is thought to enhance the uptake of glucose by adipose and muscle tissue as well as decrease the intestinal absorption of glucose and the production of glucose in the liver. All such actions would have beneficial effects on blood sugar, obesity, and the storage of body fat.

Performance benefit: GS may assist athletes in weight loss and reduction of body fat.

Research: In 2022, Turner and colleagues provided 58 healthy adults 4 mg of *Gymnema sylvestre* (75% gymnemic acids) or placebo, plus a fiber and vitamin supplement, and an associated healthy eating guide for 14 days. Among other measures, the amount of chocolate bars eaten and sensory testing were conducted before and after the 14-day intervention. After GS dosing, subjects consumed fewer chocolates on day 0 than controls, but there were no differences between groups on day 15. This mixed result leaves interpretation open. Similarly, regarding weight changes, a 2019 review of studies by

Khan and colleagues reported that ethanol extract of GS resulted in mixed findings on loss versus gain in rat models. These authors also cited a couple studies on weight loss in humans, but co-ingestion of other ingredients and the presence of disease states tend to confound any conclusions for athletes. Claims of improved body composition and fat burning have not been validated scientifically. A study performed on rats found that a dose of 100 mg of GS/kg was capable of decreasing body weight, food consumption, triglyceride levels, and total cholesterol in obese rats fed a high-fat diet (Reddy et al., 2012). A 2007 review of GS in the treatment of diabetes concluded that the clinical efficacy of GS is supported only by a small number of nonrandomized, open-label trials, and that further research is urgently needed (Leach, 2007). Currently, GS lacks enough evidence to support any of its claims.

Common usage: Open-trial diabetic studies have used doses ranging from 200 to 800 mg/day.

Health concerns: The use of GS appears to be safe; however, one report of toxic hepatitis was noted in a diabetic patient treated with GS. The German Federal Institute for Risk Assessment (2018) also noted that "human studies provided some indications that certain Gymnema extracts may enhance the glucose-lowering effects of certain antidiabetic drugs," calling for caution in this regard.

Harpagophyum Procumbens

(see *devil's claw*)

Herba Epimedii

(see *horny goat weed*)

Hericium Erinaceus (Lion's Mane)

(see *medicinal mushrooms*)

Hippophae Rhamnoides L.

(see *sea buckthorn*)

Hoodia Gordonii  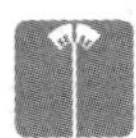 

aka *P57*

What it is: *Hoodia gordonii* is a cactus-like plant grown in South Africa. The plant was first recognized in 1932 where it was recorded as a source of food for the Khoi-San people, who consumed hoodia to suppress appetite and thirst during long hunting trips when food was scarce. In 1963 a compound known as P57 was isolated from hoodia that was believed to be responsible for the plant's appetite-suppressing affects. In 1998 a patent was granted for P57, and between 1998 and 2009 several large pharmaceutical companies such as Pharmacia, Unilever, and Phytopharm worked to develop obesity treatments containing P57. Since 2009 all companies except Phytopharm have terminated their efforts because of safety and efficacy concerns (Vermaak et al., 2011).

Function: Hoodia is believed to work by affecting the central nervous system and hypothalamus. A 2004 study showed that P57, the active constituent of hoodia, increased ATP in the hypothalamus of rats. The elevated ATP content countered decreases in ATP that would be expected from a reduced-calorie diet (MacLean and Duo, 2004).

Performance benefit: Athletes such as wrestlers or physique athletes needing to restrict calorie intake for weight loss might benefit from the appetite-suppressing affects of hoodia.

Research: The data on hoodia remain debatable. To date, no conclusive evidence from clinical studies in humans have been reported in peer-reviewed scientific journals. Private, for-profit companies have conducted the majority of the research, the results of which are often protected and unpublished. The only other published data are on animal models. These studies often compare the effects of hoodia on food intake in obese and nonobese mice and report substantial reductions in food intake when rats are fed ad lib diets. Although data on animals are positive, much more evidence is needed before hoodia is recommended as a weight-loss supplement. Consumers should be leery, considering the termination of research efforts by many pharmaceutical companies (Vermaak et al., 2011).

Common usage: Studies in rats have determined 1.8 to 2.7 g/kg to be the optimal effective dose. Human trials have typically provided 400 to 500 mg/day. It is difficult to determine a recommendation for safe and effective use without further research.

Health concerns: A history of safe use within the indigenous Khoi-San people of South Africa is known, but peer-reviewed assessments are important. Those considering supplementing with hoodia should be cautious about the quality of the product they purchase; studies on quality control have found fake products claiming to contain *Hoodia gordonii* (Vermaak et al., 2011). Bonetti and colleagues (2022) note that the use of hoodia has been questioned due to several adverse effects, including nausea and skin reactions.

Hordenine 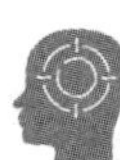 

aka: N,N-dimethyltyramine (see also *synephrine*)

What it is: According to Pellati and Benvenuti (2007), hordenine, along with synephrine, is one of the most important biologically active (stimulant) constituents of the *Citrus aurantium* (bitter orange) fruits. The alkaloid can also be isolated from germinated barley seeds as well as cacti and some algae and fungi.

Function: Depending on the route of administration, hordenine is known to stimulate the central nervous system, inducing cardiovascular changes such as increased heart rate and contractility as well as elevated blood pressure in animal studies. More recently, Hahn and colleagues (2022) have further noted that the compound has several pharmacological properties such as being a dopamine D2 receptor agonist, although the intestinal barrier may need to be circumvented for such an effect.

Performance benefit: Dietary supplement marketers may be focusing on hordenine's ability to stimulate beta-2 adrenergic receptors in skeletal muscle. Such a selective adrenalin-like effect could have effects on muscular strength or bodyfat reduction; performance-enhancing drugs like clenbuterol operate via this mechanism. However, insufficient evidence exists to support this effect.

Research: Little scientific evidence exists in humans.

Common usage: There is not enough scientific evidence to suggest an appropriate dose for athletic or weight management effects.

Health concerns: Hordenine may interact with medications such as MAO inhibitors and other stimulants such as caffeine. Consumption is best avoided.

Horny Goat Weed 

aka *epimedium, Epimedium grandiflorum, Herba epimedii, icariin*

What it is: Horny goat weed is a more common name used to refer to *Herba epimedii*, a plant used in traditional Chinese medicine; legend claims that a Chinese goat herder noticed increased sexual activity in his flock after consuming the plant. The plant has been sold as a dietary supplement for many years and is claimed to have a range of benefits, including an ability to increase sex drive, treat sexual dysfunction, increase testosterone, and improve vitality.

Function: Horny goat weed is thought by some to act as a natural testosterone booster. As men age, testosterone production begins to decline. This drop in testosterone limits the ability to build muscle and maintain strength. It also decreases sex drive, lowers vitality, and can leave many men feeling depressed. Horny goat weed contains the flavonoid icariin, which is believed to be the active flavonoid responsible for beneficial effects.

Performance benefit: Supplementation is most common among male athletes looking for a natural alternative to anabolic steroids to increase testosterone levels. Testosterone, a powerful anabolic hormone, increases muscle mass and improves strength and power.

Research: The data on horny goat weed remain debatable. Most research trials on horny goat weed, icariin, and *Herba epimedii* have used mouse and rat models. There are no readily available clinical trials on humans related to its effects on testosterone. More research has focused on its use in treating and preventing osteoporosis and erectile dysfunction. Mostly animal models have been used to test these benefits. Presently, there is no scientific research backing any claims for horny goat weed as a natural testosterone booster for athletes.

Common usage: Typically, dietary supplements sold as horny goat weed contain roughly 500 mg and recommend using 60 to 90 mg before physical exertion. These recommendations have no scientific data to validate them.

Health concerns: The safety is unknown at this time. Few human research trials exist, making it difficult to determine any potential health concerns related to use. One review by Zhang and colleagues (2022), which focused on rheumatoid arthritis and relied largely on rodent models, found that, although *Herba epimedii* is relatively safe for clinical use, it could cause drug-induced liver injury; the authors cautioned against large doses or long-term use.

⚠ SUPPLEMENT WARNING

Horny goat weed is often marketed as a natural supplement for the enhancement of sexual performance. Consumers should proceed with caution when purchasing natural products making these claims: A recent analysis of nine dietary supplements intended to improve sexual performance found four of the nine to be adulterated with analogues of Viagra. Two others were adulterated with other drugs not approved for supplemental use (Balayssac et al., 2012).

Hot Pepper

(see *capsicum*)

Huang Qi

(see *astragalus*)

Huperzine A 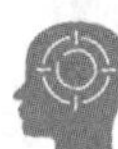 

aka *Chinese club moss (Huperzia serrata), fir club moss (Huperzia selago),*

What it is: Huperzine A is an extract derived from a Chinese moss, *Huperzia serrata*, sometimes appearing in preworkout supplements.

Function: It purportedly increases concentrations of acetylcholine in the body (acetylcholinesterase inhibitor)—enough to enhance memory, particularly in those with cognitive decline.

Performance benefit: Enhanced neuromotor or cognitive ability could conceivably enhance those aspects of sport performance (muscular force, processing of complex sensory inputs during dynamic sports).

Research: A 2013 meta-analysis by Yang and colleagues concluded that huperzine may improve cognition in participants with Alzheimer's disease but that "the findings should be interpreted with caution due to the poor methodological quality of the included trials." Among healthy participants, Morasch and colleagues (2015) reported that a single oral dose of huperzine A (100-200 mcg) significantly inhibited acetylcholinesterase (suggestive of elevated central acetylcholine concentrations) but did not enhance neurobehavioral performance. The authors posited that there may be a ceiling effect in young, healthy participants, who do not exhibit hampered cholinergic activity. A more recent direct investigation by Wessinger and colleagues (2021) studied 11 women and 4 men acutely ingesting 200 mcg of huperzine A and concluded no cognitive effects (verbal/word fluency and Stroop tests) or muscular benefit (e.g., hand grip strength, vertical jump) in these exercise-trained individuals; the authors questioned its inclusion in preworkout supplements. Longer-term use in exercisers needs further investigation.

Common usage: A common dosing regimen used by adults is 200 to 500 mcg/day for up to 6 months.

Health concerns: Huperzine A has been reported to induce oral and gastrointestinal side effects in some persons. Huperzine should be avoided by those who are also taking pro- or anticholinergic drugs.

Hyaluronic Acid (HA) 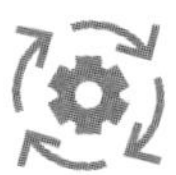 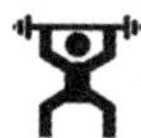 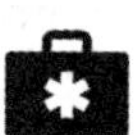

aka *hyaluronan, hyaluronate*

What it is: Hyaluronic acid (HA) is a "gooey, slippery substance that your body produces naturally. Scientists have found hyaluronic acid throughout the body, especially in eyes, joints and skin" (Cleveland Clinic, 2022). According to Stern (2004), there are 15 g of hyaluronan in a 70 kg individual. Commercially, it is made via bacterial fermentation or from rooster combs.

Function: This chain-like (polymer) polysaccharide can attract water and serve as a scaffolding in the soft tissue building processes, which could be relevant to athletes needing joint repair.

Performance benefit: HA could potentially decrease pain and inflammation, with enhanced joint lubrication and maintenance for athletes enduring the rigors of resistance training (as well as weight-bearing activities like running). The FDA approved HA injections for use in the knees. According to the Arthritis Foundation (2023), injections for osteoarthritis are typically most effective in people with mild to moderate progression of the condition.

Research: Jensen and colleagues (2015) concluded that 2 to 3 tablespoons of hyaluronan (30 to 45 mL orally, at 5 mg/mL) over 4 weeks (*n* = 72) decreased chronic pain enough to reduce the need for pain medications. The higher dose was reportedly more effective. Oliva and colleagues (2021) further stated that it has value for various tendinopathies.

Common usage: Hyaluronic acid can be taken by mouth, applied topically or, with a prescription, directly injected into joints. It is sometimes sold in a combination formula with vitamin C, glucosamine, collagen, or other joint supplements. Oral HA supplement capsules are typically 50 to 250 mg. Consumers should exercise caution when reviewing the doses in supplements, which may pertain to contents beyond HA.

Health concerns: Hyaluronic acids has been reported as safe by the Cleveland Clinic and other sources. However, it is prudent to speak with a health care provider about symptoms such as arthritis or soft tissue injuries.

Hydroxy-Beta-Methylbutyrate (HMB)

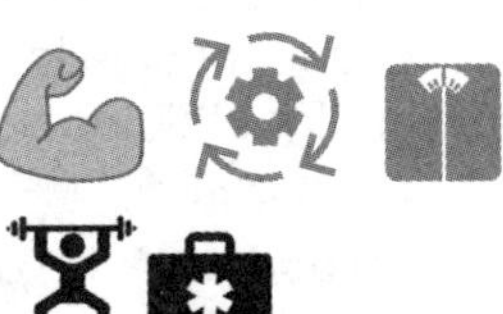

(see also *leucine*)

What it is: Hydroxy-beta-methylbutyrate (HMB) is a metabolite of the amino acid leucine. When leucine is metabolized, it is converted into alpha-ketoisocaproate (α-KIC), which is further converted into HMB. Roughly 5% of leucine is converted into HMB. HMB became popular in the 1990s when Juven—a combination of HMB, arginine, and glutamine— was developed to help prevent losses in lean body mass in cancer and AIDS patients. Juven is currently often targeted at wound healing and relies on its unique combination of ingredients toward that end.

Function: The exact mechanisms of HMB are unknown; however, a couple of theories exist. HMB is believed to upregulate (increase) the gene expression of the anabolic hormone IGF1 (insulin-like growth factor 1) in skeletal muscles, which would assist in building muscle as well as preventing muscle breakdown. Additionally, HMB might stimulate muscle building or protein synthesis directly by affecting the mTOR pathway, which is a key regulator of protein synthesis. Finally, the most promising theory involves an ability of HMB to prevent protein breakdown by inhibiting the ubiquitin-proteasome pathway, which is involved in the breakdown of proteins in the body, including in muscle (Zanchi et al., 2011).

Performance benefit: HMB has a number of potential benefits for athletes. Because of its ability to prevent protein breakdown, supplementation would lessen the catabolic effects of exercise and training on muscle, thereby assisting athletes in maintaining and building muscle mass through training. HMB might also assist injured athletes by preventing some of the losses in muscle mass experienced during immobilization or limited activity and possibly limit extreme muscle soreness experienced from heavy training and competition.

Research: Unfortunately, research studies to date have produced mixed results. A systematic review and meta-analysis by Jakubowski and colleagues (2020) found that HMB does produce a small effect on total body mass gain, but this effect does not translate into significantly greater increases in fat-free mass, strength, or decreases in body fat during periods of resistance training. They concluded that their findings did not support the use of HMB for the purpose of improving body composition or strength. It may be noted that this laboratory, the Kinesiology Department of McMaster Univeristy has reported positive muscle protein synthesis effects with HMB's parent compound, leucine. Earlier research on HMB was contentious as well. A meta-analysis conducted in 2003 concluded that HMB did produce statistically significant effects on both strength and lean body mass; however, this review was criticized for including only nine studies (Nissen & Sharp, 2003). Taken together, research continues to produce mixed results, and more research is needed to provide a better understanding of these differences. It appears that the benefits of HMB are most significant in untrained populations who experience more significant muscle damage as a result of training. In addition, HMB might benefit athletes during times of heightened training volume and intensity or when exposed to different types of physical stress or training their bodies have not adapted to (Wilson et al., 2008). Although no studies to date have been done related to injured athletes, this is another a potential area of benefit: One recent study found HMB capable of preventing muscle loss in rats during immobilization (Hao, 2011). HMB may be most promising for athletes suffering from injury or during heavy, intensified periods of training and competition.

Common usage: A 1 g dose of HMB taken 3 times/day is recommended; however, more research is needed to validate this recommendation (Gallagher et al., 2000).

Health concerns: HMB is safe for use by athletes and has been shown to decrease risk factors related to cardiovascular disease. Research found HMB to lower LDL cholesterol and blood pressure and to have no effect on HDL cholesterol (Nissen et al., 2000).

Hydroxocobalamin

(see *vitamin B$_{12}$*)

Hydroxycitric Acid (HCA) 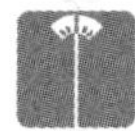

aka *Citrimax (brand name), Garcinia cambogia, hydroxicitrate*

What it is: Hydroxycitric acid (HCA) is found in plants such as *Garcinia cambogia, Garcinia indica,* and *Garcinia atroviridis*. These plants are typically native to South Asia and India. HCA is commonly found in weight-loss supplements.

Function: The mechanisms of HCA are speculative. Some scientists believe that HCA causes weight loss by inhibiting ATP-citrate-lyase, an enzyme involved in the synthesis of fatty acids, via a link with carbohydrate metabolism; others believe HCA increases the release of serotonin, leading to appetite suppression. HCA may inhibit the carbohydrate digestive enzyme alpha-amylase, thereby reducing carbohydrate absorption and metabolism. None of these mechanisms is currently proven. Most scientific studies note the ability of HCA to reduce food intake or produce an anorectic effect.

Performance benefit: If the proposed benefits of HCA are true, it would be of benefit for athletes wanting to improve body composition and lose weight.

Research: Evidence in support of use by athletes remain controversial. Some research studies in animals have been positive (Saito et al., 2005). HCA was shown to suppress food intake and prevent weight gain in rats fed high-carbohydrate diets. Human trials have also been undertaken, including a 2011 systemic review and meta-analysis of randomized clinical trials related to HCA (Onakpoya et al., 2011), which concluded that HCA can generate short-term weight loss; however, the magnitude of loss was small and only observed in less rigorous trials. When more rigorous trials are considered, HCA has not regularly produced a statistically significant amount of weight loss. Further, during exercise, data appear to be mixed: Lim and colleagues (2002) concluded "short-term administration of HCA [250 mg daily for 5 days vs. placebo] enhances endurance performance with increasing fat oxidation, which spares glycogen utilization during moderate intensity exercise in athletes." However, van Loon and colleagues (2000) concluded "HCA, even when provided in large quantities [3.1 mL/kg HCA solution (19 g/L)], does not increase total fat oxidation in vivo in endurance-trained humans." Therefore, HCA's relevance as a weight-loss supplement or an ergogenic aid is questionable. Often, scientists recommend that more rigorous, longer-duration, and better-reported studies be completed. Finally, a review of herbal weight-loss supplements concluded that "while HCA appears to be well tolerated, there is limited data with regards to its efficacy" (Egras et al., 2011). It is unknown if the source of HCA has an impact on results, and various trials have only ranged from 2 to 12 weeks in duration, highlighting the need for longer-term studies.

Common usage: The dosage, which depends on the herbal (fruit) extract of *Garcinia cambogia* versus HCA per se, typically ranges from about 0.5 g to 2.8 g/day for the herbal extract. This dosage is commonly distributed into two to three smaller doses of 300 to 1,000 mg consumed before meals. Consumers should note that the herb is often sold in a formula with other ingredients.

Health concerns: It is unclear whether the use of HCA is completely safe, with some studies reporting that subjects experienced headache, nausea, and upper respiratory and gastrointestinal tract symptoms. Further, an analysis by Zovi and colleagues (2022) addressed the "most recent literature that analysed the herb-induced liver disease due to the use of hydroxycitric acid, from the first alert coming from the European Food and Drug Administration in 2009, to the last recent European food alerts from 2020 to 2021." These authors included, "It is noteworthy that in some cases it demonstrated the relationship between hydroxycitric acid and hepatotoxicity." Athletes should also be aware that the mechanisms of HCA are related to suppressing appetite and reducing food intake, which can negatively affect performance if calorie restriction is severe. Taken together, this information suggests it is advisable to check with a health care professional.

Hydroxytyrosol (HT) 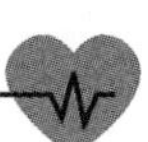  

aka *olive leaf extract, olive polyphenols*

What it is: Hydroxytyrosol (HT) is a phenolic phytochemical in olive leaves and oil that exhibits antioxidant properties. Because hydroxytyrosol is a degradation product of oleuropein, which is hydrolyzed during processing, olive oil can have greater concentrations of hydroxytyrosol than olives (Goldsmith et al., 2018).

Function: It may improve endothelial function (blood vessel health or blood flow), decrease oxidative stress, and be neuro- and cardioprotective. This latter effect appears most represented in clinical studies. This is in line with broad support for the Mediterranean diet (which focuses on olive oil) on cardiometabolic health. Very limited research in athletes suggests enhanced perceived exertion and respiratory recovery.

Performance benefit: Potential benefits for athletes may include enhanced blood flow, mitochondrial function, and perceived exertion.

Research: According to Bertelli and colleagues (2020), hydroxytyrosol is currently the most actively investigated natural phenol. Roberts and colleagues (2023) provided 28 mL of an olive-derived phytocomplex drink 2 times/day (providing ~0.8 mg/kg/day of HT) or placebo to 29 middle-aged recreationally active participants ($\dot{V}O_2$max approximately 50 mL/kg/min) for 16 consecutive days and had them complete submaximal and maximal performance tests before and after exposure. They concluded the HT and its metabolites may provide benefits for aerobic exercise (e.g., lower perceived exertion at participants' lactate turn point as well as modestly improved acute respiratory recovery). However, they concluded that "the overall change in exercise performance was not different" between the intervention and placebo and "there is a paucity of scientific research surrounding HT and exercise performance."

Common usage: As olive fruit extract, doses range from 50 to 500 mg; as hydroxytyrosol, doses range from 10 to 25 mg.

Health concerns: Noguera-Navarro and colleagues (2023) state that no untoward effects have been shown even at very high doses. Vijakumaran and colleagues (2023) reported that "hydroxytyrosol is the only phytochemical with European Food Safety Authority (EFSA)-approved health benefits with safety approval." As a guideline, EFSA suggests that a minimum of 5 mg of HT be consumed to achieve physiological benefits.

Hypoxanthine Riboside, Hypoxanthine

(see *inosine*)

Icariin

(see *horny goat weed*)

Indian Ginger

(see *ginger*)

Indian Ginseng

(see *Withania somnifera*)

Inosine

aka *hypoxanthine riboside, hypoxanthine, 9-beta-D-ribofuranosylhypoxanthine*

What it is: A member of a chemical family called purine nucleotides, inosine is a molecule that serves as one of the basic structural compounds comprising cells. It can be found dispersed in all tissues within the human body, in particular cardiac and skeletal muscle. Inosine can be derived naturally from such dietary sources as organ meats and Brewer's yeast. Supplementation use by athletes became popular in the 1990s when inosine was marketed as enhancing muscle-building capacity as well as increasing energy and endurance during training and competition.

Function: Involved in the production of 2,3 DPG (a substance that facilitates the transport of oxygen from red blood cells to the muscles and heart), inosine is purported to help promote blood flow, enhance the oxygen-carrying capacity of the blood, and increase endurance performance. In addition, as a precursor to the manufacture of adenosine (a molecule involved in the synthesis of ATP), inosine is thought to help optimize energy production and protect against muscle fatigue.

Performance benefit: Athletes may benefit from enhanced energy and endurance during training and competition.

Research: Little research in recent years has overturned the negative early findings. Well-designed studies evaluating the ergogenic benefit of inosine are limited and have not been favorable. In fact, in some cases inosine actually impaired performance: One small double-blind study of highly trained runners failed to demonstrate any performance benefit of a 2-day supplementation protocol that incorporated 6,000 mg of inosine/day leading up to a run workout that included a submaximal warm-up run, a maximal 3 mi (4.8 km) treadmill run, and a competitive 3 mi (4.8 km) treadmill run (Williams et al., 1990). In fact, the placebo group actually posted significantly faster times, suggesting actual impairment by oral inosine supplementation. Similarly, a study of 10 highly trained cyclists found that a supplementation protocol incorporating 5,000 mg/day of inosine over 5 days actually impaired the performance (compared to a placebo) of a cycling exercise protocol that incorporated a Wingate 30-second test, 30-minute time trial, and sprint to fatigue (Starling et al., 1996). Increasing the dose to 10,000 mg over 5 or 10 days during an exercise protocol that incorporated a series of bike sprints followed by a 20-minute time trial also failed to yield any performance benefit (McNaughton, Dalton, & Tarr, 1999). Indeed, Nascimento and colleagues (2021) pointed out that that inosine may contribute to or mediate adenosine's effects, a theory reinforced by studies that deem inosine to be a natural trigger of adenosine receptors. (Note that caffeine operates in an opposing way, blocking adenosine to reduce fatigue.) Consequently, the current consensus is that inosine does not seem to improve endurance performance and may even have a detrimental impact on it.

Common usage: Available in tablet or capsule form, inosine can be consumed 45 to 60 minutes before training or competition, preferably with food. Because study results have not been favorable related to performance benefits, dosing recommendations cannot be made with confidence, though study doses have generally ranged between 5,000 and 10,000 mg/day.

Health concerns: Excessive intake of inosine may increase blood levels of uric acid, increasing the risk for kidney stones. Thus, supplementation should be avoided by athletes with gout or kidney disorders. Other reported symptoms include stomach upset, nausea, and bloating.

Inositol 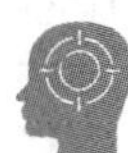 

aka *D-chiro-inositol, hexahydroxycyclohexane, myoinositol*

What it is: Inositol is a carbohydrate similar to glucose that appears in multiple forms, one of which is myoinositol. Reportedly, myoinositol and D-chiro-inositol are most common in supplements.

Function: Inositol appears to affect the production of serotonin, a neurotransmitter that affects mood. Myoinositol may also be effective for reducing insulin resistance and other symptoms of metabolic syndrome such as hyperlipidemia or blood pressure. However, more data are needed, particularly in athletes.

Performance benefit: Although some research suggests improved glucose tolerance in certain populations, this is not typically a concern with athletes. Performance applications may include reducing the anxiety of competition or treating depression, which can coincide with overtraining. This, however, is speculative.

Research: Studied populations include those with gestational diabetes and insulin-resistant postmenopausal women, as well as those with psychiatric conditions. Some data are promising but overall are mixed. Some research suggests anxiety or panic disorders may be reduced with inositol supplementation at 12 to 18 g/day for a month (Benjamin et al., 1995; Palatnik et al., 2001). It has been shown to reduce depression with a similar dosing plan and was described by Levine and colleagues (1995) as a "precursor strategy for a second messenger rather than a neurotransmitter in treating depression." Still, not all research supports the use of inositol in these conditions. Research in athletes is lacking.

Common usage: Myoinositol doses of 4 g/day, split into two doses, taken for up to 6 months have been used for blood sugar-related disorders (not common among athletes). Doses up to 18 g/day for 4 weeks have been used for psychiatric-related conditions.

Health concerns: Doses of up to 18 g/day for a month appear safe. Palatnik and colleagues (2001) stated that inositol has "few known side effects [and] it is attractive to patients who are ambivalent about taking psychiatric medication." Inositol may affect blood sugar, as noted, and thus could interact with diabetes medications or during exercise, in which blood glucose concentrations may decline over the session.

Iron (Fe) 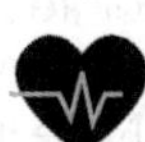 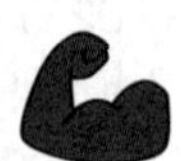     

aka *elemental iron, ferrous bisglycinate, ferrous carbonate anhydrous, ferrous fumarate, ferrous gluconate, ferrous pyrophosphate, ferrous sulfate*

What it is: Iron, a trace mineral, is a major component of hemoglobin, whose role is to transport oxygen from the lungs to the muscles via the blood. Research has shown that exercise creates an added demand for iron. Failure to meet this added demand through dietary intake and proper absorption of such whole food sources as whole grains, leafy greens, dried fruit, red meat, fish, and poultry can compromise blood iron stores and lead to iron-deficiency anemia (IDA).

Function: Without enough iron in the blood, the body becomes starved for oxygen; ATP cannot be properly synthesized, limiting work capacity and leading to pronounced feelings of fatigue. IDA occurs in three stages, with stage 3 having the most detrimental effect on athletic performance. Most athletes with iron depletion have a stage 1 deficiency, also known as nonanemia iron deficiency, which is diagnosed when ferritin, the storage form of iron, falls below normal. If stage 1 iron deficiency is left undetected for several months, an athlete may develop stage 2 deficiency when red blood cells and consequent oxygen transfer decrease, negatively affecting exercise capacity. The final stage of iron deficiency, stage 3, is detected by insufficient hemoglobin and a low concentration of red blood cells; stage 3 leads to feelings of intense fatigue, compromised physical ability, and decreased athletic performance.

ATHLETES' TIP

Sports anemia is a term applied to endurance athletes who have lower-than-normal hemoglobin levels but normal levels of other iron status indicators. This situation is a response to the increase in blood volume that accompanies training; therefore, it is not a true anemia, nor should it be treated like one.

Performance benefit: By restoring hemoglobin and the blood iron levels of iron-deficient and anemic athletes, oxygen delivery to working muscles and ATP production increase, thereby allowing the athlete to better meet the metabolic demands of aerobic activity. Iron may also help improve both short- and long-term recovery times by improving immune functionality.

Research: There have been reports showing a high number of athletes are affected by iron deficiency, particularly stage 1. One study of college athletes revealed 47% of the female participants to exhibit serum ferritin levels of 30 ng/mL or less—within the parameters of stage 1 iron deficiency (Nabeyama et al., 2023); another showed 46% of nonprofessional competitive female athletes also fell within the parameters of stage 1 iron deficiency (Sims et al., 2022). Although male athletes tend to suffer from anemia less often than female athletes, there have been reports of over 10% of male athletes falling within the parameters of stage 1 iron deficiency (Roy et al., 2022). Athletes tend to be more prone to iron deficiencies for several reasons, including increased losses brought on by microischemia, hemolysis, and sweating (Clénen et al., 2015). Furthermore, the inflammatory response that occurs with exercise can reduce iron uptake when demands are elevated to support increased erythropoiesis and rebuilding processes, triggering an imbalance (Sim et al., 2019). Poor iron status is often a side effect of low energy availability secondary to increases in hepcidin, a hormone that regulates how the body uses iron, which, in turn, inhibits iron absorption (Badenhorst et al, 2019). Insufficient dietary intake of iron is also often correlated with low energy availability, particularly in cases of disordered eating and eating disorders where energy intake is intentionally restricted (Petkus et al, 2017). Female athletes are also more prone to iron deficiency due to menstrual bleeding. Any stage of iron deficiency can negatively affect performance, with endurance, power, strength, speed, coordination, concentration, immune function, and recovery all potentially being disrupted (Sim et al., 2019). However, there remains controversy about when (i.e., at what stage of deficiency) iron supplementation becomes most beneficial. In most circumstances, there appears to be no performance benefit associated with iron supplementation without iron deficiency or with nonanemia (stage 1) iron deficiency, particularly in those athletes with ferritin levels above 30 ng/L (Borrione et al., 2011; Solberg & Reikvam, 2023). However, there are variables that may affect so-called optimal serum levels of ferritin for performance, including training environment. For athletes living or competing at moderate to high altitudes (2,500 m+), for example, hematological adaptations to hypoxia are highly dependent on adequate iron stores, with some research suggesting ferritin levels above 50 ng/mL are needed to promote optimal performance. Thus, dietary adjustments and iron supplementation may be warranted in athletes with levels falling short of this who train or compete at altitude (Clénin et al., 2015; Okazaki et al., 2019).

Common usage: The RDA for iron stands at 18 mg/day for females 19 to 50; lower levels of 8 mg/day are warranted for males 19 to 50 and males and females over 50. During pregnancy, RDA for iron increases to 27 mg. Athletes at risk for iron deficiency, including female athletes whose menstrual blood loss often affects iron or those athletes with serum ferritin levels under 30 ng/L (or <50 ng/L at altitudes 2500 m+), may increase to 20 to 30 mg/day from whole food or supplementation doses. Properly diagnosed cases of IDA, especially stage 2 and stage 3, should be treated with therapeutic doses of supplemental iron, preferably ferrous sulfate or ferrous bisglycinate due to enhanced absorption rates and in slow-release form to reduce constipation. The treatment dose will depend on the cause and severity of iron deficiency, and thus it is important to work with a health professional to determine an appropriate supplementation protocol. Therapeutic doses of elemental iron range for adult athletes are 50 to 100 mg taken 3 times/day for a total of 150 to 300 mg/day. Youth athletes are recommended to take a total of 4-6mg/kg/day yet split into 3 separate doses. 4 to 6 mg/kg/Taking 500 mg of vitamin C or drinking a glass of orange juice may help enhance absorption of the iron. Correction of anemic conditions can take anywhere from 3 to 6 months, though improvements will be seen as quickly as within a few weeks.

Health concerns: Dietary iron supplementation is not recommended for athletes with normal blood iron levels. Some researchers have linked excess iron to diabetes, cancer, increased risk for infection, exacerbation of arthritis, and heart disease. Large doses, generally indicated at levels of 20 mg/kg/day, are toxic; levels above 60 mg/kg/day can be fatal.

Isoinokosterone

(see *ecdysteroids*)

Isoleucine

(see *branched-chain amino acids*)

Isomaltulose 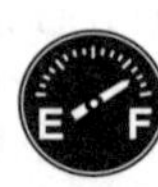  

aka *Palatinose (brand name), 6-0-a-D-glucopyranosyl-D-fructose*

What it is: A natural constituent of honey and sugar cane as well as commercially manufactured from bacterial fermentation of sucrose, isomaltulose (marketed in the supplement industry as Palatinose) causes a slower rise in blood glucose than other sugars. As a result, it may have beneficial applications for hypoglycemic and diabetic athletes as well as athletes looking for an easy-to-digest preworkout carbohydrate option that better sustains blood sugar.

Function: As a carbohydrate with a low glycemic index, isomaltulose helps keep insulin increases at bay, which helps protect against blood sugar crashes that can cause dizziness, fatigue, and diminished performance. This is especially relevant for athletes vulnerable to hypoglycemia (low blood sugar). Furthermore, studies suggest isomaltulose enhances the oxidation of fat for energy, thereby demonstrating potential benefit for glycogen sparing and enhanced endurance as well as benefits for athletes wanting to shed body fat.

Performance benefit: Athletes, especially those inflicted with diabetes or hypoglycemia, may benefit from better control of blood sugar, improved metabolic risk factors, and favorable body composition changes.

Research: Research evaluating the benefits of isomaltulose has primarily been conducted with subjects having preexisting health issues such as metabolic syndrome and diabetes. Although some results have been favorable when it comes to glycemic and insulinemic responses in this population, the translation to a healthy population, particularly athletes, is less clear (Xie et al., 2022). The applications for athletes with type 1 diabetes have shown promise after a study demonstrated consumption of isomaltulose at a dose of 0.6 g/kg in coordination with a reduced dose of rapid-acting insulin improved blood glucose responses to a high-intensity exercise protocol: Subjects maintained both speed and endurance compared to an isocaloric dose of dextrose (Bracken et al., 2012). Similarly, West and colleagues (2011) found consumption of 75 g of isomaltulose 2 hours before 45 minutes of treadmill running at 80% VO(2peak) improved the blood glucose responses of type 1 diabetics during and after exercise through reduced glycogen and improved fat oxidation during the later stages of exercise (West et al., 2011). Yet, when looking at a healthy population of recreational runners, no differences were seen in glycogen and fat oxidation rates or treadmill running performance (70-minute constant load trial at 70% maximal running speed followed by a time-to-exhaustion test at 85% Vmax (maximal running speed) after ingesting 50 g isomaltulose versus maltodextrin or glucose, though blood sugar fluctuations during the treadmill test were less pronounced (Notbohm et al., 2021). Even so, isomaltulose offers an attractive, low-glycemic (solicits steadier blood sugar response), easy-to-digest carbohydrate source for athletes, particularly diabetic athletes, to consume pre- and postworkout as well as during carbo-loading protocols (Achten et al., 2007).

Common usage: Isomaltulose is commonly added as an ingredient in meal replacement powders and shakes; it is also available as a standalone powder or liquid carbohydrate source. As a preworkout snack, 50 g or 0.25 to 0.3 g/lb (0.11 to 0.14 g/kg) can be consumed 1 hour before starting. A similar dose can be consumed immediately after workout to support recovery. Isomaltulose can also be incorporated into carbo-loading routines, which comprises 3.6 to 4.5 g carbohydrate/lb (1.64 to 2.0 g/kg) daily for 3 days leading up to an endurance event.

Health concerns: Similar to the use of any highly concentrated source of carbohydrate, risk for gastrointestinal disturbances such as stomach upset and diarrhea increase exponentially with concentrations above 10% (more than 25 g carbohydrate/8 oz [0.23 L] of water consumed).

Jamaica Ginger

(see *ginger*)

Japanese Silver Apricot

(see *Ginkgo biloba*)

Ketones 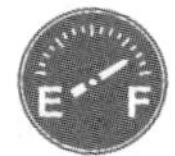

aka ketone bodies (acetoacetate, beta-hydroxybutyrate [BHB], acetone), ketone ester (KE), ketone salts

What it is: The body makes three types of ketone bodies from the partial breakdown of fatty acids: acetoacetate, beta-hydroxybutyrate (BHB), and acetone. This typically happens on very low carbohydrate diets (less than 50 g/day, which varies by individual), or more dramatically, when diabetes is uncontrolled. Exogenous (supplemental) ketone supplements on the market are typically sold as salts. Ketone esters are a more recent market development but have been used in research.

Function: These supplements are meant to be a fuel source for contracting skeletal muscle and (when fat-adapted) the brain. Researchers are still learning how providing this fuel as a supplement interacts with circulating glucose. Supplementation with ketone bodies creates a unique metabolic environment in that the body can be replete with carbohydrate yet have considerable circulating ketone bodies at the same time; that is, it does not need to be in a state of relative carbohydrate starvation for this fuel to appear, as is typical. This makes it a curious phenomenon for researchers, who hypothesize a dose-dependent 2 mM performance threshold of circulating BHB.

Performance benefit: It is feasible that elite athletes or those seeking to enhance body composition by training on a low-carbohydrate diet might benefit metabolically (e.g., muscle glycogen sparing, reduced lactate) from the alternate fuel. However, this is still under study.

Research: According to Margolis and O'Fallon (2020), ketone monoester supplementation results in a greater acute increase in BHB concentrations than ketone salts; a 20 to 40 g total dose (depending on ketone supplement formulation) is most common in their reviewed studies. From a performance perspective, work by Cox and colleagues (2016) led to bicycle ergometer time trial performance that was approximately 2% greater following ketone ester (KE) plus carbohydrate (CHO) supplementation (573 mg KE/kg, in a 40:60 ratio with CHO) versus CHO alone. This was described as representing a modest increase in physical capacity in highly trained athletes ($n = 8$) that was close to the sensitivity of measurement (i.e., questionable). In some contrast, recent data from Howard and colleagues (2023) investigated 573 mg KE/kg plus 110 g glucose, versus 110 g glucose before and during 90 minutes of steady-state treadmill exercise in 12 subjects. These researchers suggested that blood glucose utilization is similar between KE plus CHO versus CHO alone. Further, KE plus CHO supplementation results in lower physical performance compared with CHO alone. As noted in Lowery (2020), "Contrasting results from existing studies using different ketone compounds, performance tests, dosages, and analytic techniques highlight that further research is required." Similarly, Margolis and O'Fallon (2020) stated in their systematic review, "Heterogeneity across studies makes it difficult to conclude any benefit or detriment to consuming ketone supplements on physical performance."

Common usage: As noted previously, depending on the form of ketone supplement, 20 to 40 g total dose is most common in the literature, with ketone monoesters increasing circulating levels the most.

Health concerns: Ketone supplementation may cause gastrointestinal distress in sensitive persons.

Lactobacillus

(see *probiotics*)

L-Amino Succinate, L-Aspartic Acid

(see *aspartate*)

Lauric Acid

(see *medium-chain triglycerides*)

Lentinula Edodes (Shiitake)

(see *medicinal mushrooms*)

Leucine 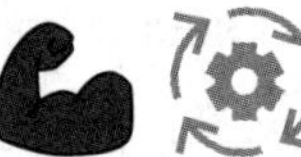 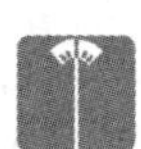 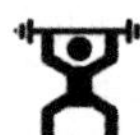 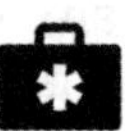 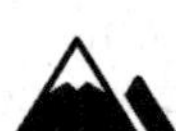

aka *L-leucine, D-leucine (see also branched-chain amino acids and hydroxy-beta-methylbutyrate)*

What it is: Leucine is an essential amino acid, meaning that it cannot be synthesized in the body and must be obtained from the diet. It is found in high-protein foods such as lentils, beef, fish, chicken, nuts, pork, eggs, chickpeas, and perhaps most abundantly in milk (whey protein). Leucine is unique in that it is also a branched-chain amino acid, which can be oxidized in skeletal muscle, unlike most other essential amino acids, which are mainly catabolized in the liver.

Function: Amino acids are often viewed as building blocks for the synthesis of proteins in the body. Leucine is much more than a building block and can signal cells to begin muscle building by acting somewhere in the cell-signaling pathway known as mTOR, which is responsible for initiating protein synthesis; it is thought to enhance this pathway's signals and cause it to increase production of proteins (Pasiakos & McClung, 2011).

Performance benefit: The role of leucine in the stimulation of protein synthesis has a number of applications for athletes. Supplementation with leucine before and during exercise may indeed prevent the breakdown of proteins and result in less muscle damage as a result of training. Postexercise leucine supplementation would signal protein synthesis, the recovery and rebuilding of tissues. Most notable is muscle protein synthesis (MPS), which should be specifically considered when reading the protein and leucine literature—as opposed to studies using whole body protein synthesis. Finally, as a branched-chain amino acid, leucine could provide a fuel source for muscles during exercise and improve performance.

Research: Although research supports the use of leucine before exercise to lessen protein breakdown and muscle damage and after exercise to stimulate and enhance protein synthesis, there is no benefit to leucine supplementation when adequate amounts of high-quality proteins are consumed either before or after exercise. It is therefore important when evaluating these results to take whole proteins into consideration. However, leucine supplementation is advantageous if adequate amounts of high-quality proteins cannot be consumed at these times. Protein synthesis is maximized in young healthy subjects with a 20 g dose of high-quality complete proteins, equivalent to roughly 9 to 10 g of essential amino acids and roughly 1.8 g of leucine (Kerksick et al., 2008; Moore et al., 2009). Older subjects are now known to exhibit anabolic resistance, however, and likely require more than 20 g of protein to optimize protein synthesis. Other studies, depending on their methods, have shown that additional leucine above 1.8 g does not further enhance protein synthesis (Pasiakos & McClung, 2011). This is not a fixed ceiling but it does illustrate an approximate dose. Phillips (2017) has stated "stimulation of MPS would require ingestion of a protein that is higher in leucine or fortification of a lower leucine-containing protein [lower quality or lower dose] with leucine." Research related to the performance-enhancing effects of leucine during exercise is less promising, and most early studies showed no benefit (Negro et al., 2008).

Common usage: To support muscle protein synthesis and recovery, 0.03 to 0.045 g/kg of body mass is recommended to be consumed pre- and postexercise. For a 165 lb (74.8 kg) athlete, this would be equivalent to 2.25 to 3.4 g of leucine before and after exercise. Note that a dipeptide of leucine (two units of this amino acid connected) is being studied for potentially superior effects.

Health concerns: Leucine supplementation within recommendations is safe and does not produce adverse effects.

Leuzea Carthamoides

(see *ecdysteroids*)

Levoglutamide, L-Glutamine

(see *glutamine*)

L-Glutathione

(see *glutathione*)

Linum Usitatissimum, Linseed Oil

(see *flaxseed*)

Lipoic Acid, Lipolate

(see *alpha-lipoic acid*)

L-Selenomethionine

(see *selenium*)

L-Tyrosine

(see *tyrosine*)

Lutein 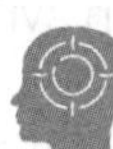 

aka *macular pigment*

What it is: Lutein is a carotenoid compound found in green leafy vegetables like kale and spinach as well as in other foods, such as egg yolks. Chicken egg yolks present a more bioavailable source of lutein (as well as zeaxanthin, a related carotenoid) compared to fruits and vegetables; a typical U.S. diet contains 1 to 3 mg/day (Abdel-Aal et al., 2013). High concentrations of lutein are found in the human retina.

Function: Lutein is commonly marketed as an antioxidant and protector of eye health. This does have some research support. According to a review by Mitra and colleagues in 2021, interest in this antioxidant compound continues to be focused on neuroprotection and vision. Indeed, there is a relationship between neural processing and vision.

Performance benefit: Enhancement of visual processing speed could potentially enhance performance in sports requiring visual tracking.

Research: According to Bovier and Hammond (2014), optical density of macular pigment is positively correlated with temporal contrast sensitivity function. Further, they reported that their intervention with lutein and zeaxanthin increased processing speed even in young healthy subjects. Similarly, in a paper exploring their potential applications to baseball players, Hammond and Fletcher (2012) stated that lutein and zeaxanthin might increase temporal processing speeds and reduce glare, concluding that "supplementation with lutein and zeaxanthin could potentially improve visual performance by increasing both hardware (optical effects within the eye) and software (cognitive and processing abilities)." These researchers also noted that baseball players are exposed to high levels of actinic (shorter-wave, blue/ultraviolet) light stress, which lutein may help reduce. Consumers should use caution when reading lutein-cognition data on very young or very old nonathletic populations—population specificity matters.

Common usage: Abdel-Aal and colleagues (2013) reported that approximately 6 mg/day has been related to decreased risk of advanced macular degeneration. Popular brands such as Ocuvite and Now include 5 to 10 mg of lutein, sometimes in combination with zeaxanthin. Athletes should note that less research exists on the sports-specific benefits of lutein than on overall health.

Health concerns: According to Shao and Hathcock (2006), evidence of safety is strong at intakes up to 20 mg/day.

Maca 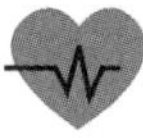 

aka *maca powder, maca root, Lepidium meyenii, Peruvian ginseng*

What it is: Maca is a root from the brassica family and traditional medication native to the Andes of Peru. It is also grown in China and around the globe.

Function: Claims about the benefits of maca range from adaptogenic effects to libido and testosterone enhancement to energy boosts, but there is insufficient evidence in humans to support these claims. However, phytochemicals like macamides and alkaloids may produce biological effects.

Performance benefit: For overreaching athletes, a mild fatigue-fighting, libido-stabilizing, or anti-inflammatory effect during periods of high-volume training could be possible, but population specificity matters and there remains a dearth of data on athletes.

Research: Most related to athletes, Lee and colleagues (2023) studied the effects of 2,500 mg black maca supplementation in 44 male elite athletes over 8 weeks and concluded that changes in aerobic energy systems, particularly in fin swimmers, provided preliminary evidence of improved inflammation and physical fitness. Studies on other populations provide suggestive but indirect evidence as well. A 2022 paper from Honma and colleagues in the journal *Functional Foods in Health and Disease* reported that maca extract containing benzyl glucosinolate (9.6 mg/day) may have antifatigue effects in young women (<45 years) after 4 weeks. Data on exercise-induced fatigue appears largely limited to rodents. Regarding well-being and sexual function, Zenico and colleagues (2009) found a small but significant effect on subjective perception of general and sexual well-being (versus placebo) when 50 Caucasian men with erectile dysfunction consumed 2,400 mg dry maca extract for 12 weeks.

Common usage: Products on the market can contain 500 to 800 mg. Periods of intake spanning of 1 to 4 months have been reported by MedlinePlus.gov.

Health concerns: Maca appears safe to consume in foods, and supplementation of up to 3 g/day for 4 months has been reported to be safe (MedlinePlus.gov). It is advisable for pregnant women to avoid it until more data emerge. Speak with a health care professional about interactions with any medications.

Magnesium (Mg)    

aka *magnesium aspartate, magnesium chloride, magnesium citrate, magnesium gluconate, magnesium oxide, magnesium sulfate*

What it is: As an essential mineral, magnesium is the fourth most abundant element in the body (behind sodium, potassium, and calcium), with a total of 50% to 60% being stored in the skeletal system and the remainder being stored in muscles and soft tissues. Magnesium can be found naturally in such dietary sources as pumpkin seeds, nuts, whole grains, and legumes.

Function: Magnesium plays an instrumental role in maintaining both structural (bone) and biochemical (muscle contraction, nerve transmission, enzyme production) homeostasis in the human body. Magnesium is responsible for 80% of all enzymatic reactions in the body; it regulates virtually every activity, making magnesium balance crucial to an athlete's overall health. Of particular importance from a performance standpoint is the fact that magnesium is required for both aerobic and anaerobic energy production. Magnesium is also involved in reactions necessary for electrolyte balance. Because prolonged exercise increases magnesium loss via sweat, it is thought that supplementation during exercise, generally in the form of a sport drink or electrolyte capsules, can protect against muscle weakness and cramping.

Performance benefit: Athletes, particularly those with poor dietary intake of magnesium, may benefit from enhanced metabolic efficiency during exercise. Magnesium also aids bone health by protecting against bone loss and consequent risk of fracture.

Research: An increased utilization of magnesium during exercise makes athletes more susceptible to magnesium deficiency (Mariño et al., 2020; Rakhra et al., 2021). Indeed, an 8-year analysis of magnesium status in elite international track and field athletes found that 22% of the athletes were identified as clinically deficient (<1.19 mmol/L) on at least one blood test during the study time. Female athletes, athletes with Black or mixed-race ethnicity, athletes with cerebral palsy, and athletes with a history of Achilles or patella tendon pain all had significantly lower magnesium levels than average (Pollock et al., 2019). Additional research has demonstrated low energy availability and menstrual irregularities to be correlated with inadequate intakes of dietary magnesium (Łagowska et al., 2022; Monedero et al., 2023). Thus, special attention might be warranted for certain subpopulations. Lukaski and Nielson (2002) previously established that a diet deficient in magnesium (112 mg/day or 36% of the RDA) over just a month significantly increased the peak oxygen uptake, total and cumulative net oxygen usage, and heart rate for a given training workload in comparison to a period when sufficient magnesium (based on the RDA) was provided through whole foods and supplementation. Furthermore, as the level of magnesium deficiency intensified, so did the metabolic cost of exercise, an established detriment to performance. This also translated similarly to a group of elite basketball, handball, and volleyball players whose performance during several isometric strength and plyometric drills was compromised when magnesium intake fell significantly below the RDA (Santos et al., 2011). A 2012 study by Matias and colleagues confirmed dietary magnesium intake to be a significant predictor of bone mineral density in elite athletes, and follow-up studies have confirmed a correlation between dietary magnesium intake, bone mineral density, and fracture risk (Rondanelli et al., 2021). This has important applications for the bone health of athletes, particularly young, growing athletes and those engaged in low-impact activities such as cycling and swimming, for whom bone mass tends to be lower. Increasing magnesium intake to the RDA and even slightly higher through dietary intervention, whole foods, and supplementation, consequently, is thought to improve variables of health and performance in athletes. Córdova and colleagues (2019) found supplementation with 400 mg/day of magnesium over a 21-day cycling stage race to help maintain serum levels in physiological ranges, elicit a modest impact in maintaining muscle integrity, and thereby facilitate muscle recovery from intense and strenuous exercise in a group of male professional cyclists. Steward and colleagues (2019) found supplementation with 500 mg of magnesium over a 7-day period prior to a 10 km downhill time trial to reduce proinflammatory IL-6 response, enhance recovery of blood glucose, and decrease muscle soreness in a group of recreationally trained male runners whose diets were deficient in magnesium; however, there was no reported benefit to actual time trial performance. There has not been support for supplementation as protection against muscle cramping, though well-designed studies on athletes are lacking (Garrison et al., 2020). It is evident based on current data that magnesium status is important for the performance and health of athletes, and therefore increased dietary intake via whole food and supplementation is encouraged in certain deficient populations.

Common usage: The current RDA is 400 to 420 mg for adult males and 310 to 320 mg for adult females. It is thought that athletes may require additional magnesium above the current RDA to accommodate the increased metabolic demands of exercise and offset sweat losses. Magnesium is generally bound with salts such as gluconate, citrate, and aspartate for supplement use and is available in tablet, capsule, powder, and liquid form. Magnesium is also commonly added as an electrolyte to sport drinks and products. As a daily supplement, typical doses range from 100 to 350 mg/day, though doses reported in studies vary greatly and often exceed the RDA. Magnesium is best taken with food to minimize adverse side effects. To offset sweat losses, athletes training or racing longer than 3 hours should replace 20 to 30 mg of magnesium/8 to 12 oz (0.24-0.35 L) of fluid ingested.

Health concerns: The most common side effect associated with magnesium supplementation is diarrhea, generally at single doses of greater than 350 mg (the current tolerable upper intake level for supplement use in adults and adolescents). Abdominal pain and nausea have also been reported at high doses.

Magnesium Pyruvate
(see *pyruvate*)

Medicinal Mushrooms 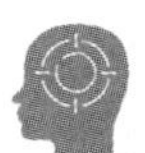 

aka *Agaricus blazei murrill, Cordyceps sinensis, Ganoderma lucidum (reishi), Grifola frondosa (maitake), Hericium erinaceus (lion's mane), Lentinula edodes (shiitake)*

What it is: Typically grown above ground on soil or on top of a food source, medicinal mushrooms are fungi that contain a wide spectrum of nutritional attributes that may enhance health and performance through cardiovascular, antiviral, antibacterial, neurotrophic, and anti-inflammatory properties. There are over 14,000 species of mushrooms; the following five types commonly appear in supplements used by athletes: *Agaricus blazei murrill, Ganoderma lucidum* (reishi), *Grifola frondosa* (maitake), *Hericium erinaceus* (lion's mane), and *Lentinula edodes* (shiitake).

TYPES OF MEDICINAL MUSHROOMS

Medicinal mushrooms comprise a broad genre of supplements, so it is important for consumers to know what biological benefit they are looking for and focus on a specific medicinal mushroom to help support it (table 3.4).

(continued)

TABLE 3.4 Most Commonly Used Medicinal Mushrooms

Mushroom Name	How It Works	Performance Benefits	Common Usage
Agaricus blazei murrill	Provides immune support Extracts can provide relief from symptoms associated with inflammatory bowel diseases such as Crohn's and ulcerative colitis	Can protect an athlete against infection as well as allergy and asthma-related symptoms	Can be consumed fresh, dried, as a tincture or an extract, and in capsule or tablet form. Although dosing recommendations are hard to make based on the available human data and the sheer variety of medicinal mushrooms, dietary use of medicinal mushrooms as whole food or a combined daily supplementation protocol incorporating 40 to 50 mg of shiitake, 50 to 60 mg of maitake, 50 to 60 mg of reishi, and perhaps 1,000 to 1,800 mg of lion's mane (depending on the extract or concentrate) may provide benefit to athletes seeking specific effects, especially those feeling run down, fatigued, stressed, or mentally foggy during training
Ganoderma lucidum (reishi)	Strengthens immune function	Prevents altitude sickness May help oxygenate the blood and prevent fatigue	
Grifola frondosa (maitake)	Stimulates the production of T cells, which help defend the body against viruses	Extracts from maitake have been shown to enhance the forced swimming capacity of mice by increasing fat usage and delaying the accumulation of plasma lactate and ammonia	
Lentinula edodes (shiitake)	Beta-glucans (sugars found in the cell walls) from this mushroom have been shown to help moderate immune response	May help reduce the incidence of illness and symptoms associated with chronic fatigue during heavy training	
Hericium erinaceus (lion's mane)	Has constituents that appear to affect nerve growth factor synthesis*	Provides potential effects on memory and speed of mental performance** Could be of interest to athletes looking for memory benefit and support of cognition	

* (Lai et al., 2013)

** (Docherty et al., 2023; Hersant et al., 2023)

Function: Certain antioxidants, such as L-ergothioneine and polyphenols, are found in abundance in mushrooms. These antioxidants play a key role in protecting an athlete's cells from oxidative damage that can occur during periods of heavy stress, ultimately helping to reduce inflammation and pain, optimize joint health, and enhance recovery. Several enzymes within mushrooms also provide added protection against oxidative damage. Beta-glucan, a polysaccharide or complex chain of glucose molecules found on the fruiting body of the mushroom, supports immune function by activating macrophage immune cells as well as T cells and B cells, which trap and consume various viral, bacterial, protozoan, and fungal invaders that can cause infection and sideline an athlete from competition. Furthermore, medicinal mushrooms contain a large number of secondary metabolites, such as terpenoids, that are involved in a variety of biological processes important for immune functionality.

Research: Although animal studies have presented some promising results, the results on a human population have not always been consistent, especially when focused on a healthy, fit population (You & Lin, 2002). Consumers should learn about a specific mushroom of interest. The bulk of human trials were originally small in nature or of poor design—but again, it is not prudent to lump all medicinal mushrooms together. For example, in a rather conservative review of dietary supplements for memory enhancement, Hersant and colleagues (2023) stated that there is some current evidence for memory benefit from supplementation with lion's mane. Note that necessarily reductionist research methodology—for example, the specific type of cognitive test (e.g., Stroop tests)—make broad conclusions difficult. It depends in part on the biological system being studied (e.g., aerobic capacity, immune function, cognition, recovery). In 2023, Docherty and colleagues, using a double-blind, randomized, placebo-controlled design, studied the acute (60-minute) and chronic (28-day) cognitive and mood-enhancing effects of 1,800 mg *Hericium erinaceus* (lion's mane) in 41 healthy young adults. They observed subjects performing quicker on the Stroop task ($p = 0.005$) at 60 minutes after dosing and a trend toward reduced subjective stress following 28 days of supplementation ($p = 0.051$). Overall, it remains evident that larger, double-blind, controlled human studies, especially on a healthy athletic population, are required for each of the many mushrooms and inherent compounds before any overall efficacy of medicinal mushrooms for purported health and performance outcomes can be confirmed.

Health concerns: Though only eight types of mushrooms in North America are considered poisonous, consumption of wild mushrooms is discouraged. A small number of allergic reactions, including anaphylactic shock, have been reported with medicinal mushrooms, as have mind-altering symptoms brought on by reactions to secondary metabolites within some mushrooms. There are also concerns of heavy metal exposure as a result of mushrooms' sponge-like absorption ability; consumption has led to reports of stomachaches, drowsiness, and confusion, as well as heart, liver, and kidney damage. Even so, the bulk of the data indicate that medicinal mushrooms are safe and well tolerated by most.

Medium-Chain Triglycerides (MCTs) 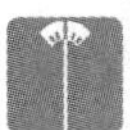

aka *capric acid, caproic acid, caprylic acid, lauric acid*

What it is: Naturally occurring in coconut oil and palm kernel oil, medium-chain triglycerides (MCTs) are a class of fatty acids that, like all triglycerides, consist of a glycerol backbone with three fatty acid molecules; in MCTs, though, the carbon chain is only 6 to 12 atoms long, far fewer than in its long-chain sibling. Because MCTs require significantly less energy for uptake and storage in the body than long-chain triglycerides

(LCTs) yet still provide 8.3 kcal/g, they make an appealing choice for athletes looking for an easy-to-digest and energy-dense fuel source.

Function: Unlike LCTs, MCTs do not require the presence of the amino acid carnitine to transport them into the mitochondria, the energy-producing factories that lie within muscle cells. The result is more rapid conversion to a molecule called acetyl-CoA, which is a key intermediate involved in the production of energy. It is thought that these attributes could produce an ergogenic effect by boosting energy output and, by sparing carbohydrate, thereby enhance endurance.

Performance benefit: Athletes may benefit from increased energy levels and enhanced endurance during moderate- to high-intensity exercise.

Research: Animal data have indicated increased levels of metabolic enzymes along with significant improvements in exercise time to exhaustion with a diet containing 80 g MCT plus 20 g LCT/kg over 6 weeks (Fushiki et al., 1995). These results, however, have failed to translate to human subjects, with the bulk of the data failing to show any benefit on glycogen sparing and consequent submaximal exercise performance of a prolonged nature at doses of 30 to 45 g over 2 to 3 hours (Berning, 1996; Clegg, 2010; Goedecke et al., 2005). Furthermore, doubling this dose over 2 hours has been shown to decrease performance in humans, likely due to increased incidence of gastrointestinal disturbances (Jeukendrup et al., 1998; Van Zyl et al., 1996). Sustained dosing at levels of 60 g/day over 2 weeks has also failed to yield any positive impact on endurance performance in humans (Misell et al., 2001). Although results from animal studies have shown some promise, human subject data have not been supportive of ergogenic purposes in athletes; thus, use is not recommended (Kerksick et al., 2018).

Common usage: Commercially available MCT supplements undergo a process called fractionation, which allows the MCT to be separated from other oils and concentrated, making the total content greater than what is naturally found in coconut oil or palm kernel oil. MCTs are also available in several medicinal food products, generally for use in a clinical setting. Taking 1 tbsp (20 g) of pure MCT or 5 tsp of coconut oil 1 to 3 times/day with food is the current research-supported supplementation protocol.

Health concerns: In one study of endurance-trained cyclists, MCT supplementation produced gastrointestinal distress, primarily intestinal cramping, in half the subjects. Additional reported symptoms include diarrhea, nausea, vomiting, and irritability. Most symptoms occur when 80 or more g (equivalent to >4 tbsp) of MCT are taken as a single dose. MCTs also contain over 100 kcal/tbsp, and thus consuming large amounts without making other dietary adjustments to achieve energy balance can lead to weight gain.

Melatonin 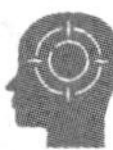 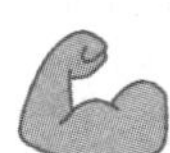 

aka *N-acetyl-5-methoxytryptamine*

What it is: Melatonin is a hormone produced naturally in the body in response to the normal circadian rhythm. The body develops this 24-hour circadian rhythm based on behavior and environmental light and secretes important hormones at particular times. Melatonin, which can affect the ability to fall asleep as well as sleep quality and duration, is released at night during sleep in dark environments. The production of melatonin declines with age, which is suspected to play a role in insomnia among older adults. In addition, melatonin and its metabolites are potent antioxidants that exhibit anti-inflammatory properties and protect mitochondria from damage by scavenging reactive oxygen species (ROS) and reactive nitrogen species (RNS), which has additional performance benefits to the athlete related to recovery (Reiter et al., 2018; Tan et al., 2016). Melatonin can also be found in foods and beverages such as cherries and red wine. Melatonin is synthesized from the sleep-inducing amino acid tryptophan.

Function: Typically, melatonin levels peak several hours after the initiation of sleep. This peak is associated with the lowest point of core body temperature, maximum tiredness, and lowest alertness. Melatonin acts on receptors found in various tissues of the body, mostly in the brain and eyes but also in peripheral tissues such as the heart, arteries, skin, small intestine, and kidneys. The exact mechanisms are not well understood; however, in theory, supplementing with melatonin either before or during sleep (if awakened) could improve the ability to fall asleep and sleep quality. The antioxidant qualities of melatonin are also purported to help offset the oxidative stress and muscle damage associated with strenuous exercise.

Performance benefit: Athletes may benefit from reduced levels of muscle damage and soreness initiated by exercise. These benefits could produce improved recovery from training and subsequent performance. Athletes may also benefit from improved quality, length, and onset of sleep. Additionally, melatonin supplementation can effectively shift the circadian rhythm of those exposed to new time zones, making melatonin a useful supplement for athletes forced to undergo extensive travel and time-zone changes for competition.

Research: A double-blind, placebo-controlled study found a nocturnal oral intake of 5 mg/day of melatonin over a 6-day intensive soccer training camp to reduce oxidative stress, postexercise leukocytosis, and markers of cellular damage, leading to improved performance of highly trained male players in a repeated sprint ability test (Farjallah et al., 2020). These results were replicated in a follow-up study by Farjallah, Ghatassi, and colleagues (2022) using the same oral dose of melatonin over the same 6-day intensive soccer training camp using modified performance parameters (squat jump, countermovement jump, 5-jump test, modified agility T-test, and 20 m sprint). An acute rapid-release dose of 6 mg of melatonin taken 30 minutes prior to a repeated (separated by 48 hours) running exercise test until exhaustion at constant maximal intensity also demonstrated favorable impacts on oxidative stress and markers of cellular damage in 13 professional male soccer players, although it failed to improve performance (Farjallah, Graja, et al., 2022). Interestingly, an acute rapid-release dose of 6 mg of melatonin taken before completing a repeated series of explosive exercises also failed to affect physical performance and recovery of handball athletes (Farjallah et al., 2018), suggesting a sustained, rather than acute, intake might be needed to elicit maximal benefit. There currently is limited data evaluating the impact of melatonin might have on the performance of active females, particularly trained athletes. There is also a lack of data evaluating the impact of melatonin on correcting sleep patterns in an athletic population, though researchers at found both a low (0.3 mg) and a high (5 mg) dose of melatonin to improve sleep efficiency in a relatively small sample (n = 24) of healthy older adults (Duffy et al., 2022). It is important to note that the higher dose affected the biological day and night sleep patterns, duration of non-REM sleep, and awakening time.

Common usage: Research-supported doses for melatonin range from 0.3 mg to 6 mg, with supplementation protocols depending on intended use. A 2017 systemic review of 12 randomized control studies revealed that 1 to 3 mg of an immediate-release formula taken 30 minutes prior to bedtime might be helpful for those suffering from insomnia, whereas the same dose of a slow-release formula can be implemented for those with sleep maintenance problems (Auld et al., 2016). To offset jet lag, doses of 0.05 mg to 5

M

mg have been indicated in the early morning prior to traveling westward or in the early evening prior to traveling eastward (Arendt, 2009).

Health concerns: No known major health concerns exist related to melatonin, and chronic use for up to 6 months appears safe based on current data (Celorrio et al., 2024). Common side effects include daytime sleepiness, dizziness, and headaches. Melatonin can interact with blood-thinning medications, immunosuppressants, diabetes medications, and birth control methods.

Meletin
(see *quercetin*)

Methylcobalamin
(see *vitamin B$_{12}$*)

Methylhexanamine
(see *dimethylamylamine*)

Methylsulfonylmethane (MSM)  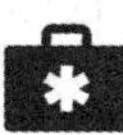

aka *dimethyl sulfone (DMSO), methyl sulfone*

What it is: Methylsulfonylmethane (MSM) is an organic compound that can be found in a variety of fruits, vegetables, grains, and animal foods. It is most abundantly found in milk, coffee, tomatoes, tea, and corn ("Methylsulfonylmethane [MSM]," 2003). MSM is most commonly used as a dietary supplement to treat joint pain and dysfunction.

Function: MSM has multiple mechanisms by which it can provide benefits for arthritic joints. First, MSM is a strong antioxidant and anti-inflammatory agent, allowing it to combat the damage done by free radicals and reduce pain and inflammation. Second, MSM is believed to enhance the activity of cortisol, a strong anti-inflammatory hormone commonly used to treat joint pain and inflammation in athletes. Finally, MSM contains sulfur, an important component of connective tissue, which is reduced in populations suffering from arthritis (Usha & Naidu, 2004).

Performance benefit: Because the physical demands of sport and daily training place a significant amount of stress on joints, many athletes experience chronic joint pain. In addition, many athletes suffer injuries to joints that require surgery or joint reconstruction. Recovery from these types of surgeries can result in changes to the joint, and MSM has potential to improve and speed rehabilitation.

Research: Unlike other popular joint supplements such as glucosamine and chondroitin, which have been studied extensively, much less research exists related to MSM. Clinical trials in humans have produced some promising results related to inflammatory conditions such as arthritis. For example, one study found supplementation with 2 g/day of MSM for 12 weeks significantly improved both knee and systemic inflammatory conditions in healthy participants with mild knee pain compared to a placebo (Toguchi et al., 2023). Another study discovered a combined supplementation protocol inclusive of 500 mg of MSM alongside 1,500 mg of glucosamine and 1,200 mg of chondroitin sulfate over 3 months to yield a significant clinical improvement, especially in terms of pain relief, in 147 patients with mild knee osteoarthritis (OA) compared with the glucosamine-chondroitin sulfate and the placebo group (Lubis et al., 2017). MSM also presents some promise in mitigating the pain and inflammation associated with exhaustive exercise. Withee and colleagues (2017) found supplementation with 3 g of MSM taken daily over 21 days prior to and for 2 days after racing a half-marathon yielded clinically significant (though not statistically significant) reductions in both muscle and joint pain compared to the placebo group. Another study of similar design found that supplementation with 3 g of MSM taken over 28 days prior to plus the 3 days following completing 100 repetitions of a knee extension exercise blunted tissue damage and resulting inflammation (van de Merwe & Bloomer, 2016). More research is needed to better understand the mechanisms of MSM and confirm positive outcomes, particularly on healthy athletic populations, since the current body of scientific research is not substantial.

Common usage: The recommended supplementation dosage of MSM is 500 to 1,000 mg 3 times/day, for a total of 1,500 to 3,000 mg.

Health concerns: MSM is on the FDA's Generally Recognized as Safe (GRAS) list and is well tolerated by most individuals at dosages of up to 4 grams daily, with few known and mild side effects (Butawan et al., 2017).

Milk Protein

(see *casein*)

Montmorency Cherry

(see *tart cherry*)

Mother's Milk

(see *colostrum*)

Mucuna Pruriens  

aka *black cohosh, cowhage seed extract, velvet bean*

What it is: A leguminous plant growing worldwide in tropical regions, *Mucuna pruriens* contains levodopa (L-dopa) as well as coenzyme Q10 (CoQ10) and NADH, both molecules that are part of aerobic metabolism. L-dopa is a precursor to dopamine, a neurotransmitter in the brain that helps regulate mood and libido.

Function: *Mucuna pruriens* may affect both dopamine and growth hormone. Dopamine is known to play a role in many bodily functions as a neurotransmitter and as a hormone, affecting reward centers, memory, attention, movement, motivation, and gastrointestinal transit. Growth hormone is a known anabolic and lipolytic agent that, in sufficient amounts over time, positively affects body composition. Traditionally, *Mucuna pruriens* has been used as treatment for neurodegenerative disorders such as Parkinson's disease due to its L-dopa content.

Performance benefit: There may possibly be neuroprotective and attention or mood-enhancing effects, as well as theoretically enhanced recovery and body composition from elevated levels of testosterone or growth hormone. However, more research is needed in athletes.

Research: *Mucuna pruriens* is sometimes co-supplemented with other herbs, making conclusions challenging. Santos and colleagues(2019) analyzed available evidence and concluded that moderate evidence supports the use of *Mucuna pruriens* (e.g., 5,000 mg/day powdered seed, plus ashwagandha root) to increase total testosterone over 12 weeks in patients with oligospermia. Earlier work by Alleman and colleagues (2011) administering *Mucuna pruriens* together with *Chlorophytum borivilianum* (safed musli) to 15 exercise-trained men reported an acute increase in circulating growth hormone.

Note that factors such as age, sleep, exercise, nutrition, and alcohol intake all influence growth hormone release patterns.

Common usage: According to Cohen and colleagues (2022), the prevalence of *Mucuna pruriens* use in the United States is unknown, but 7% of patients with Parkinson's disease use it. When testing a sample of *Mucuna pruriens* supplement products, these same researchers reported L-dopa doses from 2 to 241 mg per recommended serving size. This wide range makes accurate dosing unpredictable and makes comparisons to prescription L-dopa virtually impossible. At the time of this writing, Amazon listed products claiming 500 to 1500 mg of *Mucuna pruriens* (not L-dopa, per se), often in combination with the amino acid tyrosine, ashwagandha, and other nutrients and herbs.

Health concerns: The L-dopa content in *Mucuna pruriens* could induce cardiac, neurological, or gastrointestinal symptoms, among others. Anyone with heart disease, irregular heartbeat, low blood pressure, dizziness, fainting, liver disease. or a mental condition should check with a health care provider before using *Mucuna pruriens*. Those taking medications for Parkinson's disease should also avoid it without the advice of a physician.

Muskat

(see *grape seed*)

Mycoprotein 

What it is: According to Monteyne and colleagues (2020), "mycoprotein is a fungal-derived sustainable protein-rich food source, and its ingestion results in systemic amino acid and leucine concentrations similar to that following milk protein ingestion."

Function: Mycoproteins are emerging as a complete protein source that may be comparable to milk protein (Coelho et al., 2020; Monteyne et al., 2020; West et al., 2023).

Performance benefit: Mycoprotein can provide a vegan protein source that may be superior to plant proteins, which are typically hampered by one or more limiting amino acids or lower digestibility. Indeed, when taking into account the importance of leucine within a protein source, mycoprotein could be equal to or superior to even milk proteins (often considered the highest quality protein type) for muscle building.

Research: Testing 21 resistance-trained males (averaging 22 years old) in a double-blind, randomized, parallel-group isotope model, Monteyne and colleagues (2020) concluded that consuming a single bolus of mycoprotein (containing 31.5 g protein and 2.5 g leucine) stimulates resting and postexercise muscle protein synthesis rates to a greater extent than a leucine-matched bolus of milk protein (containing 26.2 g protein and 2.5 g leucine). Building on this, in 2023 West and colleagues hypothesized that ingestion of mycoprotein as part of its whole food matrix, or the combination of compounds in the whole fungi, would stimulate muscle protein synthesis rates in 24 males who took part in resistance exercise to an even greater degree than a leucine-matched bolus of protein concentrated from mycoprotein—however, they concluded that that there was an equivalent stimulation of myofibrillar protein synthesis with whole food and concentrated mycoprotein.

Common usage: Not all fungi are mushrooms, but foods and supplements can contain either or both. From a food product perspective, mycoprotein is commonly used as a meat substitute in products like cutlets, nuggets, and patties. Single-cell fungi and mushroom protein powders are available at online retailers, with suggested per-serving protein doses similar to other proteins (20-25g per scoop). Consumers should note these can appear in blends with plant proteins or carry claims regarding the specific mushrooms that are included.

Health concerns: According to Finnegan and colleagues (2019), "In 2002, the US FDA designated mycoprotein as "Generally Recognized as Safe" and 7 Quorn products were introduced into the US food supply." (Quorn is a common brand.) Mycoprotein products do typically carry allergy warnings, however. Allergy symptoms could range from hives to swelling of the tongue or throat, or rarely, anaphylaxis. Consumers should consult their physician if they have allergy concerns.

N-Acetylcysteine (NAC)

(see *acetylcysteine*)

N-Acetyl-5-Methoxytryptamine

(see *melatonin*)

Na-Citrate

(see *sodium bicarbonate and sodium citrate*)

N-(Aminoiminomethyl)-N-Methylglycine

(see *creatine*)

Naringin

aka *naringenin (see also quercetin)*

What it is: Naringin, along with quercetin, is a flavonoid found in citrus fruits and is the main cause of their bitter taste. For decades consuming grapefruit has been used as a popular weight-loss method. Naringin is converted into naringenin in the body, which is alleged by some to be the component in grapefruit responsible for this effect. As a result, naringin has become a popular ingredient in weight-loss and fat-burning supplements.

Function: Naringin is known to affect the cytochrome P450 enzyme complex, which is responsible for the metabolism of many drugs within the liver. It is speculated that naringin can act synergistically with other dietary supplement ingredients that are known to affect resting metabolic rate and metabolism, such as caffeine. Through its impact on cytochrome P450, such compounds may slow the metabolism of caffeine and other stimulants, potentially giving them a more potent effect and further increasing their impact on resting metabolic rate, weight loss, and fat oxidation.

Performance benefit: Athletes wanting to improve body composition, decrease body fat, or lose body weight may be interested in supplementing with naringin.

Research: As of 2024, research using in vitro and animal models outnumber the few human clinical trials using naringin. These preclinical studies have looked at effects on fat metabolism and other anti-metabolic-syndrome effects but are limited in applicability to athletes. In their investigation of grapefruit and weight loss, Dow and colleagues (2012) found that subjects who consumed one-half of a fresh grapefruit with each meal 3 times/day for 6 weeks resulted in no significant decreases in body weight, blood lipids, or blood pressure compared to the control group. This is in contrast to a 2006 study of obese patients in which the consumption of one-half of a grapefruit before meals resulted in significant weight loss compared to a placebo (Fujioka et al., 2006). Further, effects of grapefruit constituents like naringin on caffeine metabolism have been found to vary. A study in 2006 found that 200 mg of naringin did not alter caffeine metabolism nor affect resting metabolic rate, despite hypothesizing that naringin would act synergistically with caffeine and increase its effects on resting metabolic rate (Ballard et al., 2006). Currently, there are insufficient and inconclusive data related to the effectiveness of naringin. More evidence is needed before naringin supplements are recommended.

Common usage: The amount of naringin found in a grapefruit can vary depending on where the fruit is grown and is also dependent on the size of the grapefruit; however, the average is roughly 40 mg/grapefruit (~250 g), or about 16 mg of naringin/100 g of grapefruit. Most research trials have used a dose of 60 to 200 mg of naringin. Naringin is commonly added to weight-loss supplements in pill form with claims to increase fat and weight loss.

Health concerns: As noted, naringin as well as other components found in grapefruit can affect drug metabolism. The list of drugs affected is vast, so athletes should consult a physician before taking supplements containing naringin to ensure safety.

Nicotinamide Riboside (NR) 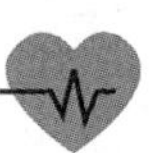  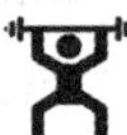

aka *Niagen (brand name)*

What it is: Nicotinamide riboside (NR) is a controversial niacin (vitamin B_3) compound purported to support cellular energy metabolism. Famous researchers have joined commercial entities promoting these expensive supplements, to such a degree that conflict of interest concerns have arisen. Some human data are positive, but this body of knowledge is still emerging.

Function: These products are purported to increase levels of nicotinamide adenine dinucleotide (NAD+)—a coenzyme central to energy metabolism—in circulation and arguably in other tissues like muscle, aiding cellular energy metabolism, including DNA repair and mitochondrial health. Animal-versus-human study results and the tight regulation of NAD+ within cells are common points of contention. These products are primarily sold as antiaging products but some emerging literature suggests they may also support physical performance, perhaps depending on age or fitness level.

Performance benefit: A potential for an increase in endurance exercise performance remains plausible, given the mechanism of increasing NAD+ or related actions in cells, but this remains controversial. NAD+ is one of the reducing equivalents critical to coupling the Krebs cycle to the electron transport chain for ATP production.

Research: After encouraging reports in rodents, this body of science is still emerging in humans. A brief investigation of 8 moderately fit males who took 1,000 mg NR/day for a week before a session of moderate-intensity cycling led to a conclusion that acute supplementation did not alter fuel metabolism nor mitochondrial adaptation signaling pathways in human skeletal muscle (Stocks et al., 2021). In some contrast, an industry-sponsored 2023 study by Yi and colleagues reported that healthy middle-aged participants given 300, 600, or 900 mg nicotinamide mononucleotide (NMN) per day increased circulating NAD+ levels after 30 and 60 days of treatment (all doses, but highest at 600-900 mg/day). They reported this to be safe and well-tolerated and to benefit physical performance (6-minute walking test), especially at 600 to 900 mg/day versus placebo.

Common usage: Based on label claims from two of the biggest sellers of NAD supplements, Elysium Health and Chromadex, a daily dose of 250 to 300 mg of NR is common. These products sometimes include antioxidants such as pterostilbene.

Health concerns: A concerning hypothesis exists that boosting NAD+ could worsen tumorigenesis or cancer growth; according to Shen (2019), early work suggested an increased number of cancerous pancreatic growths in genetically predisposed mice that consumed NMN. More research is needed on these potential effects and their applicability to humans.

9-Beta-D-Ribofuranosylhypoxanthine

(see *inosine*)

N-3 Fatty Acids

(see *omega-3 fatty acids*)

Oat Bran, Oat-Derived Beta-Glucan

(see *beta-glucan*)

Olibanum

(see *Boswellia serrata*)

Omega-3 Fatty Acids 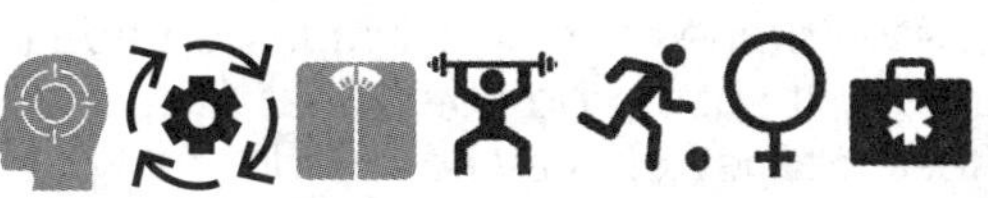

aka *alpha-linolenic acid (ALA), docosahexaenoic acid (DHA), eicosapentaenoic acid (EPA), n-3 fatty acids, omega-3s*

What it is: Omega-3 fatty acids, one of the major classes of polyunsaturated fats, can be found naturally in some nuts and seeds and their accompanying oils as well as fatty fish. Although several forms of omega-3s exist, those considered essential to human health include plant-derived alpha-linolenic acid (ALA) and marine-derived eicosapentaenoic acid (EPA) and docosahexaenoic acid (DHA), both of which are produced in small amounts from ALA. (See tables 3.5 and 3.6.)

TABLE 3.5   Best Food Sources of ALA Omega-3s

	Serving size	ALA (grams)
Canola oil	1 tbsp	1.3
Chia seeds	1 tbsp	2.4
English walnuts	1 oz (28 g)	2.6
Flaxseed, ground	1 tbsp	1.6
Flaxseed, oil	1 tbsp	7.3
Walnut, oil	1 tbsp	1.4

TABLE 3.6   Best Food Sources of EPA/DHA Omega-3s

	Serving size	EPA (grams)	DHA (grams)
Herring, Pacific	3 oz (85 g)	1.06	0.75
Oysters, Pacific	3 oz (85 g)	0.75	0.43
Salmon, Chinook	3 oz (85 g)	0.86	0.62
Salmon, Atlantic	3 oz (85 g)	0.28	0.95
Salmon, Sockeye	3 oz (85 g)	0.45	0.60
Sardines, Pacific	3 oz (85 g)	0.45	0.74

Function: Dietary fats have strong effects in the body, in part because they can incorporate into cell membranes, which affect fluidity and intracellular pathways. Thus, an imbalance in intake can lead to serious consequences. Westerners underconsume omega-3 fatty acids and overconsume omega-6 fatty acids, an imbalance leading, among other things, to overproduction of prostaglandin E2 (PGE2), an inflammatory molecule. (To provide some context on antiinflammatory potency, aspirin blocks PGE2 production.) Correcting a dietary imbalance such as this may be one reason why omega-3 fats—particularly fish oils—demonstrate such potent effects. Further, physical stress triggers the release of harmful compounds known as free radicals, which can penetrate the protective membrane of any cell in the body, leading to cell damage and a consequent inflammatory response. Although the body has defense mechanisms to deal with acute inflammation, severe injury or extreme exercise stress can lead to chronic inflammation and the activation of nerves responsible for the sensation of pain, thereby compromising recovery. It is currently thought that the benefits of omega-3s originate, in part, from two compounds that are derived specifically from EPA and DHA; these compounds—appropriately named protectins and resolvins—protect the structural integrity of cell membranes and fight tissue degradation, resolve inflammation, and significantly ease pain. It should be noted that EPA and DHA, although commonly supplemented and tested together, may have individual or even sex-specific effects.

Performance benefit: Omega-3s may help facilitate quicker recovery times as well as serve as a viable treatment option for a wide range of inflammatory-based conditions, including asthma, arthritis, and traumatic brain injury. Research shows promise for several other potential performance benefits:

- Improved cognitive parameters, such as reactivity and focus, important for such sports as baseball and golf
- Increased blood and oxygen flow to working muscles, including the heart, as a result of reduced blood viscosity, thereby aiding aerobic endurance
- Improved fuel usage with an increased ability to burn fat for energy, body composition improvements, and antidepressive effects

Research: According to a review by Thielecke and Blanin (2020), "Overall, studies of EPA/DHA supplementation in sport performance are few and research designs rather diverse. Several studies suggest a potentially beneficial effect of EPA/DHA on performance by improved endurance capacity and delayed onset of muscle soreness, as well as on markers related to enhanced recovery and immune modulation." This is in line with earlier work evaluating the impact of omega-3s on inflammation caused by exercise or sport injury. Animal and human data have shown promise. For example, a small, double-blind, randomized human study found that a daily supplementation protocol of 324 mg EPA and 216 mg DHA from fish oil (1.8 g total omega-3) over 30 days had some effect in countering chronic inflammation and associated delayed-onset muscle soreness (DOMS) in untrained individuals after a single 40-minute session of eccentric loading exercise (Tartibian, Maleki, & Abbasi, 2009). The same supplementation protocol was found to ameliorate exercise-induced markers of inflammation associated with eccentric exercise in untrained men (Tartibian, Maleki, & Abbasi, 2011). Whether this would hold true for trained athletes is unknown. According to researchers from Indiana University, however, highly trained athletes with exercise-induced asthma (EIA) may benefit from omega-3's anti-inflammatory attributes by following a daily supplementation protocol of 3.2 g EPA and 2.0 g DHA from fish oil over 3 weeks. This protocol was shown to significantly reduce airway inflammation and enhance overall lung function in highly trained subjects affected by EIA (Mickleborough et al., 2003). Finally, regarding inflammation, a daily supplementation protocol incorporating 10 or 40 mg/kg of omega-3s over 30 days was shown to be effective in countering the neural inflammation and damage caused by concussive injuries in rats; the higher dose demonstrated an astounding 98% reduction in neural damage tested (Mills et al., 2011). Further research needs to confirm this benefit in human subjects. Also likely related to anti-inflammatory effects, body composition enhancements may take place when addressing the insufficiency of omega-3 fatty acids in the diet relative to omega-6 intake. Noreen and colleagues (2010) supplemented 44 healthy men and women with 4 g/day of a safflower oil control or 4 g/day of a fish oil intervention (comprising 1,600 mg EPA and 800 mg DHA) for 6 weeks. These investigators reported that compared to the common safflower oil group, there was a significant increase in fat-free mass following treatment with fish oil, a significant reduction in fat mass, and a tendency for a decrease in body fat percentage. However, they reported no significant differences in body mass, resting metabolic rate, or respiratory exchange ratio. There was also a tendency for salivary cortisol to decrease in the intervention group. Note that subjects were healthy and active, but not engaged in consistent, systematic exercise training; application to highly trained athletes should take this into account. Collectively, some but not all studies suggest body composition enhancement. Lastly, brain health beyond the cognitive effects listed above may benefit. A meta-analysis based on 26 studies by Liao and colleagues (2019) reported an overall beneficial effect of omega-3 polyunsaturated fatty acids on depression symptoms. EPA appeared to be the beneficial fatty acid in this review, and a dose of up to 1 g daily was suggested. DHA has also received the attention of researchers as a distinct entity that may be particularly helpful for certain populations. DiNicolantonio and O'Keefe (2020) concluded "DHA plays a significant role in mental health throughout early childhood and even into adulthood. In the brain, DHA is important for cellular membrane fluidity, function and neurotransmitter release." It is not known whether the mood-stabilizing effects of omega-3 fats apply to athlete-specific depressive symptoms such as those seen with overtraining.

Common usage: For anti-inflammatory benefit, target daily consumption is 1 to 2 g of EPA and DHA in an approximate 2:1 ratio, as is common in fish oil, krill, and algae supplements. Fard and colleagues (2019) report a "distinctive ratio" of 18:12 of EPA to DHA is typically the most abundantly available and commonly studied. ALA omega-3s, present in plant-based supplements such as flaxseed oil, are weaker and should be taken at a dose 3 to 5 times higher due to conversion rates to EPA and DHA, which are estimated at only 36% for women and 16% for men. A dose–response effect, particularly when considering the overall ratio of omega-6 to omega-3 in the diet, is something to discuss with a physician. Omega-3 supplements are best taken with food.

Health concerns: Use of omega-3s is generally recognized as safe, although reported side effects include indigestion and gas, especially at doses above 3 g of EPA and DHA. Note that such high-dose omega-3 intake could reduce blood clotting and may interact with drugs like aspirin, which also affects such pathways.

1,3-Dimethylamylamine, 1,3-Dimethylpentylamine

(see *dimethylamylamine*)

Ornithine 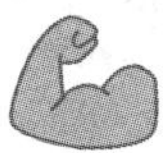

aka *L-ornithine, ornithine hydrochloride,* *ornithine alpha-ketoglutarate (OKG)* (see also *arginine*)

What it is: Ornithine is a nonprotein amino acid, meaning it is not naturally part of protein structure. It can, however, be found to some extent in protein-rich foods such as meats, fish, dairy, and eggs. Some researchers note that as a free amino acid, L-ornithine is not particularly rich in meats or fish, making supplementation attractive if an antifatigue effect is desired (Sugino et al., 2008). As a nonessential amino acid, it can also be synthesized in the body from other amino acids. Ornithine alpha-ketoglutarate (OKG) is a salt that is formed from ornithine and alpha-ketoglutarate. OKG is more bioavailable than ornithine alone and is metabolized differently. As noted by Cynober (2004):

> There is evidence that OKG activity is not the simple addition of the effects of ornithine (Orn) and α-ketoglutarate (αKG) . . . the main feature of Orn at the whole-body level is to be metabolized through the Orn aminotransferase-dependent pathway, whereas the simultaneous administration of Orn and α-KG saturates this pathway, diverting Orn toward metabolism into Arg[inine].

Function: L-ornithine plays an important role in ammonia metabolism via the urea cycle in the liver. Ornithine and OKG are also precursors of the amino acids proline and arginine. Proline is an important amino acid found in connective tissues such as collagen. Arginine is important in the production of nitric oxide, a powerful vasodilator that can improve blood flow. In addition, arginine is involved in the production of growth hormone, although large intravenous dosing may be required for this mechanism to be relevant. It is speculated that ornithine supplementation can increase concentrations of both arginine and proline. Ornithine supplementation could indirectly promote the availability of both arginine and proline. There is also evidence that OKG supplementation has a better effect on both arginine and proline compared to ornithine alone.

Performance benefit: For athletes, an antifatigue effect may be possible, at least with cycling exercise. Also, supplementation with ornithine or OKG could improve the availability of arginine, which would promote blood flow and delivery of oxygen and nutrients to muscles, as well as proline, which would increase the strength and density of connective tissues. Ornithine and OKG may increase levels of growth hormone, a powerful anabolic hormone, which in clinically relevant amounts could increase gains in lean body mass and strength.

Research: An antifatigue effect, perhaps due to enhanced ammonia metabolism, has interested some researchers. In a placebo-controlled, crossover design, Demura and colleagues (2010) concluded that ornithine hydrochloride supplementation (0.1 g/kg) in 14 trained, healthy young adults before performing incremental exhaustive ergometer bicycle exercises cannot be expected to improve performance, but it does increase the ability to buffer ammonia, both during and after exercise. Demura and colleagues (2011) then tested the effect of L-ornithine hydrochloride ingestion (0.1 g/kg) on ammonia metabolism and performance using a different maximal exercise protocol (5 sets/30 seconds each); here they reported peak cycling rpm was significantly greater with L-ornithine hydrochloride ingestion than with placebo. Serum ornithine level after exercise was also significantly greater with L-ornithine hydrochloride ingestion than with placebo, suggesting it was sufficiently absorbed. This time the investigators concluded that although maximal intermittent anaerobic performance may be improved by L-ornithine hydrochloride ingestion, it may not depend on increase of ammonia metabolism with the supplement. These two studies came after other scientists (Sugino et al., 2008) suggested L-ornithine (2 g/day for 7 days) and L-ornithine hydrochloride (6 g/day for 1 day) may reduce fatigue. Studies have also looked at ornithine and OKG supplementation in various populations, finding positive results in clinical settings for patients with burns and other wounds (De Bandt et al., 1998; Donati et al., 1999). These trials found OKG to be superior to ornithine in promoting the availability of arginine and proline. However, this improved availability did not prove to be beneficial for the promotion of nitric oxide, growth hormone, or connective tissues in healthy, well-nourished populations.

Common usage: Because the efficacy of ornithine and OKG supplementation depends on the intent and because data are mixed, even for cycling fatigue, it is difficult to establish recommendations. As noted, 0.1 g/kg of L-ornithine hydrochloride has been used in research. This would equal 8 g for a typical 80 kg individual. Successful research studies for burn and other wound-healing patients have used a daily intake of 10 g. A range of 0.04 to 0.17 g/kg of has also been used; however, intakes above 0.17 g/kg are not recommended.

Health concerns: According to Takeda and Takemasa (in Bagchi et al., 2019), acute toxicity tests in rodents have shown that 50% lethal dose of ornithine and arginine is more than 10 and 12 g/kg, respectively. This is challenging to equate to human intake and an upper limit of ornithine to avoid toxicity has not been established; more research in this area is needed. However, when used within recommended doses such as those noted previously, supplementation appears safe.

Palatinose

(see *isomaltulose*)

Panax Ginseng

(see *ginseng*)

Pantothenic Acid 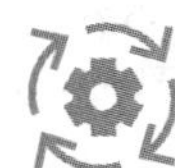 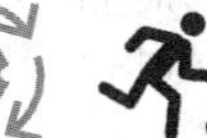

aka *calcium pantothenate, pantethine, pantothenol, sodium D-pantothenate, vitamin B_5*

What it is: Derived from the Greek word *pantos* meaning "everywhere," pantothenic acid, also known as vitamin B_5, is an essential nutrient that is naturally found in a wide variety of plant and animal foods such as peanut butter, liver, wheat bran, cheese, lobster, Brewer's yeast, and royal jelly. It is also available in supplement form, often as part of a multivitamin and multimineral formula. Although deficiencies are rare, it is thought that athletes may benefit from increased intake as a means to better support the metabolic demands of exercise.

Function: As a participant in a wide array of key biological roles, including the synthesis of coenzyme A, a key compound involved in the production of energy from carbohydrate, fat, and protein, pantothenic acid is considered essential to all forms of life. Animal studies have found deficiencies in pantothenic acid to compromise storage of glycogen in the muscle and liver, causing decreased exercise tolerance and endurance. In addition, decreased synthesis of heme, the component of hemoglobin that carries iron, has been shown to contribute to anemia in deficient monkeys, and low blood sugar, rapid breathing, and elevated heart rates have been reported in deficient dogs (Plesofsky-Vig, 1999). It is hypothesized that supplementation with pantothenic acid may help optimize oxygen usage, reduce lactate accumulation and consequent muscle fatigue, and promote optimal glycogen storage for enhanced endurance during exercise. The refining, freezing, canning, and cooking of food causes pantothenic content to drop, making dietary deficiencies an increased likelihood in athletes eating primarily processed foods.

Performance benefit: Athletes, especially those with poor dietary intake of pantothenic acid, may benefit from supplementation through reduced muscle fatigue and enhanced endurance. Animal evidence suggests supplementation with pantothenic acid, especially when dietary intake is suboptimal, may help enhance the body's adrenal response to stress, which may help protect an athlete against adverse hormonal and blood sugar changes and immune suppression that can cause performance to suffer.

Research: Although clinical deficiencies have rarely been reported in humans, suboptimal dietary intake of pantothenic acid is not all that uncommon, especially among athletes consuming a highly processed diet. For example, a recent nutritional analysis of highly trained adolescent soccer players determined over half failed to meet Dietary Reference Intake (DRI) goals for pantothenic acid (Gibson et al., 2011). Supplementation may therefore be helpful, especially for athletes eating primarily processed foods. One study of elite distance runners that found a supplementation protocol providing 2 g/day of pantothenic acid over 2 weeks lowered lactate buildup by 17% and the oxygen cost of prolonged, strenuous exercise by 7% (Litoff, Scherzer, & Harrison, 1984). However, Whitfield and colleagues (2021) failed to find any performance benefit in trained cyclists with a supplementation protocol that included 6 g/day of pantothenic acid taken over 16 weeks. Indeed, the bulk of human research has not demonstrated any performance benefit from supplementation, suggesting most athletes are better off focusing on improving intake of whole foods rich in pantothenic acid (Nice et al., 1984; Wall et al., 2012; Webster, 1998).

Common usage: Pantothenic acid is available in capsule, liquid, and tablet form and is included in multivitamin and multimineral formulas, generally as the derivative pantothenol. Pantothenic acid is also available as salts (calcium pantothenate and sodium D-pantothenate) to promote better absorption. Doses of pantothenic acid typically range from 10 to 50 mg/day in multivitamin and multimineral supplements and 100 to 500 mg in single-ingredient tablets and capsules. The current DRI for adult men and women aged 14 and older is 5 mg/day.

Health concerns: Although pantothenic acid is generally well tolerated by most in doses up to 1,200 mg per day, gastrointestinal side effects such as nausea and heartburn have been reported with doses of 1,000 mg/day.

Piascledine

(see *avocado soybean unsaponifiables*)

P57

(see *Hoodia gordonii*)

Phosphate Salts 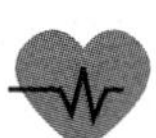 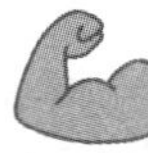 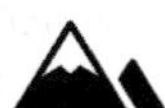

aka *phosphates, calcium phosphate, potassium phosphate, sodium phosphate*

What it is: Phosphorus, which is found naturally in a wide array of foods such as milk, cheese, grains, beans, peas, and nuts, is an essential mineral. It must be obtained from the diet; after consumption, it is distributed throughout the body's tissues in the form of phosphate, the bulk of which is stored in bone. Phosphate salts, a combination of phosphate and minerals such as calcium, potassium, and sodium are commonly included in sport foods, drinks, and supplements for the purpose of helping protect athletes against premature muscle fatigue during sport competition.

Function: Phosphates play three key roles that are believed to contribute to their performance-enhancing potential. First, they are relied on metabolically to generate adenosine triphosphate (ATP), the chemical form of energy within cells, as well as phosphocreatine, an immediate energy source that also can be used to recycle used ATP. Consequently, it is thought that phosphate supplementation may help provide a boost to the energy stores required to propel performance. Second, phosphates serve as an effective buffer against hydrogen ions and lactate, which accumulate during exercise (especially high-intensity exercise) and cause a burning sensation that contributes to muscle fatigue and failure. Finally, phosphates increase the concentration of a chemical in red blood cells called 2,3-diphosphoglycerate (2,3-DPG), which helps release oxygen from hemoglobin, promoting quicker delivery of oxygen to muscles for enhanced endurance and recovery.

SUPPLEMENT FACT

The use of phosphates to improve physical performance dates back to World War I, when German soldiers reportedly used sodium phosphate to reduce combat fatigue.

Performance benefit: Phosphate loading may help reduce fatigue and the sensation of pain during exercise, extending endurance and enhancing recovery.

Research: Studies investigating the benefit of phosphate loading across the performance spectrum, including anaerobic, power-oriented, and endurance-focused performances, have been equivocal. For example, Pope and colleagues (2022) failed to find an ergogenic benefit of taking 3.5 g/day of dibasic sodium phosphate for 4 days prior to a 30 km time trial compared to the placebo in 16 highly trained cyclists. Similarly, two previous double-blind, placebo-controlled studies evaluated the performance benefit of 4 g of sodium phosphate divided into 4 1-g feedings for 4 consecutive days leading to either a 30-second all-out effort or an incremental $\dot{V}O_2max$ test using 3-minute stages on a cycle ergometer; these studies failed to identify any improvement on such parameters as $\dot{V}O_2max$, blood lactate levels, and overall performance (Brennan & Connolly, 2001; Tourville, Brennan, & Connolly, 2001). However, another double-blind, randomized study of trained cyclists identified a favorable impact on performance with the same supplementation dose of sodium phosphate taken over 6 days rather than 4 days before completing a more endurance-focused 16.1 km (10 mi) time trial (Folland & Brickley, 2008). The phosphate loading yielded a 10% boost to mean power output, allowing the cyclists to complete the time trial significantly faster than the placebo trial. Though not a significant change, the study investigators noted a tendency toward higher maximal oxygen uptake ($\dot{V}O_2max$) after phosphate loading versus the placebo, which was a proposed reason for the improved performance. In another randomized, placebo-controlled crossover study, a supplemental dose of 50 mg/kg sodium phosphate over 6 days prior to two incremental cycle tests to exhaustion under acute hypoxic conditions spread out by 21 days failed to demonstrate an ergogenic effect on aerobic exercise in trained male cyclists—namely, there was no significant changes in 2,3-DPG levels, buffering capacity, myocardial efficiency, or aerobic capacity (Płoszczyca et al., 2022). Study investigators did note that there were a small number of subjects with lower levels of central and peripheral training adaptations who saw 3% to 5% improvements in maximal oxygen uptake and power output at submaximal and maximal exercise intensity following phosphate loading and, as a result, hypothesized that supplementation might be most beneficial in less-trained athletes or those competing at altitude when not acclimated. The discrepancy in results indicate more research is needed, particularly evaluating the impact of phosphate loading during varying phases of training and environmental conditions, before definite conclusions for use can be made.

Common usage: Research-supported doses for phosphate loading are 50 mg/kg body mass or 3 to 6 g/day of sodium or potassium phosphate, split into several 1 g doses throughout the day, taken over 6 days leading up to competition.

Health concerns: Because stomach upset, diarrhea, and general GI discomfort have been reported with loading periods of phosphate salts, athletes who choose to supplement should experiment while training before using the salts in competition. It is also important to note that excessive intake of phosphate, especially over the long term, can drive blood levels abnormally high, increasing the risk for electrolyte imbalances.

Phosphatidic Acid (PA) 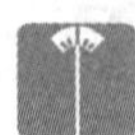

What it is: Phosphatidic acid (PA) is a phospholipid component of cell membranes involved in cellular signaling processes. Its presence in the diet is negligible, making supplementation necessary for any intended effects.

Function: Phosphatidic acid has been reported to activate the mTOR signaling pathway, potentially enhancing the anabolic effects of resistance training (Hoffman et al., 2012).

Performance benefit: Although dose appears to be an issue in the relatively few studies on PA, the intent is an increase in muscle mass and strength.

Research: According to a review by Bond (2017): "A small number of studies carried out with resistance-trained men suggest that PA supplementation might be a useful dietary strategy to increase muscle mass and possibly strength in this population, although only one study has found a statistical significant effect on these parameters." This author also concluded that approximately 750 mg/day would be an appropriate dose for effects; this is an amount larger than that used in some negative studies. Still, that same year (2017) Gonzalez and colleagues concluded that PA supplementation at 750 mg/day, in combination with a 3 days/week resistance-training program, did not have a differential effect on changes in muscle thickness or 1RM strength compared with placebo over 8 weeks.

Common usage: Doses range from 250 to 1,000 mg/day, with some quasi-lay Internet sites suggesting the higher end of this range on particularly intense training days.

Health concerns: According to a review by Bond (2017), research investigating the safety of PA supplementation is lacking. No subjects in human trials at the time of this review reported side effects, but detailed long-term data need to be collected and analyzed.

Phosphatidylserine (PS) 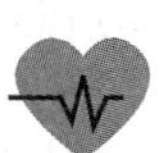 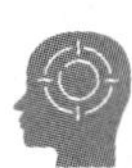  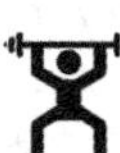 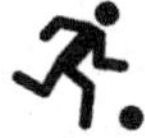

What it is: Phosphatidylserine (PS) is a phospholipid nutrient found in the cell membrane of a variety of tissues, including the brain, lungs, heart, liver, and skeletal muscle. The best dietary sources of PS are organ meats such as brain, liver, heart, and kidney. Fatty fish, meats, and white beans can also provide PS in smaller amounts. PS supplements were first derived from the brains of cows; however, concerns about infectious disease have resulted in the development of soy-derived PS supplements (Starks et al., 2008).

Function: It is believed that PS affects the actions of receptors and signaling molecules in cell membranes in much the same way that diets high in omega-3 fatty acids alter phospholipid membrane composition and create positive physiological changes. to suppress cortisol, a major catabolic hormone that becomes elevated during periods of physical exertion and overtraining. In addition, PS may enhance mood, improve memory, and prevent dementia.

Performance benefit: Possible benefits of PS for athletes include the ability to speed recovery, prevent muscle soreness, improve well-being, and enhance performance in endurance and strength sports.

Research: Scientists completed multiple studies on PS in 2005 and 2006. In both studies PS was ineffective in decreasing markers of muscle damage, oxidative stress, inflammation, cortisol, and creatine kinase in response to exercise (Kingsley et al., 2005, 2006). In one of the two studies PS was shown to increase exercise capacity during cycling until exhaustion (Kingsley et al., 2006). Another group of scientists measured the impact of PS on cortisol during a short-duration (15-minute) moderate-intensity exercise session. Although the number of subjects was small (10), PS did lower cortisol and increase testosterone (Starks et al., 2008). Overall, results are inconclusive, and more research trials are needed to clarify potential benefits for athletes.

Common usage: Research studies with athletes have typically used doses of 300 to 800 mg/day of soy-derived PS; however, these trials were short in duration (10-15 days). A 300 mg/day dose is recommended for treatment of mental stress, and doses as low as 100 mg/day are common for enhancement of cognitive function (Jager, Purpura, & Kingsley, 2007).

Health concerns: The use of PS appears to be safe: 300 to 600 mg/day provided for up to 120 days for older patients did not result in any adverse effects, and 800 mg doses over 10 to 12 days have been tolerated without adverse effects in healthy adults.

Pine Bark Extract 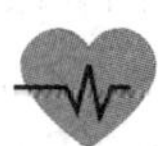 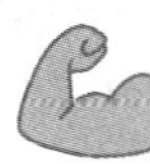 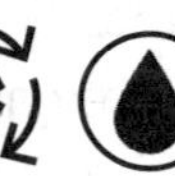 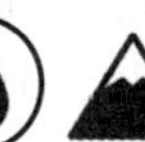 

aka *Pycnogenol, Pinus pinaster*

What it is: An herbal extract derived from the bark of the French maritime pine tree and sometimes referred to by the trade name Pycnogenol, pine bark extract contains plant compounds called oligomeric proanthocyanidin complexes (OPCs), which that carry strong antioxidant qualities of potential benefit to human health and physical performance.

Function: The metabolic demands of sport, reflected by a 10- to 20-fold increase in inhaled oxygen, generate detrimental molecules called free radicals. Although athletes have natural antioxidant defenses to suppress free radicals and protect cells from damage, it is not uncommon to see levels of free radical production exceed natural defenses during high-volume training, leading to increased muscle damage, inflammation and soreness, and reduced performance. Pine bark extract increases the production of antioxidant enzymes and scavengers, strengthening the body's ability to fight off free radicals and prevent such problems, thereby allowing an athlete to recover more efficiently during cycles of heavy training. Of further benefit to recovery and performance is the apparent ability of pine bark extract to shut down the production of proinflammatory enzymes such as COX-2 and enhance nitric oxide production, which helps increase blood and oxygen flow to muscles and encourage muscle tissue growth and repair as well as better support aerobic endurance. Pine bark extract also may help inhibit the enzymes responsible for the destruction of lung tissue in chronic bronchitis and decrease the amount of circulating inflammatory substances in the bloodstream, thereby helping provide relief from symptoms associated with asthma and chronic bronchitis (Shin et al., 2013).

Performance benefit: Athletes may benefit from improved recovery times during periods of increased training stress as well as boosts to endurance performance.

Research: Supplementation with pine bark extract has been shown to improve physical performance and protect against postexercise oxidative stress in both a healthy nonathletic population as well as in trained athletes. In one placebo-controlled study, healthy male subjects who consumed 800 mg/day of pine bark extract over 14 days prior to exercise and 2 days after exercise were found to have significantly greater protection from oxidative stress generated from a $\dot{V}O_2$peak exercise test (Aldret et al, 2020). In another study, untrained healthy participants who took a lower supplemental dose of 100 mg/day of pine bark extract over 8 weeks were found to have a significant improvement not only in exercise-induced oxidative stress but also performance in an Army Physical Fitness Test (APFT) protocol (2 mi run, sit-ups, push-ups) compared to the placebo group (Vinciguerra et al., 2013). In the same study, a supplementation protocol consisting of 150 mg/day of pine bark extract over 4 weeks significantly decreased cramps and postexercise pain levels, lowered exercise-induced oxidative stress, facilitated better triathlon performances, and sped recovery compared to a placebo group of healthy trained participants (Vinciguerra et al., 2013). Applications for use may also extend to those with mild osteoarthritis, with a dose of 120 mg of pine bark extract supplemented over 12 weeks being shown to provide relief from pain and improve mobility as compared to a placebo group in an extensive clinical study including 358 subjects suffering from mild knee osteoarthritis (Heffernan et al., 2020).

Common usage: Pine bark extract is available in tablet and capsule forms in a wide variety of dosing strengths. To help reduce muscle pain and inflammation during heavy training cycles, a range of 100 to 200 mg/day for up to 3 months is recommended. Higher doses up to 800 mg/day over 14 to 16 days have been used to help mitigate exercise-induced oxidative stress and promote optimal postworkout recovery.

Health concerns: There have been reports of dizziness, gut problems, headache, and mouth ulcers, especially at doses above 450 mg.

Piperine 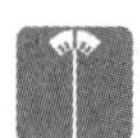

aka *BioPerine (brand name), black pepper, piperdine*

What it is: Piperine is an alkaloid-amine component of the commonly used spice black pepper, as well as of green and white pepper, (Tripathi, et al. 2022) among other sources. *Piper nigrum* is a flowering vine, and its fruits, known as peppercorns, are dried and ground to produce black pepper. The vine is native to Southeast Asia, China, and Vietnam, which are the world's largest producers of pepper. As a traditional medicine, black pepper has been used to treat upset stomach and diarrhea. Recent evidence suggests that black pepper might reduce triglycerides, blood sugar, and cholesterol. Piperine is believed to play an important role in this reduction. Piperine is also included in various supplements with poor bioavailability in an effort to enhance their uptake or maintain concentrations in the blood. Lastly, piperine alkaloids are becoming a common ingredient found in so-called fat-burning and weight-loss supplements.

Function: Many of the mechanisms behind piperine as a sole intervention are unknown; however, recent studies suggest that it works at the cellular level by influencing gene transcription. Specifically, piperine influences a number of genes that are downstream targets for PPARγ, which is involved in the regulation of genes involved in stimulating adipogenesis (development of fat cells). Piperine alkaloids found in black pepper can inhibit PPARγ, decreasing adipogenesis and the negative effects of body fat accumulation such as high blood cholesterol and triglycerides. As an adjunct to other supplements—which may be its most common application—piperine appears to increase intestinal absorption and decrease hepatic clearance of botanicals that have low bioavailability, although evidence is mixed.

Performance benefit: Piperine may benefit athletes wanting to improve body composition, reduce body weight, maximize strength-to-mass ratios, or enhance the bioavailability of co-consumed herbal supplements. However, more research on human athletes is necessary.

Research: Preclinical and clinical evidence suggest piperine's absorption-enhancing effects hold some promise. For example, a 2011 study of mice found that the addition of piperine significantly increased resveratrol bioavailability (Johnson et al., 2011). According to a review by Tripathi and colleagues (2022), "Piperine is a natural bioenhancer to increase the bioavailability of phytochemicals including curcumin and resveratrol." Piperine was also reported to enhance the bioavailability of EGCG from green tea 1.3-fold and increase the serum response of beta-carotene 60% (Tripathi et al., 2022). However, a double-blind, randomized pilot study with participants receiving a single dose of resveratrol (2.5 g) along with piperine in 0 mg, 5 mg, or 25 mg doses found no significant relationships between dose and pharmacokinetic values (Bailey et al., 2021); in a sex-stratified analysis, however, maximum serum concentration for resveratrol in women showed a trend ($p = 0.057$) toward an increase with piperine. It should be noted that when searching the National Library of Medicine, most studies using piperine as an absorption adjunct do so with curcumin. Two animal studies completed in 2011 also found piperine to be beneficial in preventing adipogenesis and a number of the negative side effects associated with it (Diwan, Poudval, & Brown, 2011). Piperine supplementation at 100 mg/kg, 300 mg/kg, and 375 mg/kg in mice that were fed an obesity-inducing diet reduced adiposity and weight gain and improved lipid profiles (Jin Kim et al., 2011). Other animal studies have found a beneficial effect of piperdine on antioxidant status, suggesting the compound can reduce oxidative stress and increase activity of antioxidant defense enzymes (Srinivasan, 2007). More human research is needed before strong conclusions can be made. Currently, there is a lack of evidence to recommend piperine supplementation on its own.

Common usage: Not enough research is available to develop a definite supplementation dose or usage for humans. Existing human studies tend to combine curcumin with 5 mg piperine. Dietary supplements commonly contain 10 mg of piperine.

Health concerns: There does not appear to be any risk of toxicity or consensus over adverse effects of piperine. Consumers should nonetheless exercise caution and discuss use with a health care professional about the possibility of increasing circulating levels of drugs or other supplements.

Potassium (K) 

aka *potassium acetate, potassium bicarbonate, potassium chloride, potassium citrate, potassium gluconate*

What it is: Found naturally in such dietary sources as bananas, potatoes, tomatoes, prunes, and milk, potassium is an essential mineral stored alongside carbohydrate within the muscles; it is also the primary electrolyte in body cells. Because significant amounts of potassium are lost via sweat during exercise, increased dietary or supplementation intake may be warranted in athletes to support optimal muscle function.

Function: Potassium plays an active role in metabolism, facilitating the synthesis of protein from amino acids in the cell, thereby promoting normal growth and muscle building, and aiding the conversion of glucose to glycogen to enhance the storage of carbohydrate essential for energy production. In addition, as an electrolyte, potassium works with sodium and chloride to control fluid and electrolyte balance and assist in the conduction of nerve impulses critical for optimal muscle contraction and a regular heartbeat. Deficiencies in potassium can trigger nausea, vomiting, slowed reflexes, muscle weakness and cramping, and racing heartbeat.

Performance benefit: Athletes will benefit from improved muscle function, including protection against muscle cramps and enhanced muscle endurance.

Research: During exercise, especially at high intensities, potassium is released from the muscles at an accelerated rate, causing potassium concentrations to rise outside the cell as well as in the bloodstream. This activity, according to several studies, is a significant contributing factor to the development of fatigue in human muscle during exercise (Juel, 2007; Knochel, 1978, 1982; McKenna et al., 2008; Nielson et al., 2004). Therefore, scientists agree that maintenance of potassium balance in and outside the cells is a relevant factor in muscle performance. Human sweat data have demonstrated an average potassium loss of 100 to 200 mg/L of fluid. Most athletes lose 0.5 to 1 L of fluid/hour during physical exertion, making replacement of potassium, often via electrolyte replacement beverages such as sport drinks or electrolyte supplements, especially beneficial to athletes when performing activities lasting longer than 1.5 hours.

Common usage: An update on Dietary Reference Intake (DRI) for potassium was released in 2019, with adequate intakes being indicated at 3,400 mg/day and 2,600 mg/day for adult (age 19+) men and women, respectively. During pregnancy and lactation, adequate intake (AI) increases to 2,900 mg and 2,800 mg, respectively. To maintain electrolyte balance and optimize muscle function, athletes should replace 75 to 150 mg of potassium/L of fluid consumed during physical exertion. Potassium supplements are available as a number of salts, including potassium chloride, potassium citrate, and potassium gluconate; all are available in powder, pill, capsule, and effervescent form. The most common way to replenish electrolytes for most athletes is through use of a sport drink.

SUPPLEMENT FACT

Use of diuretics, laxatives, alcohol, and large doses of caffeine (>6 mg/kg); prolonged diarrhea or vomiting; and excessive sugar intake can increase the risk for potassium deficiency.

Health concerns: Excessive potassium intake, generally at doses of 18 g or more, alters sodium balance and can lead to gastrointestinal distress, electrical impulse disturbance, irregular heartbeat, and possibly death. Therefore, large doses of potassium beyond what is commonly found in supplements should never be consumed without the direct supervision and advice of a physician. Athletes engaged in contact sports where blunt-force trauma damages muscle tissue, such as football and hockey, may be at increased risk for abnormally high serum potassium levels due to rapid movement of potassium from the cells into the bloodstream during injury.

Potassium Phosphate

(see *phosphate salts*)

Potassium Pyruvate, Proacemic Acid

(see *pyruvate*)

Potassium (K)

Probiotics 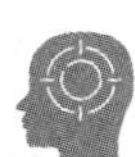  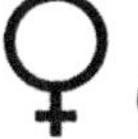 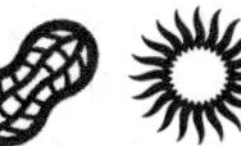

aka *Bifidobacterium, Enterococcus, Escherichia, Lactobacillus, Saccharomyces*

What it is: Probiotics are live microorganisms found naturally within the digestive tract that, when maintained at adequate levels, are thought to support intestinal health and enhance immune function. Most probiotics are of bacterial nature, thus the nickname "friendly bacteria," and originate from the Lactobacillus (L.) or Bifidobacterium (B.) family. Over 500 types of bacterial species exist, each exerting a unique health benefit by helping fight the growth of harmful bacteria and yeast. Strains of the Bifidobacterium family account for nearly 25% of all probiotics in the body and are found primarily in the large intestine; species of Lactobacillus are generally found in the small intestine. Probiotics can be added to the diet via such foods as yogurt, cultured milk products, and beverages as well as taken in capsule, tablet, and powdered form.

SUPPLEMENT FACT

Probiotics should not be mistaken for prebiotics, which are complex sugars such as fructooligosaccharides that serve as fuel for bacteria already present in the digestive tract. Products containing both pre- and probiotics are often labeled as synbiotics.

Function: Immune functionality has been shown to be suppressed after intense exercise, making the athlete more vulnerable to upper respiratory tract infections and gastrointestinal illness. Because recovery can take away significant time from training and competition, reducing the occurrence of these illnesses is a high priority. Probiotics may provide added nutritional support in the intestines, where more than 70% of the body's immune defenses work to fight against harmful microbes that can contribute to infection, thereby helping reduce the incidence of illness during heavy training and competition.

Performance benefit: Probiotics may aid the overall health of an athlete, helping to protect against and reduce symptoms of gastrointestinal and upper respiratory tract illnesses.

Research: Results examining the efficacy of probiotic supplementation as it relates to immune and gut support in an athletic population have shown promise. Multistrain Lactobacillus and Bifidobacterium probiotic cocktails, for example, have been shown to improve or preserve gut barrier function during exercise training and competition, helping to reduce GI symptom frequency and severity (Miles, 2020). Pugh and colleagues (2019) discovered that a supplementation protocol entailing consumption of a probiotic cocktail containing 25 billion colony-forming units (CFU) of *L. acidophilus*, *B. bifidum*, and *B. animalis* subsp. *Lactis* over 28 days reduced both the incidence and severity of symptoms associated with GI distress in training as well as on marathon race day in a group of long distance runners. It is important to note both the placebo and supplement group in this study used standardized, recommended carbohydrate loading as well as in-race carbohydrate and hydration strategies, yet only the supplement group was able to sustain running speed toward the end of the marathon, suggestive of a potential performance benefit. A supplementation protocol that implemented a cocktail of 15 billion CFU of *L. helveticus Lafti* L10, *B. animalis* ssp. *lactis Lafti* B94, *E. faecium* R0026, *B. longum* R0175, and *Bacillus subtilis* R0179 over 90 days in a group of trained male cyclists yielded significantly less incidences of heartburn, nausea, belching, and vomiting at rest and in training compared to a control group (Schrieber et al., 2021). In addition, the supplement group reported lower ratings of perceived exertion during exercise, likely due to improved overall GI health, though there was no significant difference between the two groups when looking at $\dot{V}O_2$max values. As for respiratory diseases, the results are also encouraging for multispecies probiotic administration. Strasser and colleagues (2016) found a supplementation protocol that included daily administration of probiotic cocktail inclusive of 1 × 10^{10} CFU of *Bifidobacterium bifidum* W23, *Bifidobacterium lactis* W51, *Enterococcus faecium* W54, *L. acidophilus* W22, *L. brevis* W63, and *Lactococcus lactis* W58 over 3 months to significantly reduce postexercise levels of tryptophan, which lead to a 2.2-fold lowered risk of experiencing one or more upper respiratory symptoms compared to the placebo group of male and female endurance-trained athletes. Once again, there were no significant differences in the groups as it related to athletic performance as measured by a cycle ergometer test to exhaustion. A supplementation protocol consisting of daily administration of another multistrain cocktail inclusive of 1 billion CFU each of *L. acidophilus* LB-G80, *L. paracasei* LPc-G110, *L. subp. Lactis* LLL-G25, *B. animalis* subp. *Lactis* BL-G101, and *B. bifidum* BB-G90 over 30 days prior to running a marathon helped preserve the functionality of monocytes and significantly lowered incidence of respiratory infections in trained male runners compared to the placebo group (Tavares-Silva, 2021). Future research should continue to focus on the impact of both single- and multistrain probiotic cocktails on variables important to athletes' health and performance. Research exploring the impact during various phases of training as well as differences seen in female versus male athletes is also needed.

Common usage: Commonly used probiotics include Lactobacillus, Bifidobacterium, Streptococcus, and Bacillus. The most potent probiotic supplements will contain more organisms, expressed in terms of billions of organisms or CFUs per serving. Dosing regimens typically fall in range between 1 × 10^9 to 1 × 10^{11} CFU. Though both single-strain and multistrain products are commonly used, the optimal combination and individual dosing recommendation for each strain remains unclear (Jäger et al., 2019).

Health concerns: Probiotics are considered safe for use, with minimal side effects reported. However, athletes with milk allergies should be aware that some probiotic products, especially those made with Lactobacilli or Bifidobacterium, may contain trace amount of milk proteins and thus may trigger allergic symptoms.

Provitamin A

(see *beta-carotene*)

Prunus Cerasus

(see *tart cherry*)

Pterostilbene 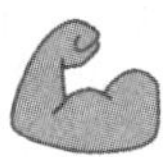 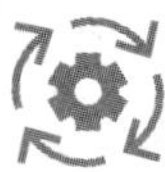 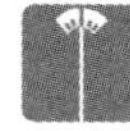

aka *trans-3,5-dimethoxy-4-hydroxystilbene* (see also *nicotinamide riboside* and *resveratrol*)

What it is: Pterostilbene is a phenolic antioxidant compound found in grapes, wine, and blueberries. It is related to resveratrol and included in some NAD+ supplements.

Function: Produced by plants in response to microbial infestation or exposure to ultraviolet light, this antioxidant shares qualities with resveratrol but is more bioavailable and may have its own therapeutic potential (Belviranli et al., 2015). Due to its antioxidant and anti-inflammatory effects, pterostilbene may help prevent or treat a variety of conditions from cancer to cardiovascular disease, but few investigations exist examining its effects on exercise performance or exercise-induced oxidative stress and inflammation. Interestingly, by itself, it may play a role in dissipating energy as heat, which could potentially lead to fat loss, but this needs more study.

Performance benefit: Antioxidant and anti-inflammatory effects may help promote nerve or muscle recovery or protect an athlete from the increased oxidative stress induced during exercise. However, this is speculation from preclinical literature. Potential for thermogenic and fat-reducing effects are also possibilities (Özyalçın and Sanlier, 2023) that require more data.

Research: Again, data on pterostilbene alone in athletes are scarce to absent. As reported by Nagarajan and colleagues (2022), a small number of studies have been logged at ClinicalTrials.gov, with one suggesting that pterostilbene in combination with other ingredients "improved strength and power output in the lower body"; however, pterostilbene-specific effects are hard to discern from this work. One potential benefit lies in pterostilbene's effects on adipose tissue, and perhaps over time, body composition. According to Milton-Laskíbar and colleagues (2020), "studies, carried out in cell cultures and animal models, show that both resveratrol and pterostilbene induce thermogenic capacity in interscapular BAT [brown adipose tissue] by increasing mitochondriogenesis, as well as enhancing fatty acid oxidation and glucose disposal."

Common usage: There is no established recommended dose for pterostilbene. Typical doses sold are 50 to 250 mg.

Health concerns: According to Nagarajan and colleagues (2022), in humans, pterostilbene has been observed to exhibit safety at doses up to 250 mg/day. This is in alignment with the conclusion from Riche and colleagues (2013). More research needs to be done regarding food and drug interactions. At this time, it is advisable to discuss interactions with anticoagulant medications (among others) with a health care practitioner.

Pycnogenol

(see *Pine Bark Extract*)

Pyruvate 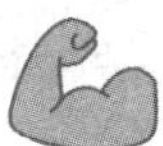

aka *acetylformic acid, alpha-keto acid, alpha-ketopropionic acid, calcium pyruvate, calcium pyruvate monohydrate, creatine pyruvate, magnesium pyruvate, potassium pyruvate, proacemic acid, pyruvic acid, sodium pyruvate, 2-oxopropanoate, 2-oxypropanoic acid*

What it is: Naturally synthesized in the body from glucose (sugar) as well as found naturally in such dietary sources as red wine, dark beer, and red apples, pyruvate, which is the salt derivative of pyruvic acid, is thought to help facilitate body fat loss and enhance endurance performance, making it a popular supplement choice among athletes.

Function: It is thought that pyruvate increases the uptake of glucose from the blood into working muscles, enhancing the fuel available for immediate use and providing a boost to energy reserves (muscle glycogen) for future use. This helps improve muscle endurance and consequent performance. In addition, as a participant in the Krebs cycle of metabolism, pyruvate is thought to increase the body's use of fat for energy as well as resting metabolic rate, thereby helping to facilitate body fat loss.

Performance benefit: Pyruvate supplementation may benefit athletes wanting to optimize body composition and boost endurance capacity.

Research: Although early studies showed some promise, the bulk of current data have not been supportive. For example, in a double-blind, placebo-controlled study, a supplementation protocol providing 6 g/day of pyruvate over 6 weeks was shown to significantly decrease body weight, body fat, and percentage body fat in healthy, overweight men and women participating in a fitness program 3 days a week (Kalman et al., 1999). However, a similar supplementation protocol providing 5 g/day of calcium pyruvate over 30 days failed to demonstrate any significant body composition changes in healthy, untrained women engaged in an exercise program compared to a placebo group (Koh-Banerjee et al., 2005). Furthermore, no significant differences were observed between groups in the metabolic responses to and overall performance during an aerobic exercise routine. Similar void results were identified in soccer players, though the supplementation protocol incorporated only 2 g/day of pyruvate over 4 weeks (Ostojic & Ahmetovic, 2009). The current consensus is that pyruvate appears to be an ineffective strategy for body fat and weight loss (Onakpova et al., 2014). The body of evidence on pyruvate supplementation and various performance parameters, particularly in a human population, is limited. Although there is some evidence to suggest a supplementation protocol containing both pyruvate and the simple carbohydrate dihydroxyacetone may enhance muscle endurance, the applications evaluating pyruvate as a solo ingredient or in combination with creatine have not demonstrated positive results (Ivy, 1998; Morrison, Spriet, & Dyck, 2000; Stanko et al., 1990a, 1990b; Van Schuylenbergh et al., 2003). More recently, Yang and colleagues (2022) revealed a supplementation protocol consisting of 0.1 g/kg/day of sodium pyruvate taken over 7 days to significantly improve repeated sprint exercise performance compared to a placebo group of trained soccer players of which was attributed to accelerated restoration of the acid-base balance and ATP-PC regeneration. Additional research is needed on a human athlete population before conclusions can be made on the efficacy of use for performance.

Common usage: Pyruvate supplements are available in capsule, tablet, and bulk powder form; pyruvate is also commonly included as an ingredient in so-called fat-burning supplements as well as paired with creatine as a sports supplement. Doses used in research have been highly variable, ranging from 2 to 30 g taken daily either before exercise or with a meal, or based on body weight (0.1 g/kg/day over 7 days), with conflicting outcomes. It is evident more research is needed before standardized supplementation protocol recommendations are established.

Health concerns: Acute doses of pyruvate above 25 g may trigger gastrointestinal symptoms such as stomach upset, bloating, gas, and diarrhea.

Pyruvate Oxidation Factor

(see *alpha-lipoic acid*)

Pyruvic Acid

(see *pyruvate*)

Quercetin 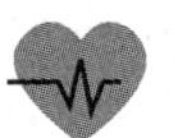  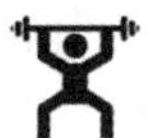 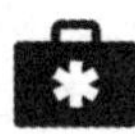  

aka *meletin, sophretin* (see also *naringin*)

What it is: Quercetin is an antioxidant found naturally in the pulp of many citrus fruits and in apple skins, buckwheat, red onions, red grapes, wine, and tea. It is estimated that the average adult diet provides up to 50 mg of quercetin each day; athletes, especially those enjoying healthy amounts of fruits and vegetables, will accumulate significantly more due to higher calorie intakes to support the demands of training.

Function: Quercetin has recently garnered a lot of attention among athletes for its ability to reduce exercise-induced oxidative stress, thereby helping to improve sport performance and recovery. This compound may also slow the metabolism of other drugs or supplements in the liver.

Performance benefit: Lowering the oxidative stress associated with intensive exercise helps facilitate optimal sport performance by delaying the onset of muscle fatigue and decreasing muscle damage, which, in turn, will improve recovery. There has also been scientific evidence demonstrating significant immune-enhancing and anti-inflammatory benefits that aid recovery and may even present promise for athletes with allergies or asthma (Aghababaei & Hadidi, 2023).

Research: The health benefits of polyphenols, particularly quercetin, are substantial. Emerging evidence from human studies have also shown a wide range of potential applications related to sport performance in sprint and endurance exercises as well as resistance training (Somerville et al., 2017). A 2011 meta-analysis of 11 studies and 254 human subjects, for example, found a statistically significant increase in $\dot{V}O_2max$ and endurance performance (2%) with supplementation of 1,000 mg/day of quercetin over 11 days compared to a placebo (Kressler, Millard-Stafford, & Warren, 2011). A 2% boost can have huge performance implications, especially for the elite or professional athlete—for reference, it would be equivalent to a 40-minute 10K runner dropping their time to 39:20. A small, double-blind, randomized study using the same 1,000 mg/day dose over 6 weeks was found to lower exercise-induced oxidative stress in trained runners compared to the placebo group but failed to enhance peak oxygen consumption or running economy measured by oxygen consumption during a 10 km running time trial (Scholten & Sergeev, 2013). Another small study of similar design found an acute 1 g dose of quercetin taken 3 hours prior to a resistance-training session improved the neuromuscular performance of healthy male subjects by improving the torque–velocity curve of knee extensors and significantly increasing the total volume of resistance exercises completed compared to the placebo group. Study investigators also noted that the quercetin facilitated a more favorable postexercise neuromuscular response compared to the placebo group (Patrizio et al., 2018). In another double-blind, randomized, crossover study, a supplementation protocol using 1 g/day over 14 days significantly increased the isometric strength in maximal voluntary isometric contraction and attenuated muscle weakness severity compared to baseline (Bazzucchi et al., 2019). A larger clinical study of similar design utilizing a 500 mg dose of quercetin over 8 weeks found a significant increase in basal metabolic effect, lean body mass, total body water, and overall energy expenditure, yet no improvements in maximal oxygen consumption compared to the placebo group of male students with an athletic history (Askari et al., 2013). Overall, quercetin has shown promise in its ability to regulate multiple pathways associated with sport performance, though additional research further exploring dosage and timing of intake for optimal outcomes in an athletic population is warranted.

Common usage: Quercetin is available in tablet, powder, softgel, or capsule form in a variety of strengths and often combined with other nutrients, such as vitamin C, to form an antioxidant cocktail. Depending on the formulation and bioavailability, the daily dose of quercetin used in human studies have ranged from 50 mg to upwards of 2,000 mg. An average daily dose of 200 to 400 mg is taken up to 3 times/day, preferably 20 minutes before meals. There is no RDA for quercetin.

Health concerns: Because quercetin is found naturally in several common foods, it is thought to be generally safe and well tolerated through usual dietary intake. Hypersensitive individuals may experience headaches or tingling. Though rare, other reported side effects include gastrointestinal discomfort, hematoma, and kidney toxicity. Children and those who are pregnant or lactating should consult with a health care professional before supplementing with quercetin.

Raspberry Ketone

aka *European red raspberry (Rubus idaeus) extract, 4-(4-hydroxyphenyl) butan-2-one, frambinone, rheosmin*

What it is: Raspberry ketone is an aromatic compound found within red raspberries, kiwifruit, peaches, apples, maple, and pine. It defines the characteristic fragrance and taste of raspberry. It is used in cosmetics and as a flavoring agent and appears widely in foods and beverages. Consumers may also see it associated with weight loss claims from marketers.

Function: Li and colleagues (2022) have stated that the mechanism for potential weight loss is largely unknown. It may include lipolysis (fat breakdown) or antioxidant and lipogenic gene interactions, but Rao and colleagues (2021) state: "Raspberry ketone-mediated activation of peroxisome proliferator-activated receptor-α (PPAR-α) stands out as one of its main modes of action. Although rodent studies have demonstrated the efficacious effects . . . its mechanism remains largely unknown."

Performance benefit: Controversially, raspberry ketone may enhance weight (fat) loss. Note that raspberry ketone does not induce ketosis, as is sometimes suggested in marketing.

Research: According to Rao and colleagues (2021), "A single clinical study showed that a multi-ingredient supplement containing [raspberry ketone] was able to reduce body weight, metabolic lipid, and inflammatory parameters in 45 obese individuals after an 8-week exercise and weight loss program. Although the supplement consisted of different concentrations of other herbs in addition to RK." Evidence is currently weak.

Common usage: There is no recommended dosage for raspberry ketone, but it is sold in a broad range of doses from 100 to 1,000 mg, sometimes with other ingredients in a blend. Simply eating more raspberries within one's individual tolerance is suggested.

Health concerns: Raspberry ketone is on the FDA's Generally Recognized as Safe (GRAS) list. GRAS status suggests low toxicity for intended uses, but there have not been well-designed clinical trials involving supplementation in humans. Drug interaction data are also limited.

Radix Astragali (RA)

(see *astragalus*)

Red Beet

(see *beetroot*)

Red Pepper

(see *capsicum*)

Red Yeast Rice  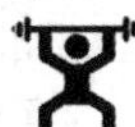

What it is: Red yeast rice is the product of yeast (*Monascus purpureus*) that has been grown on white rice. It contains compounds such as monacolin K, which is part of the prescription cholesterol-lowering drug lovastatin. It should be noted that the FDA has sent warning letters to companies selling red yeast rice products that contain added lovastatin. Further, the amount of monacolin K has been reported to vary hugely in red yeast rice products, and contamination with the mycotoxin citrinin could be an issue with some brands.

Function: It is principally sold as an LDL-lowering supplement for cardiovascular health. Application to sport performance appears minimal at the time of this writing. The potential for anti-inflammatory effects could potentially support recovery, but this needs further study. Patel (2016) has also alluded to osteogenic effects. Indeed, based on preclinical animal studies, Wu and colleagues (2020) concluded that red yeast rice can promote bone formation and may be useful for the treatment of osteoporosis.

Performance benefit: Applications of red yeast rice to athletes with low bone density remain largely speculative. Beneficial effects in clinical populations such as those with metabolic syndrome (e.g. dyslipidemia, hypertension, fatty liver, central body fat) cannot be extrapolated to athletes.

Research: In 2016, Patel reported that based on mechanistic studies, red yeast rice may interact with functional agents such as astaxanthin, berberine, coenzyme Q10, folic acid, policosanol, and vitamin D. Most research has been done on cardiometabolic benefits in nonathletes.

Common usage: In 2015, Gerards and colleagues stated that in clinical trials, red yeast rice doses varying from 200 mg to 4,800 mg/day have been studied. Products on the market may contain 600 to 1,800 mg, often with other ingredients such as coenzyme Q10.

Health concerns: According to the Mayo Clinic (2023), red yeast rice supplements are generally considered safe, but could carry the same potential side effects, such as liver stress and muscle disorders, as with statin drugs. Other side effects could include abdominal discomfort and gas, heartburn, headache, or dizziness. Drug interactions with prescription statins, antidepressants, antibiotics, and other medications that interact with statins could also occur, so speaking to a physician is important.

Resveratrol 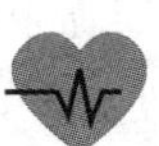 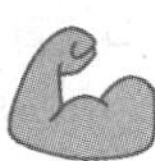  

aka *3,4'5-stilbenetriol, 3,4'5-trihydroxystilbene*

What it is: Found in greatest concentration in the skin of grapes as well as on the vine, root, seed, and stalk of a grapevine (also found naturally in peanuts and mulberries), resveratrol is a naturally occurring molecule called a stilbenoid that carries strong anti-oxidant qualities and is marketed to enhance athletes' health, endurance, and recovery.

Function: Animal data suggest that resveratrol may help enhance endurance by significantly increasing the size and number of mitochondria within muscle. Mitochondria, also known as the powerhouse of the cell, are responsible for breaking down carbohydrate, fat, and protein in the presence of oxygen to generate the ATP needed to propel performance. Increasing the size and number of mitochondria therefore allows more energy to be generated during exercise, thereby enhancing endurance. Furthermore, with its strong antioxidant properties, resveratrol is purported to help offset some of the damage caused by the release of highly reactive oxygen species (ROS) that often are generated at a rate faster than the body's natural defense system can control during heavy training. In combination with its anti-inflammatory properties—resveratrol inhibits the activity of the enzyme cyclooxygenase-2 (COX-2) to fight acute inflammation, much like nonsteroidal anti-inflammatories (NSAIDs) do—resveratrol is thought to enhance recovery and may also serve as a natural treatment option for inflammatory-based conditions such as arthritis that are common among athletes.

Performance benefit: Athletes may benefit from improved muscle strength and fatigue tolerance as well as muscle recovery after use and regeneration after disuse.

Research: Although animal studies have demonstrated promise for several performance variables, including aerobic capacity, exercise time to fatigue, improved mitochondrial function, and lower levels of oxidative stress (Lagouge et al., 2006; Murase et al., 2009), the translation to a human population, particularly athletes, is limited and conflicted. One small study using a supplementation protocol of 160 mg of oral resveratrol 3 times/day over 4 consecutive days failed to improve postexercise muscle glycogen resynthesis and related glucose uptake and mitochondrial biosynthesis gene expression in healthy men compared to placebo (Huang et al., 2020). In another small study, oral supplementation with 480 mg of resveratrol over 4 days failed to demonstrate any effect on high-intensity cycling exercise performance or exercise-induced fatigue; however, it did significantly reduce the proinflammatory IL-6 response, helping prevent muscle stress and damage (Tsao et al., 2021). A larger double-blind, placebo-controlled study found a daily intake of 500 mg or 1,000 mg of resveratrol over 7 days leading up to a plyometric test to reduce levels of muscle damage, inflammation, and soreness caused by exercise and significantly improve the recovery of power and anaerobic performances in a healthy untrained male population (Huang et al., 2021). It is evident that more human data from an athletic population is needed before recommendations for use as it relates to sport performance can be made.

Common usage: Resveratrol is available in capsule and tablet form containing extracts of red wine and giant knotweed, a plant found in China; it is also commonly seen as an ingredient in a combined antioxidant or phytonutrient blend that often sold in a wine bottle. Several functional food products also advertise various strengths of resveratrol. Supplements vary in purity and can contain anywhere from 50% to 99% resveratrol. The human studies reported using a daily dose ranging from 480 mg to 1,000 mg per day. For reference, fresh grape skin contains about 0.1 to 0.5 mg of resveratrol/g, whereas a glass of wine provides 0.6 to 0.7 mg per glass. Dietary supplements generally provide 250 to500 mg of resveratrol.

Health concerns: Use of resveratrol appears to be well tolerated by most, but long-term safety has yet to be established.

Rhaponticum Carthamoides

(see *maral root*)

Rhodiola Rosea (RR) 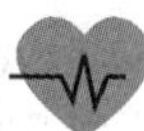 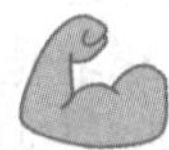 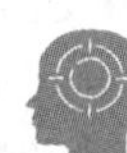 

aka *Aaron's rod, Arctic root, golden root, Rhodiola arctica, Rhodiola iremelica, rose root, R. rosea, Sedum rosea*

What it is: Commonly marketed as an adaptogen that enhances the body's resistance to physiological stress, including exercise, *Rhodiola rosea* (RR) is an herb that grows in the mountainous regions of central and northern Europe, Asia, and North America as well as in the cold climate of the Arctic. Active components of Rhodiola rosea that are commonly studied and extracted for supplemental use include rosavins and salidroside.

Function: RR is believed to enhance performance through several mechanisms; the most relevant for the athlete is its apparent impact on energy usage. As demonstrated in animal studies, RR improves energy usage by increasing essential energy metabolites, ATP, and phosphocreatine within muscle and brain mitochondria, thereby stimulating protein and amino acid synthesis and boosting fat metabolism. In addition, RR seems to moderate levels of cortisol during physical stress, helping to limit muscle damage as well as protect the immune system, thus optimizing both short- and long-term recovery.

Performance benefit: RR is purported to enhance many areas of athletic performance, including speed, strength, stamina, muscle building, energy reserves, and recovery time.

Research: The ergogenic benefits of acute RR supplementation have not been consistently demonstrated in well-designed human studies. A further evaluation of data specifically evaluating RR dosing patterns confirms a bell-shaped curve, indicating the bulk of negative results have been seen in subjects taking low or high doses of RR. A daily dose of 170 mg taken over 4 weeks, however, seems to demonstrate favorable changes in exercise-related blood markers that are consistent with results of well-designed animal studies, according to a double-blind, placebo-controlled study of 14 trained male athletes (Parisi et al., 2010). After the athletes completed an exhaustive cardiopulmonary test at 75% of $\dot{V}O_2$max, significant reductions in plasma free fatty acid (indicating increased fat metabolism), blood lactate levels (key to extending endurance), and plasma creatine kinase (a parameter of skeletal muscle damage) were seen. A similar dose of RR (3 mg/kg or ~170 mg) taken acutely 60 minutes prior to exercise significantly reduced heart rate during a standardized 10-minute warm-up as well as decreased ratings of perceived exertion and significantly improved time trial performance in a 6 mi (9.6 km) bicycle ergometry test compared to the placebo group of recreationally active females (Noreen et al., 2013). In contrast, a double-blind, randomized, placebo-controlled trial failed to find any significant improvements in the physical performance of physically healthy men in a $\dot{V}O_2$peak test when given an increased dose of RR supplementation (600 mg/day) over 4 weeks (Jówko et al., 2018). However, it is important to note that, although statistically insignificant, there was a noted improvement in both maximal cycling power and time to exhaustion, which might hold some promise for those competing at high levels. Similarly, a supplementation protocol of 600 mg/day in the 30 days prior to running a marathon failed to exert any performance benefit in a group of experienced runners, with no significant differences being reported in postmarathon decrease in muscle function, increases in muscle damage, DOMS, or plasma cytokines compared to a placebo group (Shanely et al., 2014). Interestingly, higher doses of RR seem to elicit a favorable response on more explosive resistance-focused exercise. One recent trial of resistance-trained males found short-term supplementation with 1,500 mg/day of RR over 3 days to significantly improve bench press velocity compared to a placebo group, although repetition volume decreased (Williams et al., 2021). Recent research has shown a synergistic effect of caffeine (3 mg/kg) plus 2,400 mg of rhodiola rosea, yielding significant improvements on training adaptations seen with resistance training in untrained subjects compared to a placebo (Liu et al., 2023). Additional research is needed to establish the conditions in which RR supplementation facilitates exercise performance and adaptations before practical guidelines for use in an athletic population can be made. Furthermore, more data needs to include female athletes to determine if applications can be made across sexes.

R

Common usage: Most commonly available in tablet or capsule form, RR supplements generally contain 100 mg of a standardized amount of 3% rosavins and 1% salidroside, which matches the natural ratio of the most active compounds found in the root of the plant. The research-supported doses of RR range from 170 mg to 600 mg/day, with higher doses often split into a couple doses throughout the day and generally taken in the morning and early afternoon; some reports of sleep disturbances have been reported with evening use over a period of a few days to 4 weeks. Doses upwards of 2,400 mg, have been used to yield favorable effects on resistance-trained athletes.

Health concerns: RR appears to be safe for supplementation use with no severe adverse effects (Tao et al., 2019). Even so, comprehensive safety studies are lacking; the safety of its use in young children, pregnant or nursing women, and people with liver or kidney disease has not been established, making supplementation ill-advised for these populations.

Riboflavin   

aka *riboflavin-5-phosphate, vitamin B$_2$*

What it is: Playing a key role in the production of energy, riboflavin is an essential nutrient and member of the B-vitamin family that must be obtained from such key dietary sources as organ meats, shellfish, dairy foods, eggs, green leafy vegetables, legumes, and almonds. It is thought that exercise increases the requirements for riboflavin, making supplementation of potential benefit to athletes, especially those restricting energy intake or following fad diets where intake often falls short of recommendations.

Function: Along with its vitamin siblings thiamine (B$_1$) and pyridoxine (B$_6$), riboflavin (B$_2$) plays a key role in the energy-producing metabolic pathways of the body, helping break down carbohydrate, fat, and protein for conversion into available energy. Physical training puts additional stress on these metabolic pathways, which raises the question of whether athletes might benefit from supplementation to help accommodate these increased demands and protect against deficiency, which has been correlated with a lower tolerance to high-intensity exercise and consequent reduced performance.

Performance benefit: Athletes may benefit from enhanced endurance during high-intensity competition, with the greatest results likely to be seen in those whose diets are deficient in riboflavin.

Research: The intentional implementation of a riboflavin-deficient diet (55% of the RDA) over 11 weeks has been shown to have a detrimental impact on performance, with healthy men demonstrating a significant decrease in $\dot{V}O_2$max (−12%) and peak power (−9%) from a baseline nondeficient state (van der Beek et al., 1988, 1994); however, athletes who maintain riboflavin status are unlikely to benefit from supplementation with riboflavin regardless of training volume and intensity. One study failed to discover any change in blood riboflavin in collegiate swimmers despite a dramatic increase in the intensity, volume, and energy expenditure during a heavy training cycle (Sato et al., 2011). Similarly, an evaluation of riboflavin blood concentration in a cross-section of athletes from multiple sports found that 90% fell above the normal range, with a direct correlation being noted for riboflavin blood level and intake over 7 days (Rokitzki et al., 1994). Janssen and colleagues (2021) has also reported no differences in riboflavin status between highly fit ($\dot{V}O_2$peak \gte\47 mL/kg/min) and less fit (≤37 mL/kg/min) females after 60 minutes of maximal exercise. Research suggests that female athletes, especially those restricting calories or following fad diets that limit intake of specific food groups or macronutrients, are at greater risk for riboflavin deficiency, making supplementation of possible benefit for this population (Woolf & Manore, 2006).

Common usage: Available in capsule and tablet form, riboflavin can be supplemented by itself; however, it is commonly added to multivitamin and multimineral supplements as well as B-complex preparations. The RDA for riboflavin is 1.3 to 1.1 mg/day for adult (19+) men and women, respectively. For those who are pregnant or breastfeeding, RDA increases to 1.4 mg and 1.6 mg, respectively. Typical supplementation doses range from 1.7 to 10 mg/day. Doses above 30 mg/day should be taken in several smaller amounts throughout the day.

Health concerns: Use of riboflavin supplements appears to be safe, though there have been reports of diarrhea and polyuria (harmless yellow-orange coloring to urine) with long-term daily use of doses greater than 400 mg. Deficiency symptoms, which generally manifest after several months of failing to consume the RDA, include cracked lips as well as a sore tongue. Child athletes may also experience stunted growth patterns.

Ribose 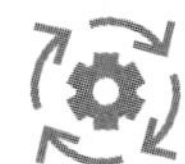

aka *beta-D-ribofuranose, D-ribose*

What it is: Ribose is considered a sugar or monosaccharide. Its chemical formula is $C_5H_{10}O_5$, which is similar to that of glucose ($C_6H_{12}O_6$). Ribose is not commonly found in food but can be synthesized in the body; phosphorylated ribose can become a subunit of ATP and DNA. It is this relationship with ATP that sparked the interest in ribose as a dietary supplement. Ribose became popular in the 1980s as creatine became popular in the mainstream and research supporting the use of creatine more substantiated. Both ribose and creatine are involved in the synthesis of ATP.

Function: Essentially, ribose works in the synthesis of ATP (adenosine triphosphate), the high-energy molecule used by muscles during contraction. During high-intensity exercise, muscles use ATP at high rates. The breakdown of ATP results in adenosine diphosphate (ADP) and adenosine monophosphate (AMP). The muscles can recycle some of these ADP and AMP molecules back into ATP through phosphocreatine stores. Unfortunately, during this process some AMP molecules are removed from the cell, at which point they can no longer be recycled back into useful ATP. Ribose prevents AMP from leaving the cell, keeping more AMP available to be recycled back into useful ATP.

Performance benefit: Athletes engaged in high-intensity strength and power sports would benefit most from ribose supplementation. Higher levels of ATP in muscles would enable athletes to train for longer periods of time at higher intensities as well as improve recovery.

Research: Early data evaluating the impact of D-ribose on various performance variables in athletes were conflicting. Favorable studies found intravenous administration of ribose to aid replenishment of ATP stores in tissues exposed to ischemia (Peveler et al., 2006), yet other studies reported no performance benefit with ribose (Berardi & Ziegenfuss, 2003; Hellsten, Skadhauge, & Bangsbo, 2004; Kerksick et al., 2005; Kreider et al., 2003). More recent results have found a positive response of oral D-ribose supplementation on recovery variables, yet such results have been found in healthy untrained subjects versus athletes. For example, Cao and colleagues (2020) found oral administration of 15 g of D-ribose 1 hour before and 1, 6, 12, and 36 hours after a lower-limb plyometric exercise session to reduce lower limb muscle soreness, improve the degree of knee extensor function, lower muscle damage and the degree of lipid peroxidation, and accelerate the recovery of DOMS, with some numbers reaching statistical significance, in untrained healthy males compared to a placebo group. Similarly, Seifert and colleagues (2017) found a supplementation protocol of 10 g of D-ribose/day over 5 days, which included 3 days of 60-minute high-intensity interval training, to yield significantly higher mean and peak power outputs from day 1 to day 3 as well as significantly lower ratings of perceived exertion and significantly lower creatine kinase levels compared to the placebo group—but only for the less fit group ($\dot{V}O_2$max 39.9 ± 4.1 mg/kg/min). There were no performance benefits discovered for the group with a higher $\dot{V}O_2$max (52.2 ± 4.3 mL/kg/min), suggesting that oral intake of D-ribose may only provide benefit to athletes who are detrained and rebuilding fitness.

Common usage: A wide variety of supplementation strategies for ribose have been employed, with the majority of research trials using 10 to 20 g/day. The maximum safe oral dose of D-ribose has been indicated at 200 mg/kg/hour.

Health concerns: Supplementation with ribose appears safe, though doses of more than 200 mg/kg/hour of D-ribose has been shown to elevate diarrhea risk.

Rose Root, *R. Rosea*

(see *Rhodiola rosea*)

Russian Leuzea

(see *maral root*)

Rutaecarpine

aka *evodia fruit, evodiamine, Evodia rutaecarpa, wu-chu-yu*

What it is: A nitrogen-containing compound called an alkaloid, rutaecarpine is derived from the fruit of an *Evodia rutaecarpa,* a small tree native to China and Korea. Rutaecarpine has been widely used in Chinese medicine for over 100 years and more recently has emerged as a dietary supplement marketed to naturally treat inflammatory-based conditions.

SUPPLEMENT FACT

Evodia rutaecarpa is a natural source of synephrine, a common ingredient found in weight-loss drugs due to its purported ability to boost metabolism, enhance fat burning, and decrease appetite.

Function: Although acute inflammation is a normal physiological response that is critical to protecting muscle tissue and cells from damage, inflammation that lingers is suggestive of an overactive inflammatory response that is detrimental to recovery, sport performance, and overall health. Animal data suggest rutaecarpine helps mediate the activity of the proinflammatory enzyme COX-2, helping to protect against such chronic inflammation (Moon et al., 1999). Additional animal studies have shown that rutaecarpine promotes the release of nitric oxide, which opens up the blood vessels for enhanced delivery of nutrients to support muscle performance and recovery (Wang et al., 1999). As a sympathomimetic agent, rutaecarpine potentially has thermogenic properties, meaning it may have the ability to increase the production of body heat, which may enhance overall calorie and fat burning (Kim et al., 2009). Alternatively, rutaecarpine stimulates the production of natural molecules called vanilloids that, in animal studies, have demonstrated the ability to reduce the uptake of fat as well as increase the rate of fat burning (Kobayashi et al., 2001).

Performance benefit: Athletes may benefit from enhanced protection against chronic inflammation that can hurt performance and slow recovery. It has also been proposed that rutaecarpine may facilitate favorable body composition changes in athletes, although human studies have not confirmed this theory.

Research: Little research specific to rutaecarpine and sports nutrition exists in the National Library of Medicine. As a potential human sympathomimetic (Kim et al., 2008), it may induce contractile force and speed effects on heart function (Jia & Hu, 2010), but this has yet to be established as beneficial to athletes. As a potential metabolism enhancer while low-calorie dieting, Kim and colleagues (2008) were unable to show an effect with evodia extract (evodiamine 6.75 mg, rutaecarpine 0.66 mg) over 8 weeks in obese women. Claims marketed to athletes have been drawn primarily from results of animal-based or in vitro studies, with human data on healthy, fit subjects essentially nonexistent. As a result, applications and recommendations for rutaecarpine use in humans are impossible to make.

Common usage: There are not sufficient data to confirm optimal doses for supplementation use, though available doses generally range from 10 to 100 mg, often in combination with other ingredients. Rutaecarpine can be prepared as an extract by boiling 1.5 to 12 g of the dried fruit in water for 5 to 10 minutes and then straining. Athletes can then drink the extract up to 3 times daily, including 1 hour before workouts.

Health concerns: Rutaecarpine appears to be safe when consumed in recommended doses, though studies evaluating adverse effects are limited. The aforementioned study by Kim and colleagues (2008) did conclude it was safe for short-term use. Because rutaecarpine slows blood clotting, athletes undergoing surgical procedures are advised to avoid its use for at least 2 weeks leading up to a surgery.

Saccharides (Mono-, Di-, Poly-, Oligo-)

(see *carbohydrate*)

Saccharomyces

(see *probiotics*)

S-Adenosyl Methionine (SAMe) 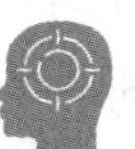  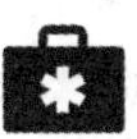

What it is: S-adenosyl methionine (SAMe) is produced naturally in the body from the amino acid methionine. Since its discovery in 1952, it has been known to play an important role in cellular biochemistry and has become a popular supplement for the treatment of depression. Recently, the use of SAMe as a treatment of joint pain and osteoarthritis has become more common.

Function: SAMe has a role in the biochemical pathways that influence the body at the cellular level. The mechanisms of SAMe are not known; however, a number of theories exist. Some speculate SAMe decreases the production of inflammation-promoting cytokines such as TNF-α and alters gene expression of enzymes involved in degenerative pathways. In addition, SAMe may stimulate the production of proteoglycan.

Performance benefit: Many athletes experience chronic joint pain and degeneration as a result of training or injury to cartilage. SAMe could offer a safe alternative to nonsteroidal anti-inflammatories (NSAIDs), which are commonly used to treat pain and inflammation but are also associated with heartburn, ulcers, bleeding, liver and kidney dysfunction, and skin reactions.

Research: Some short-term studies have found SAMe to be more effective than a placebo and just as effective as many commonly prescribed anti-inflammatory drugs such as ibuprofen, naproxen, and Celebrex in the treatment of osteoarthritis. It was noted that although NSAIDs typically offered immediate relief, 2 weeks of supplementation with SAMe were required before beneficial effects were reported (Najm et al., 2004). A 2002 meta-analysis of 11 studies concluded that SAMe appeared to be as effective as NSAIDs in reducing pain and improving functional limitation in patients with osteoarthritis without the adverse effects often associated with NSAIDs (Sofken, 2002). Follow-up data evaluating the efficacy of SAMe for pain associated with arthritic conditions, however, has lacked overall quality, and certainty of evidence is low (Crawford et al., 2019), making additional research, particularly on a healthy, fit population, warranted before practical recommendations for use in this population can be made.

Common usage: A dose of 400 mg taken 3 times/day for a total of 1,200 mg is most commonly used in research trials for treatment of osteoarthritis.

Health concerns: An oral dosage of SAMe is readily safe up to 1,600 mg, with no serious adverse concerns, though minor side effects such as headaches, restlessness, insomnia, and diarrhea have been reported (Ullah et al., 2022).

Salicin, Salicylates, Salix, *Salix Daphnoides, Salix Fragilis, Salix Purpurea*

(see *willow bark*)

Sallowthorn

(see *sea buckthorn*)

Salt 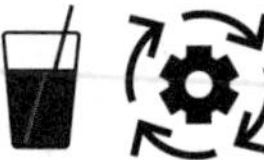 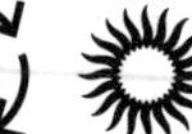 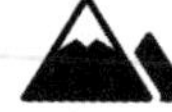

aka *sodium chloride (NaCl), table salt*

What it is: Comprised of the elements sodium and chloride, salt is an ingredient commonly included in sport foods and drinks to help offset sweat losses and promote hydration. Also known as electrolytes, sodium and chloride carry and transmit electrical charges important to muscle and nerve function.

Function: Salt helps maintain optimal fluid levels outside the body's cells, with sodium in particular being the key determinant in how much water will be retained within the body versus excreted as urine. Failure to replenish at least a portion of salt losses during exercise, which generally range between 2.25 and 2.4 g/L of fluid loss, can lower blood volume and cause the heart to work overtime trying to pump sufficient blood and oxygen to the brain and muscles for peak performance.

SUPPLEMENT FACT

The concentration of salt within human sweat decreases with increased fitness levels as well as with heat acclimatization, a process in which an athlete regularly trains and competes in heat.

Performance benefit: Athletes may benefit from enhanced hydration status and consequent muscle and nerve function when supplementing with salt during exercise, especially when exercise is conducted in extreme environmental conditions or at altitude over prolonged periods, which tends to increase losses.

Research: The amount of sodium needed to support athletic performance is a subject under much dispute, mainly due to the fact that the human body has defense mechanisms to protect against sodium deficiency during exercise, including the release of sodium from internal body stores. There is evidence that supplementation with additional sodium during exercise does nothing to affect serum electrolyte and hydration status or affect the incidence of muscle cramping. For example, a randomized prospective study of Ironman athletes found the consumption of 3.6 g of sodium during the 140.6 mi (226.3 km) race produced no significant difference in finishing time, serum sodium concentration before and after the race, weight change during the race, rectal temperature, or systolic and diastolic blood pressure after the race compared to placebo and no supplementation groups (Hew-Butler et al., 2006). In a review by Grozenski and Kiel (2020), however, the consumption of drinks with 20 to 50 mEq-L of sodium (460-1,150 mg) or small amounts of salted snacks helped to stimulate thirst, promote reabsorption of fluids and, by extension, support osmotic balance and performance during endurance events. Thus, current recommendations support sodium supplementation during exercise, particularly sessions lasting longer than 2 hours (Veniamakis et al., 2022).

SUPPLEMENT FACT

Milliequivalents per liter (mEq/L) is a unit of measurement used to express the concentration of ions in a solution, particularly electrolytes. It accounts for the chemical activity of the ions, with one milliequivalent representing one-thousandth of an equivalent, which is based on the ion's charge and the amount of substance that can react with a specific number of hydrogen ions.

Common usage: Although the recommended ceiling intake for salt, and more specifically sodium, is 1,500 mg/day for the general public, athletes may need more to offset sweat losses during training and competition. Current guidelines from the Academy of Nutrition and Dietetics (AND), Dietitians of Canada (DC), and the American College of Sports Medicine (ACSM) recommend sodium intake during exercise for athletes with high sweat rates (>1.2 L/hour) or subjectively "salty sweat" (white salt crystals on clothing, skin) and during prolonged exercise (>2 hours). Average sweat rates range from 0.3 to 2.4 L/hour, and the average sweat sodium content is 1 g/L (50 mmol/l); however, these can vary greatly from athlete to athlete and are highly dependent on environmental conditions. ACSM guidelines for sodium intake are 300 to 600 mg/hour (1.7-2.9 g salt) during prolonged exercise (Kersick et al., 2018). During exercise, sodium is most commonly replaced in the form of sport drinks, though energy gels, energy chews, and salty foods such as pretzels can be used. A sport drink containing sodium in the range of 230 to 690 mg/L (10-30 mmol/L) results in optimal absorption and prevention of hyponatremia and is encouraged over water during prolonged exercise (>2 hr) or extreme heat conditions (Jeukendrup et al., 2009; Veniamakis et al., 2022). If water is used for hydration and the carbohydrate used for fueling (e.g., energy gels, chews) fails to meet sodium replacement guidelines, athletes may benefit from supplementation with electrolyte capsules that contain sodium and chloride as well as other key minerals lost in sweat, such as potassium, magnesium, and calcium.

Health concerns: To maintain proper functioning of cells, tissues, and organs, sodium levels within extracellular fluid should remain within a range of 130 to 160 mmol/L. Low levels of sodium, also known as hyponatremia, generally are caused by excessive intake of fluids or inadequate replacement of salt. Initial symptoms include confusion, nausea, fatigue, muscle cramps, and weakness. As the condition worsens, the nervous system becomes affected; seizures, coma, and even death can occur. Because nonsteroidal anti-inflammatory agents (NSAIDs) such as aspirin, ibuprofen, and acetaminophen (Tylenol) interfere with kidney function and seem to increase risk for hyponatremia, using these in and around competition is discouraged. On the opposite end of the spectrum, excessive dietary salt intake can contribute to a variety of health problems, including high blood pressure, stroke, heart disease, edema (water retention), and osteoporosis (brittle bones). Bloating and GI discomfort are also common symptoms in athletes consuming too much salt (>920 mg of sodium/L of water consumed).

Salvia Hispanica

(see *chia seeds*)

Sambucus Nigra

(see *elderberry*)

Sandthorn

(see *sea buckthorn*)

Sea Buckthorn 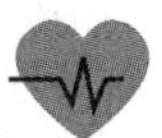 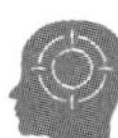 

aka *Hippophae rhamnoides L.*, sallowthorn, sandthorn, seaberry

What it is: A plant with distinctive orange berries that grows in mountainous regions of China and Russia as well as coastal regions of Europe, sea buckthorn has long been used as a medicine. It has more recently garnered attention for its purported ability to fight fatigue and reduce inflammation that can hurt performance.

Function: Although every part of the sea buckthorn plant has historically been used for medicinal purposes, it is the nutrient-packed orange berry and its seeds that are thought to provide anti-inflammatory and energy-boosting qualities of potential benefit to athletes. The sea buckthorn berry is recognized as a potent dietary source of antioxidants, including vitamins C and E, beta-carotene, lycopene, and flavonoids. Animal studies have shown sea buckhorn to limit the production of damaging free radicals and reduce oxidative stress, helping to maintain the integrity of the mitochondria, the cell's energy-producing factory. In addition, sea buckhorn has been shown to provide a boost to the body's natural antioxidant defense system by restoring levels of such key antioxidants as reduced glutathione (GSH) and glutathione peroxidase (GPx), which may help an athlete better withstand heavy cycles of training and competition. Furthermore, sea buckthorn seems to help reduce levels of creatine kinase and C-reactive protein, two markers of inflammation that can negatively affect the overall health and performance of an athlete.

Performance benefit: Athletes may benefit from enhanced endurance during competition as well as quicker postcompetition recovery.

Research: Data evaluating the potential performance benefits of sea buckthorn are primarily limited to animal studies; however, these studies present some promise. In one study of male rats, sea buckhorn leaf extract (SBT) provided at doses of 200 and 800 mg/kg/day over 1 week was shown to significantly extend swim time to exhaustion as well as counter the oxidative stress associated with the exercise protocol (Zheng et al., 2012). In addition, markers of inflammation were lowered in the treatment group versus the control group. Similarly, another study of rats found that administration of sea buckthorn juice, also known as hippophae juice, over 6 weeks of training extended exercise time to exhaustion, significantly enhanced levels of antioxidant enzymes in skeletal muscle, reduced oxidative stress within skeletal muscle, and significantly reduced inflammation as indicated by levels of creatine kinase compared to the nontreatment group (Qiao & Pan, 2010). Investigators from these two studies concluded that SBT, either in extract or juice-concentrate form, can enhance exercise capacity, boost the antioxidant capacity of skeletal muscle, and protect against oxidative damage and exercise-induced inflammation in rats. A double-blind study of healthy humans confirmed the anti-inflammatory benefits of SBT with 28 g/day of frozen sea buckhorn puree over 90 days, demonstrating significantly lower levels of C-reactive protein than the placebo group (Larmo et al., 2008). According to several studies, the fatty acids within sea buckthorn may also have many important functions in the human body, including protecting against cardiovascular disorders, stimulating the immune system, and promoting cognitive functions and bone health (Olas, 2018; Żuchowski, 2023; Olas, 2018). Additional human studies, particularly evaluating the potential impact of the constituents of sea buckthorn on various performance parameters in a healthy, fit population, are needed before conclusions can be made for this population.

Common usage: Sea buckthorn can be consumed in whole food form, either frozen or fresh, and is also used in juices, jams, and teas. As a dietary supplement, it is commonly available in capsule, tablet, seed oil, powder, and extract form. Although only limited human clinical trials are currently available to draw dosing conclusions from, a daily intake of 28 g of a frozen berry puree or 300 mL of a juice concentrate has shown some benefit.

Health concerns: No adverse effects have been documented, and thus it appears that use of sea buckthorn as a whole food is safe. However, the safety of sea buckthorn oil has yet to be established, so extra caution should be exercised with its use.

Sedum Rosea

(see *Rhodiola rosea*)

Selenium (Se) 

aka *L-selenomethionine, selenium chelate, selenium proteinate, selenium yeast, selenomethionine, sodium selenite*

What it is: An essential trace mineral of the sulfur family, selenium is required by the body in small amounts and can be found naturally in variable amounts in plant foods as well as some meats and seafood. The actual content of selenium in food is dependent on the soil the plants were grown in and where the animals were raised. In the United States, for example, soils in the high plains of northern Nebraska and the Dakotas have typically demonstrated high selenium content, whereas it is low in parts of China and Russia. In the body, selenium is concentrated in the lining of the GI tract and in the lungs, liver, and skeletal muscle. As with many minerals, it is thought that physical sport training increases the body's requirement for selenium.

Function: Through its antioxidant qualities, selenium is believed to help protect an athlete against cellular damage that can negatively affect immune function, recovery from sport, and overall performance. In particular, selenium is essential to the production of glutathione peroxidase (GPx), an enzyme that is responsible for a portion of the antioxidant actions within the body. Animal research has shown increased levels of muscle damage and fatigue during prolonged exercise are associated with declines in GPx production, suggesting that selenium supplementation may help offset some or all of this detrimental effect and have a favorable impact on endurance as well as recovery.

Performance benefit: Athletes may benefit from reduced muscle damage, better endurance, and enhanced recovery during heavy cycles of training and competition. Athletes with gastrointestinal disorders such as Crohn's disease or who have undergone gastric bypass surgery are at greater risk for selenium deficiency due to impaired absorption and thus may benefit from supplementation. There is also some evidence that supplementation with selenium may help alleviate joint stiffness and pain associated with arthritis (Huang, Rose, & Hoffman, 2012). Furthermore, of special interest to master athletes, there is favorable evidence regarding the use of selenium for prevention and treatment of sarcopenia and related performance declines (van Dronkelaar et al., 2018).

Research: Studies evaluating the efficacy of selenium supplementation on a healthy, athletic population have brought mixed results. One study of long-distance runners, for example, failed to find a significant or clinically relevant drop in blood selenium levels or activity of GPx upon completion of running a marathon (26.2 mi [42.17 km]), suggesting that endurance exercise, in itself, does not warrant supplementation with selenium (Rokitzki, Logemann, & Keul, 1993). Furthermore, a cross-sectional study of 118 athletes discovered that only 2.6% demonstrated low blood selenium levels despite 23% of the men and 63% of the women failing to achieve recommended dietary allowances for selenium (Margaritis et al., 2005). Nonetheless, a recent meta-analysis of randomized control trials published from January 1988 to December 2010 (Jiang et al., 2012) concluded that supplementation with organic selenium does have a significant impact on GPx activity in healthy adults, which may be of benefit to athletes. A more recent systematic review of five studies found selenium supplementation might actually blunt some of the favorable muscle mitochondrial adaptations to exercise, though some reduction in postexercise oxidation was also reported with selenium supplementation (Heffernan et al., 2019). Overall, the present evidence is not supportive of selenium supplementation in athletes.

Common usage: Selenium supplements are available in capsule and tablet form, with selenomethionine being considered the best absorbed and used form of selenium. The current RDA is 55 mcg/day for adult men and women (ages 19 and up).

Health concerns: Prolonged intake of selenium at doses above 900 mcg/day increases the risk for toxicity, which is marked by symptoms of hair loss, skin rash, horizontal streaking and loss of nails, bad breath, fatigue, irritability, nausea, and vomiting. To avoid selenium toxicity, the Institute of Medicine of the National Academy of Sciences has established an upper intake level (UL) for selenium at 400 mcg per day.

Siberian Ginseng

(see *ginseng*)

6-0-a-D-Glucopyranosyl-D-Fructose

(see *isomaltulose*)

Sodium Ascorbate

(see *vitamin C*)

Sodium Bicarbonate, Sodium Citrate

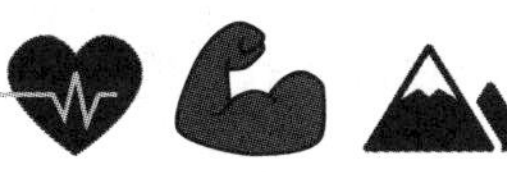

aka *baking soda, Na-citrate*

What it is: Although stored in limited amounts, sodium bicarbonate ($NaHCO_3$) is one of the body's most important natural buffering agents; it is commonly known as baking soda and is used as a leavening agent in baked goods. Sodium citrate ($Na_3C_6H_5O_7$) is a byproduct of mixing sodium bicarbonate and citric acid. Having been used by athletes for over 70 years, both sodium bicarbonate and sodium citrate serve as effective buffering agents, offsetting variations in muscle pH triggered by high-intensity exercise.

Function: To keep up with the extreme demand for energy to support muscle contraction during sustained high-intensity exercise as well as explosive bursts common in team sports, the body breaks down glucose (carbohydrate) to form ATP. The capacity for energy production is limited, however, by the formation of lactate and hydrogen ions, two metabolic byproducts that progressively increase muscle acidity (i.e., the burn), which impairs muscle contraction, contributes to fatigue, and diminishes performance. Sodium citrate and sodium bicarbonate enhance the body's natural buffering system by facilitating a faster release of fatigue-inducing hydrogen ions from exercising muscles, thereby reducing acidity as well as aiding the recycling of lactate for energy production.

SUPPLEMENT FACT

Scientific evidence has shown the natural buffering system involved in controlling acidity within muscle cells is about 20% lower in women than in men, making supplementation potentially of greater benefit to female athletes.

Performance benefit: Athletes competing in continuous or repeated periods of explosive, high-intensity activity lasting 1 to 7 minutes may experience a delay in the onset of muscle fatigue, thereby providing benefit to anaerobic endurance and overall performance.

Research: Numerous studies have explored the supplementation impact of sodium bicarbonate and sodium citrate on human performance. For example, a 2021 umbrella review by Grgic and colleagues looked at eight reviews of moderate and high methodological quality. They concluded that "sodium bicarbonate supplementation acutely enhances peak anaerobic power, anaerobic capacity, performance in endurance events lasting ~45 s to 8 min, muscle endurance, 2000-m rowing performance, and high-intensity intermittent running." They did note, however, that more research is needed on women. This sweeping 2021 review is in general agreement with a 2011 meta-analysis of current data concluding that an acute dose of 0.3 to 0.5 g/kg of sodium bicarbonate helped improve 1-minute sprint performance by 1.7%, a margin that often determines whether an athlete earns a spot on the podium (Carr, Hopkins, & Gore, 2011). Adding five additional sprinting sessions still translated to improved performance, though the benefit was not as large at 0.6%. An acute dose of 0.5 g/kg of sodium citrate has been shown to enhance 5 km performance in well-trained college-aged female runners (Oöpik et al., 2003). Interestingly, the same study investigators failed to find the same benefit for trained male runners, a result that falls in line with evidence that the natural buffering system in female athletes is 20% lower than in men (Oöpik et al., 2004). Neither buffering agent appears to have a significant impact on prolonged endurance performance; however, the results of one small study, where 10 trained cyclists completed significantly more work during a 60-minute time trial after ingestion of sodium bicarbonate at a rate of 0.3 g/kg, suggests additional research may be warranted (McNaughton, Dalton, & Palmer, 1999).

Common usage: Sodium bicarbonate or sodium citrate can be taken at an acute dose of 0.3 to 0.5 g/kg, split into five relatively even doses and consumed in a staggered fashion starting 3 hours before competition so that loading is complete 1 hour before competition. They can also be taken as a chronic dose of 0.5 g/kg, split into four equal doses and consumed every 3 to 4 hours throughout the day for 5 to 6 days before competition. Although both protocols are effective, the chronic loading protocol may help provide an added boost to the body's bicarbonate stores as well as eliminate some of the negative side effects commonly experienced with the acute dosing protocol.

Health concerns: It is not uncommon for athletes to experience nausea, water retention and bloating, vomiting, and diarrhea with sodium bicarbonate loading. Splitting the doses and drinking plenty of fluids seem to help reduce symptoms as does using gelatin capsules. Supplementing with sodium citrate instead of sodium bicarbonate can further reduce adverse GI symptoms.

Sodium Chloride

(see *salt*)

Sodium D-Pantothenate

(see *pantothenic acid*)

Sodium Metavanadate, Sodium Orthovanadate

(see *vanadium*)

Sodium Phosphate

(see *phosphate salts*)

Sodium Pyruvate

(see *pyruvate*)

Sodium Selenite

(see *selenium*)

Sophretin

(see *quercetin*)

Sour Cherry

(see *tart cherry*)

Soy Protein 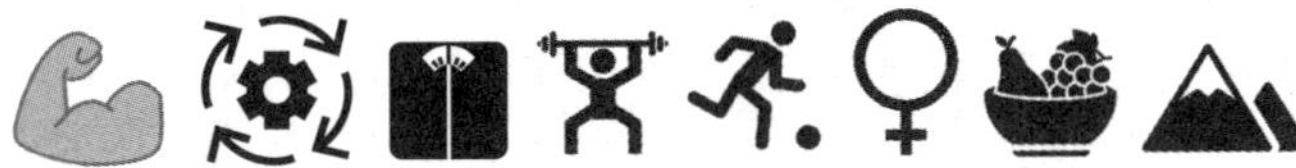

aka *soy protein concentrate, soy protein isolate*

What it is: The soybean, comprised of 38% protein plus all nine essential amino acids, provides a quality plant-based alternative to animal protein for vegetarian athletes and any athlete looking to enhance cardiovascular health. Regarding protein quality specifics, the digestible indispensable amino acid score (DIAAS) for soy is 0.90, compared to whey protein isolate at 1.09 and milk protein at 1.18. During soybean processing, the protein is separated from other nutrients, including carbohydrate and fat, and dehydrated to form either a soy protein isolate or concentrate, the dry ingredients commonly used in soy foods and supplements. Soy protein, particularly isolates, contains natural bioactive substances called isoflavones (genistein, daidzein) that may enhance plasma antioxidant activity, potentially minimizing damage to muscle tissue and cells important to immune function and aiding overall recovery and performance in sport.

Function: Soy protein is purported to improve muscle adaptations to exercise for multiple reasons. First, soy protein isolate is a rich source of leucine (8.0 g/100 g of protein), which helps activate anabolic metabolism as well as muscle protein synthesis (Drummond & Rasmussen, 2008; Norton et al., 2012). When consumed postexercise, this effect is enhanced (Drummond & Rasmussen, 2008). In addition, it has been shown that soy protein and its peptides enhance the sensitivity of pancreatic beta cells, stimulating insulin secretion and in turn increasing the cellular uptake of amino acids and initiating muscle protein synthesis (Buczkowska & Jarosz-Chobot, 2001; Hu et al., 2023; Timmerman et al., 2010). Intake of soy protein also may improve antioxidant status and reduce oxidative stress, thereby aiding recovery and promoting health (Zare et al., 2023).

Performance benefit: Athletes may benefit from better endurance, reduced muscle breakdown, and enhanced lean body weight gains.

Research: A fair amount of existing data evaluating soy protein and performance has focused on the influence of absorption rates and consequent delivery of amino acids to muscles on performance and recovery. One double-blind, randomized study determined that postexercise consumption of a protein blend consisting of 25% soy protein isolate (4.5 g), 25% whey protein isolate (4.5 g), and 50% casein (9.5 g) significantly enhanced the body's ability to build muscle compared to whey protein isolate (17.5 g) alone (Reidy et al., 2012). Study investigators attributed this recovery boost to the varying rates at which protein sources are delivered to the muscles—although whey protein is delivered rapidly, soy protein and especially casein take longer for the body to process. Similar results have been seen with a postexercise blend of soy plus whey, with reports of considerably longer and more favorable net phenylalanine balance and a slower initial increase of plasma branched-chain amino acids, thus maintaining higher levels during postexercise recovery (Reidy et al., 2013, 2014). Consuming a blend of protein sources after workout therefore extends the rate at which essential amino acids are delivered to the muscles, prolonging an anabolic effect for up to 5 hours, helping an athlete maximize lean body weight gains, and supporting recovery. It is important to note that rates of muscle protein synthesis have been shown to be significantly lower with a pre-exercise consumption of 20 g of soy protein compared to an equal dose of whey protein in both exercised and nonexercised muscle (Yang et al, 2012). Integrating a 25 g dose of soy protein isolate twice a day over 4 weeks, however, has been shown to be a valid means to mitigating reductions in isometric muscle strength and muscle force following exercise-induced muscle damage (Shenoy et al., 2016). Overall, while soy protein doesn't quite stack up to the performance of whey protein as it relates to muscle protein synthesis and recovery, it remains a valid option for plant-based athletes to boost daily protein intake as well as promote muscle strength and mass accrual, particularly when a high protein intake (1.6 g/kg/day) is followed (Hevia-Larraín et al., 2021).

Common usage: Recommendations for protein intake typically range from 1.2 to 2.0 g/kg/day, but have more recently been expressed in terms of regularly spacing intake of modest amounts of high-quality protein (0.3 g/kg) after exercise and throughout the day (Thomas et al., 2016). Adequate energy is needed to optimize protein metabolism, and when energy availability is reduced (e.g., to reduce body weight), higher protein intake is needed to support muscle protein synthesis and retention of fat-free mass. Whole food (e.g., tofu, tempeh, edamame, soy milk), bars, sport drinks, powders, and meal replacement shakes are all common ways athletes incorporate soy protein into their training menus to help meet daily intake recommendations as well as enhance performance (see table 3.7 for total protein intake recommendations). Because soy isolates carry greater protein potency than soy concentrates (containing 90%-95% versus 65%-70% protein) and are stripped of dietary fiber that can be gas forming, soy isolates are generally the preferred supplementation form for athletes.

Health concerns: Soy protein is well tolerated by most, although athletes with allergies to soy should avoid its use. There have also been reports of contamination with potentially dangerous fillers like melamine and lead in some soy protein supplement products. Protein toxicity, which is marked by unexplained vomiting, loss of appetite, and an ammonia-like smell to the breath or sweat, does not seem to be a concern at recommended daily intake levels.

TABLE 3.7 Recommended Daily Protein Intake Levels (From All Sources)

	Endurance athletes	Strength athletes
Daily protein goal	1.2-1.4 g/kg	1.2-1.7 g/kg
1-2 hours before exercise	10-40 g	10-40 g
During exercise (hourly)	2-5 g	None needed
Immediately after exercise	10-40 g	10-40 g

Spirulina 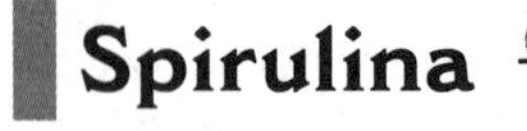 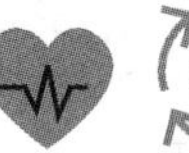 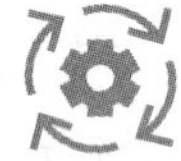

aka *blue-green algae, filamentous cyanobacterium*

What it is: Sometimes referred to as a superfood (a term with no agreed-on definition), spirulina is a type of algae and a source of vitamin B_{12} among other B-vitamins, minerals, and antioxidant compounds.

Function: In addition to vitamins B_1, B_2, and B_3 and the minerals copper, iron, and magnesium, spirulina contains the antioxidant phycocyanin, which may contribute to performance benefits from increased aerobic performance to postexercise heart rate recovery. Antioxidant and possibly blood flow effects may also be at work.

Performance benefit: Benefits may include increased time to exhaustion, higher maximal oxygen consumption, or improved heart rate recovery after exercise. More research is needed on these effects.

Research: In their recent review, Gurney and Spendiff (2022) reported that studies have documented that spirulina may improve time to exhaustion during running and maximal oxygen use ($\dot{V}O_2$max) when cycling, as well as enhanced recovery heart rate after cycling to $\dot{V}O_2$max—but that "there appears to be a distinct lack of consensus on what primary mechanism may cause the efficacious results following supplementation for exercise performance." Antioxidant effects appear to be distinct ergogenic mechanisms, but early animal work suggests vasodilation may also be at work.

Common usage: In early research, dose and duration are still be studied. Existing spirulina research in exercise science has ranged from 1.5 to 7.5 g/day for 7 to 60 days.

Health concerns: Grover and colleagues (2021) stated that their evaluation of in vivo toxicity, immunomodulatory and antioxidant effects of C-phycocyanin—one of spirulina's likely mechanisms of action—suggests that C-phycocyanin is very safe for consumption. More cautiously, Grosshagauer and colleagues (2020), suggested "The regular intake of spirulina, and very likely other algae products as well, as a dietary supplement in the gram range demands a closer monitoring of potentially harmful constituents."

(S)-2

(see *glutamine*)

Sugars

(see *carbohydrate*)

Superoxide Dismutase (SOD) 

(see also *glutathione*)

What it is: Like glutathione, superoxide dismutase (SOD) is generally considered an endogenous (originating in the body) antioxidant enzyme. It is also consumed naturally in the diet from such green foods as barley grass, broccoli, brussels sprouts, cabbage, and wheatgrass. As a family of enzymes, SOD can be found bound to several metals, including copper, zinc, manganese, iron, and nickel. In the supplement industry, SOD is marketed as an antioxidant that counters the damaging impact that stress, including exercise stress, can have on the body.

Function: Exercise triggers the production of chemically reactive molecules known as reactive oxygen species (ROS) that, when produced at a rate that exceeds the body's natural antioxidant defenses, can cause damage to DNA, cell membranes, proteins, and carbohydrates that are important to the overall health and performance of an athlete. It is thought that supplementation with SOD may decrease the production of ROS, and more specifically superoxide, the most common ROS in the body. Although there are several types of SOD, with each type playing a different role in keeping cells healthy, manganese SOD is of particular interest to athletes due to its role in protecting the mitochondria from damage that could negatively affect the production of ATP necessary for peak performance.

Performance benefit: Athletes may benefit from enhanced endurance and recovery, especially during periods of heavy training or competition.

Research: It is well established that physical training naturally enhances an athlete's antioxidant capacity, allowing the athlete's body to counter the damage associated with exercise stress. However, there is controversy over whether supplementation with antioxidants such as SOD can further enhance this activity. In fact, results from some studies suggest antioxidant supplementation, especially taken in high doses over the long term, may actually hinder this favorable training adaptation, leaving the athlete more vulnerable to the detrimental effects of ROS. Nonetheless, a small, double-blind, randomized study found a supplementation protocol of 500 mg/day of plant SOD extract during a 6-week training camp to significantly enhance SOD antioxidant activity in a group of elite rowers compared to a placebo group (Skarpanska-Stejnborn et al., 2011). In addition, levels of C-reactive protein, a marker of inflammation, were significantly reduced immediately after and 24 hours after completion of a maximal 2,000 m rowing trial, supporting the theory that SOD has strong anti-inflammatory properties. Two additional studies of similar design have confirmed these findings. One demonstrated significantly lower creatine kinase (CK) and interleukin-6 (IL-6) as well as significant improvements in power output during a 2-minute row-to-exhaustion test with supplementation with 500 mg/day of Glisodin (concentrated melon extract naturally rich in SOD) over a 6-week period compared to a placebo group of elite-level international rowers (Dudašova et al., 2022). The second study found the same supplementation protocol to significantly increase metabolic efficiency as well as significantly elevate maximal effort in a rowing-to-exhaustion test compared to the placebo group. Study investigators over the two studies concluded supplementation with SOD-rich extract promotes lower oxidative stress and better antioxidant protection, protecting against inflammation and muscle damage, thereby leading to better work performance of highly trained athletes (Dudašova et al., 2023). Future research should evaluate these applications to athletes in a variety of different sport settings.

Common usage: Available by injection, sublingual administration, topical creams, and in capsule form, current dosing recommendations suggest a daily oral dose of 500 mg taken in capsule form during a 6-week competitive or heavy training cycle to elicit anti-inflammatory and recovery benefits as well as improved training cycles and performance. Because SOD is absorbed in the small intestine, enteric-coated pills are essential to avoid destruction by stomach acids before reaching the intestines.

Health concerns: SOD is recognized as a nontoxic substance and presumed safe for supplementation use.

Sweet Pepper

(see *capsicum*)

Synephrine

aka *bitter orange, Citrus aurantium, p-synephrine (see also hordenine)*

What it is: Synephrine is a protoalkaloid found in bitter orange extract, derived from the fruits of *Citrus aurantium* and other citrus species. It can be found in a diverse range of citrus foods such as Seville, mandarin, and Marrs sweet oranges as well as clementines, tangerines, and grapefruits. Although distinct in its effects, synephrine is structurally very similar to ephedrine, a weight-loss supplement banned by the FDA in 2003 because of health concerns. There are also a variety of synephrine isomers, which have the same molecular formula; however, they are structurally different and have different physiological effects. The isomeric derivative found in citrus species is p-synephrine, whereas m-synephrine is not naturally found in plants. It is important to differentiate p-synephrine from m-synephrine and ephedrine when evaluating the health concerns associated with synephrine use (Stohs, Preuss, & Shara, 2011).

Function: A variety of cells within the body have alpha and beta adrenal receptors. These adrenoceptors are targets for stress hormones (catecholamines) released in response to exercise, such as epinephrine and norepinephrine, which initiate the sympathetic fight-or-flight response: increased heart rate, heightened alertness, and increased force production within the muscles. This response increases metabolic rate and potentially fat oxidation. Alkaloids such as synephrine and ephedrine, like catecholamines, can bind these various receptors and induce a sympathetic response, potentially increasing resting metabolic rate and fat oxidation. As a result, synephrine and other alkaloids are commonly added to weight-loss supplements.

Performance benefit: Synephrine is most commonly found in weight-loss and so-called fat-burning supplements. It may assist athletes in reducing body fat and weight, although data are mixed. In addition, its heightened sympathetic actions may potentially aid in force production, delay fatigue, or enhance performance.

Research: Two groups of scientists in 2004 and 2006 reviewed the scientific evidence of synephrine for weight loss. In 2004 it was concluded that synephrine was ineffective in aiding weight loss and was only lipolytic (fat burning) at high doses (Fugh-Berman & Myers, 2004). This was followed by conclusions made by Haaz and colleagues in 2006 that "while some evidence is promising, more rigorous clinical trials are necessary." Studies often use synephrine in combination with caffeine, green tea extract, and other speculated weight-loss ingredients, making it difficult to conclude that synephrine alone promotes body fat and weight loss. These same studies have suggested that synephrine is lipolytic and can induce increases in resting metabolic rate of roughly 6.7% without inducing any negative effects on heart rate or blood pressure (Seifert et al., 2011; Stohs et al., 2011). Regarding synephrine's impact on exercise performance, a narrative review by Ruiz-Moreno and colleagues (2021) stated: "Previous investigations have demonstrated that the acute intake of p-synephrine does not modify running sprint performance, jumping capacity, or aerobic capacity. However, the acute intake of p-synephrine, in a dose of 2-3 mg/kg of body mass, has been effective to enhance the rate of fat oxidation during incremental and continuous exercise." Additionally, one study that used a combination of caffeine and synephrine during low- to moderate-intensity exercise showed an improvement in exercise tolerance among the subjects (Haller, 2008). Taken together, synephrine isn't promising as an ergogenic aid, but some data are suggestive of acute fat burning. This may or may not translate to enhanced body composition over time, however.

Common usage: Research trials have used a range of 13 to 50 mg.

Health concerns: Scientists have found that p-synephrine does not act on alpha and beta adrenal receptors, unlike ephedrine and m-synephrine. As a result, p-synephrine does not induce the same negative effects on heart rate and blood pressure. In 2004 the FDA concluded that bitter orange extract or p-synephrine was not directly related to adverse events. This conclusion was corroborated at least in part by Ruiz-Moreno and colleagues (2021), who stated that the occurrence of adverse effects is negligible. Although p-synephrine appears safe when used within recommended doses, consumers should proceed with caution—weight-loss and fat-burning supplements are often adulterated with additional stimulants and alkaloids that might not be listed on product labels (Stohs, Preuss, & Shara, 2011).

Table Beet

(see *beetroot*)

Table Salt

(see *salt*)

Tart Cherry 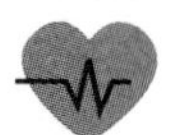   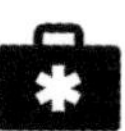 

aka *Balaton cherry, Montmorency cherry, Prunus cerasus, sour cherry, tart cherry juice*

What it is: Containing higher concentrations of naturally occurring plant compounds called phenolics, and in particular anthocyanin, than its sweet sister, tart cherries are the smallest member of the stone fruit family, which also includes plums, apricots, nectarines, and peaches. Tart cherries are grown primarily in Michigan in the United States. There are two varieties of tart cherries, Montmorency and Balaton, both of which are touted as natural alternatives to aspirin and nonsteroidal anti-inflammatory drugs (NSAIDs) for pain relief.

Function: Anthocyanins help block two enzymes, COX-1 and COX-2, that are responsible for the production of inflammatory compounds called prostaglandins. In addition, the antioxidant actions of tart cherries may help ameliorate some of the oxidative tissue damage that can trigger further production of free radicals, inflammation, and muscle soreness. Both Balaton and Montmorency tart cherries also contain melatonin, a hormone with antioxidant qualities that may aid sleep.

Performance benefit: Decreasing oxidative stress and inflammation after strenuous exercise facilitates faster recovery times, allowing the athlete to accumulate the benefits of more training. Tart cherry may also aid sleep, an essential component of overall health and necessary for efficient recovery from exercise.

Research: Data generated from a 2021 meta-analysis of 14 studies revealed tart cherry supplementation may have a small to moderate effect on reducing muscle soreness, improving recovery of muscle strength (particularly recovery of jump height), and decreasing C-reactive protein and interleukin-6, markers of inflammation and muscle damage after strenuous exercise (Hill et al., 2021). Wangdi and colleagues (2022) further confirmed these results, finding supplementation with Montmorency cherry concentrate to conserve isometric muscle strength while upregulating antioxidant gene and protein expression in parallel with increased phenolic acid concentrations, thereby enhancing functional recovery from exercise. Hooper and colleagues (2021) determined a supplementation protocol of 500 mg of tart cherry extract taken over 7 days leading up to intense resistance exercise significantly reduced oxidative stress and markers of muscle and cardiac damage as well as significantly improved recovery of handgrip strength compared to a placebo group of healthy strength-trained men. A meta-analysis of 10 studies evaluating the impact of tart cherry on endurance performance revealed tart cherry concentrate to significantly improve endurance exercise performance when used in juice or powdered form with anthocyanin content ranging from 40 to 270 mg/day and ingested for 7 days to 1.5 hours before exercise performance testing (Gao & Chilibeck, 2020). The authors concluded tart cherry concentrate may enhance endurance exercise performance due to its low glycemic response, anti-inflammatory and antioxidative qualities, and blood flow–enhancing effects (Gao & Chilibeck, 2020). Using a similar supplement dose of 1,200 mg tart cherry capsule containing 100 mg of anthocyanin 2 times/day over 4 days and once on the final day 2 hours before exercise, Horiuchi and colleagues (2023) found cycle exercise time to exhaustion in hypoxic conditions (3,800 m) to significantly improve, likely due to lower levels of deoxygenated hemoglobin and higher blood oxygen saturation compared to the placebo group of recreationally trained healthy adults. Furthermore, significantly lower levels of urinary 8-hydro-2′-deoxyguanosine excretion, a marker of oxidative stress, were also reported, making tart cherry of potential benefit to unacclimated athletes training or competing at altitude in the short term (Horiuchi et al., 2023). A double-blind, placebo-controlled study of 20 healthy men and women found that a 30 mL serving of tart Montmorency cherry juice concentrate (equivalent to 90-100 cherries) taken both in the morning and again before bed significantly increased circulating melatonin while improving sleep efficiency by 5% to 6% and overall duration of sleep by 34 minutes per night; the placebo group had no change or a negative change in sleep patterns (Howatson et al., 2011). Although the bulk of current data has shown some favorable impact of tart cherry usage on performance and recovery parameters in both an untrained and trained healthy population including competitive athletes, it is important that future research explore why some studies have not (Abbott et al., 2020; Ortega et al., 2023).

Common usage: Tart cherries can be consumed fresh, frozen, dried, or as a juice. They are also available in supplement form as an extract, tablet, or capsule. Optimal dose for reported performance benefits will include 40 to 270 mg/day of anthocyanins. This would be achieved by consuming 45 to 100 cherries or 12 oz (0.35 L) of a tart cherry juice concentrate taken 1 to 2 times/day.

Health concerns: Cherries contain sorbitol, a sugar alcohol that has natural laxative qualities that can trigger gastrointestinal distress in some, especially those with irritable bowel syndrome (IBS).

Taurine 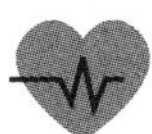 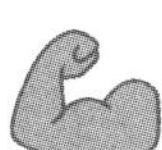 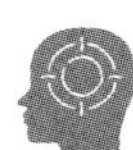 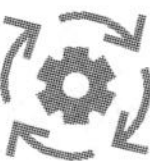  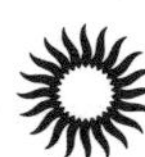

aka *2-ethanesuflonic acid*

What it is: Taurine is a sulfur-containing nonessential amino acid. It is one of the most abundant amino acids in the body and is found in muscle and organ tissues such as the heart and liver. Taurine is found naturally in fish, beef, poultry, and lamb. Taurine has become a popular ingredient in many energy drinks, such as Red Bull, which contains roughly 1,000 mg of taurine per 8 oz (0.24 L) serving.

Function: Taurine has a number of mechanisms that may aid in athletic performance. Most significant, taurine is believed to affect cellular excitability by increasing the release of calcium from the sarcoplasmic reticulum, which would ultimately improve muscle contractility and force production. Secondly, taurine is a powerful antioxidant capable of combating oxidative free radicals produced during exercise.

Performance benefit: Supplementation with taurine before and during exercise could be advantageous in delaying fatigue and improving performance in endurance athletes and those engaged in high-intensity, prolonged-duration team sports. In addition, taurine may improve strength and power production during muscle contraction.

Research: Animal data has revealed exercise to significantly deplete muscle taurine levels; administration of taurine helps to offset these losses, leading to lower levels of muscle fatigue, improved force production, enhanced muscle endurance, and decreased muscle damage (Goodman et al., 2009; Hamilton et al., 2006; Yatabe et al., 2009). Applications to a healthy human population have shown some promise as well. Compared to a control group, Carvahlo and colleagues (2020) found supplementation with 6 g of taurine taken 90 minutes before a single session of fasting aerobic exercise (on a treadmill at 60% of $\dot{V}O_2max$) to increase lipid oxidation by 38% and decrease the respiratory coefficient by 4%, which is of significance—particularly for endurance-focused athletes—because increased lipid oxidation has a glycogen-sparing effect that helps extend endurance performance. Indeed, a 2018 meta-analysis of 10 peer-reviewed studies concluded that a single oral dose consisting of 1 to 6 grams of taurine taken pre-exercise can enhance endurance performance (Waldron et al., 2018). In addition to significantly improving time to exhaustion (+10%) and lowering ratings of perceived exhaustion in a fixed-intensity cycling test in heat compared to a control group of healthy males, Page and colleagues (2019) found supplementation with 50 mg/kg of taurine taken 2 hours before exercise to also elicit favorable effects of thermoregulation, significantly increasing local sweating (+12.7%) and significantly reducing core body temperature in the later stages of exercise. Post-exercise blood lactate levels also were significantly lower compared to the control group. There is also some evidence showing a synergistic effect of taurine when consumed with caffeine. In a double-blind, placebo-controlled study, Ozan and colleagues (2022) demonstrated that 6 mg/kg of caffeine along with 3 g of taurine consumed 60 minutes before exercise yielded statistically significant results as it relates to agility, balance, and cognitive function in elite male boxers. The current human data evaluating taurine and its impact on different parameters of performance has been promising but limited, thus more research on a wide spectrum of athletes is needed before definite conclusions can be made.

Common usage: Current research-supported doses of taurine range from 3 to 6 g, generally taken in an acute fashion in the 2 hours leading up to exercise. The benefits of taurine might be enhanced when consumed with caffeine, with research-supported doses for each standing at 3 g of taurine and 6 mg/kg of caffeine consumed 60 minutes before exercise.

Health concerns: The use of taurine appears to be safe. The only noted side effect is diarrhea.

Theacrine 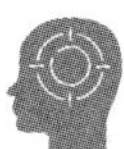

aka *bitter tea, Camellia kucha tea extract*

What it is: Theacrine is a plant chemical similar to caffeine found in coffees and teas, in particular being one of the major purine alkaloids found in the leaf of the wild tea plant species *Camellia kucha*.

Function: The mechanism of action of this proposed stimulant-like compound is similar to caffeine.

Performance benefit: Theacrine may work as a caffeine alternative when taken prior to exercise. This could mean effects ranging from a sense of energy, alertness, and focus, to increased muscular strength and endurance, to enhanced aerobic performance.

Research: Cerqueira and colleagues (2022), in a paper focused on preworkout supplementation, reported that studies on this compound are scarce. These investigators studied 22 flag footballers (19-24 years old) who consumed 200 mg of theacrine or a placebo 60 minutes before a battery of tests (sextuple jump, agility T-test, 30 m sprint, 40-second run test, and 12-minute run test). There was no difference between the groups in any of the tests. Earlier work (Cesareo et al., 2019), using a synthetic version of naturally occurring theacrine (1,3,7,9-tetramethyluric acid) called TeaCrine, similarly concluded that neither 300 mg TeaCrine, 300 mg caffeine, their combination, nor placebo (consumed 90 minutes before exercise) improved muscular strength, power, or endurance performance in resistance-trained men. In this study, only 300 mg caffeine improved measures of focus, energy, and motivation to exercise. It should be noted that these researchers found no effects with a dose of caffeine (3.6 mg/kg) that may be effective for some aspects of performance. More research is needed.

Common usage: 200 to 300 mg has been used in the scant sport nutrition research available.

Health concerns: Concerns may be similar to caffeine, although some information does exist that theacrine may differ in some regards (e.g. habituation, anti-inflammatory effects, analgesia). The median lethal dose (810.6 mg/kg) for animals is higher than that of caffeine, according to Wang and colleagues (2010). In 2016, Taylor and colleagues reported clinical safety for TeaCrine supplementation over 8 weeks of daily use at up to 300 mg/day. More research is needed, and consumers should consult their health care professional regarding potential drug interactions.

Theine

(see *caffeine*)

Theobroma Cacao

(see *cocoa*)

Thiamine 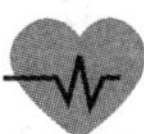 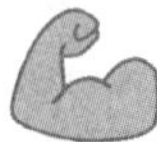 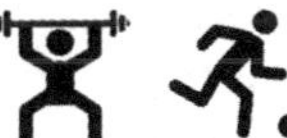

aka *antiberiberi vitamin, B-complex vitamin, vitamin B₁*

What it is: A member of the B-vitamin family, thiamine, otherwise known as vitamin B_1, aids the breakdown of carbohydrate for conversion into energy and can be found naturally in such foods as cereal grains, beans, nuts, meats, and yeast. As a sport supplement, thiamine is proposed to help combat the stress of physical training and increase energy, thereby improving performance.

Function: Thiamine plays a key role in several reactions important to the metabolism of carbohydrate, including the activation of pyruvate dehydrogenase (PDH), a mitochondrial enzyme that serves as the gateway for the production of ATP. A deficiency in thiamine has been shown to reduce the activity of PDH and consequent energy production as well as increase the production of fatigue-inducing lactate, thereby compromising performance.

SUPPLEMENT FACT

Are you a coffee or tea drinker? Frequent consumers may be at greater risk for thiamine deficiency—chemicals called tannins found in both beverages trigger a reaction that converts thiamine to a form more difficult for the body to process.

Performance benefit: Athletes may benefit from enhanced energy levels and endurance during training and competition.

Research: Although most studies have shown the thiamine intake of athletes is sufficient to meet the RDA, athletes may benefit from increased dietary intake or supplementation to offset the heightened level of stress that exercise places on thiamine-driven metabolic pathways. A 2011 study found that the blood thiamine concentration of collegiate swimmers dropped significantly during a heavy training cycle as compared to a preparatory low-volume period; this was in spite of an increased energy intake and sufficient thiamine intake, suggesting a cycle of thiamine supplementation may be beneficial at a certain point during a competitive season (Sato et al., 2011). A well-designed study of nondeficient male athletes, for example, found administration of 1 mg/kg of thiamine pyrophosphate (TPP) enhanced aerobic capacity during exercise while lowering heart rate as well as postexercise levels of blood lactate in comparison to a placebo (Bautista-Hernández et al., 2008). Similarly, an animal study found supplementation with thiamine tetrahydrofurfuryl disulfide (TTFD) over 5 days attenuated the decrease in ATP within skeletal muscle caused by a weighted swimming exercise protocol, which helped to significantly delay the onset of fatigue and enhance exercise time to exhaustion compared to a placebo group (Nozaki et al., 2009). Another animal study found supplementation with TTFD over 6 weeks to significantly increase endurance and grip strength and demonstrate beneficial effects on lactate production and clearance rate after an acute exercise challenge. Furthermore, the TTFD supplementation significantly mitigated blood urea nitrogen and creatine kinase indices after extended exercise and elevated glycogen content in the liver and muscle tissues, having implications for recovery (Huang et al., 2018). Of interest to master athletes, there are data showing higher intakes of vitamin B_1 to be associated with a 22% lower risk of early-onset sarcopenia, which is of statistical significance (Yang et al., 2024). It is clear that thiamine is an essential component of an athlete's diet, and supplementation may be of benefit, particularly during heavy training cycles and for athletes who struggle to meet the heightened caloric and nutritional demands of competition as well as master and senior level athletes.

Common usage: The RDA for thiamine in men and women aged 18 and older is 1.2 and 1.1 mg/day, respectively. Supplemental doses generally fall between 100% and 200% of the RDA and are commonly included in B-complex and multivitamin or multimineral supplement blends as well as sold individually in tablet, softgel, and lozenge form. Athletes engaged in heavy training cycles or with mild dietary deficiencies may benefit from elevated doses up to 100 mg taken daily for up to 1 month, preferably split into two to three doses throughout the day.

Health concerns: Severe deficiency, also known as beriberi, is rare in developed countries, but mild deficiencies have been reported in those who exercise intensely, are affected by Crohn's disease, follow poor dietary habits (high intake of refined carbohydrate and sugar), or drink a lot of alcohol, coffee, or tea. Symptoms of deficiency include fatigue, irritability, and muscle cramps. Supplementation with thiamine appears to be safe, even at high levels, although rare reports of allergic reactions and skin irritations have been reported.

Thiotic Acid

(see *alpha-lipoic acid*)

3-Aminopropanoic Acid

(see *beta-alanine*)

3,4'5-Stilbenetriol, 3,4'5-Trihydroxystilbene

(see *resveratrol*)

Tribulus

aka *Tribulus terrestris*

What it is: *Tribulus terrestris* is an herb native to temperate and tropical climates in Africa, Australia, southern Europe, and Asia. There have been claims that as an herbal supplement, it has provided performance enhancement for many top Bulgarian weightlifters.

Function: Tribulus supplementation is believed by some to increase levels of testosterone in athletes. Tribulus contains steroidal saponins, which supposedly block central testosterone receptors, thereby increasing circulating levels of luteinizing hormone and testosterone. The anabolic properties of testosterone would equate to gains in muscle mass and improvements in strength and power.

> ## ⚠ SUPPLEMENT WARNING
>
> Most banned substance drug testing uses a testosterone/epitestosterone (T/E) ratio as a means of detecting banned supplement use. Although tribulus does not affect the T/E ratio, and the NCAA and WADA do not consider tribulus a banned substance, supplements containing impurities and ingredients not listed on product labels may affect this ratio and result in a failed test. Athletes should be extremely cautious if considering taking a tribulus supplement.

Performance benefit: If claims are true, tribulus would benefit strength and power athletes by aiding in the development of lean body mass, strength, and power through increased levels of anabolic hormones.

Research: Data in support of tribulus supplementation are still lacking. In 2019 Santos and colleagues sought to critically analyze evidence surrounding men's health in the phytotherapeutic literature, including the effects of tribulus on testosterone concentration. They concluded that the use of tribulus and maca (*Lepidium meyenii*) were not scientifically supported to improve serum testosterone levels in men. This echoes earlier work. In 2007 Rogerson and colleagues studied the effects of tribulus supplementation on strength and body composition in rugby players. The 5-week study found tribulus to be ineffective in increasing strength or improving body composition, and it did not affect any levels of anabolic hormones. Similar results were found in a 2000 study involving 8 weeks of supplementation in resistance-trained men (Antonio et al., 2000). Additionally, a 2001 study evaluated the effectiveness of a supplement containing a cocktail of tribulus as well as androstenedione, dehydroepiandrosterone, saw palmetto, chrysin, and indole-3-carbinol. The supplement cocktail was concluded to be ineffective in promoting levels of testosterone (Brown, 2001). No evidence currently exists to support the use of tribulus as an ergogenic aid for strength and power athletes.

Common usage: Three of the research studies previously mentioned used a range of 450 to 750 mg or 3.21 mg/kg of body mass (equivalent to 240 mg for a 165 lb [75 kg] athlete). Most supplement labels recommend 750 to 800 mg of tribulus be consumed 3 times/day—in the morning, about noon, and before bed.

Health concerns: Tribulus is also marketed for sexual enhancement. Many supplements sold for sexual enhancement contain ingredients not listed on the label and other impurities.

Trigonella Foenum-Graecum

(see *fenugreek*)

Trimethylglycine (TMG)

(see *betaine*)

Turmeric

(see *curcumin*)

20-Beta-Hydroxyecdysterone, 20-Hydroxyecdysone

(see *ecdysteroids*)

25(OH)D

(see *vitamin D*)

2-Aminoglutaramic Acid

(see *glutamine*)

2-Ethanesuflonic Acid

(see *taurine*)

2-Oxopropanoate, 2-Oxypropanoic Acid

(see *pyruvate*)

Tyrosine 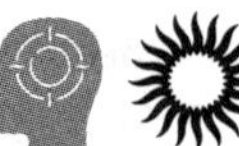 

aka *L-tyrosine*

What it is: Tyrosine is a nonessential amino acid, meaning it can be synthesized within the body and is not required from dietary sources. However, it can also be found in soy, chicken, turkey, fish, peanuts, almonds, and dairy. Tyrosine is used in the production of proteins; it also has an important function as a precursor of neurotransmitters such as dopamine, epinephrine, and norepinephrine.

Function: Tyrosine is an important precursor of the neurotransmitter dopamine. Dopamine and another neurotransmitter, serotonin, function antagonistically. When levels of serotonin are high in relation to dopamine, feelings of fatigue, tiredness, and reduced motivation result; when dopamine levels increase, feelings of fatigue are reduced and motivation increases. It is speculated that supplementation of tyrosine during prolonged exercise will help improve the dopamine-to-serotonin ratio, thereby reducing fatigue and improving performance. As noted, tyrosine is also a precursor to epinephrine (adrenaline) and norepinephrine (noradrenaline). Its potential effects on production of these catecholamines may also make it attractive to so-called fat-burner and preworkout supplement formulators.

Performance benefit: Supplementation with tyrosine during exercise could improve performance for endurance athletes and for strength and power athletes engaged in long-duration, high-intensity sports.

Research: A 2024 systematic review and meta-analysis by Solon-Júnior and colleagues stated that tyrosine supplementation is well recognized to improve cognitive function, but its impact on endurance performance is less established. These researchers reviewed 10 interventions from 8 studies. The subgroup analysis revealed no significant differences between tyrosine and placebo conditions for time to exhaustion ($p = 0.94$) and time trial performance ($p = 0.85$). They concluded that "tyrosine supplementation is ineffective on endurance performance in the physically active population, independently of the endurance task." This is in relative agreement with earlier work. In 2002 Chinevere and colleagues studied the effect of tyrosine supplementation in cyclists during a 90-minute steady-state ride followed by a time trial in temperate conditions. The athletes were provided with 25 mg of tyrosine/kg, which had no significant effects on performance. And although dopamine alterations are not the only potential mechanism of effect, other studies have used a pharmaceutical drug known as bupropion (e.g., Wellbutrin and other brand names) to increase dopamine levels during exercise and produced similar results. Interestingly, when bupropion was provided in warm environments (30°C [86°F]), a significant improvement in exercise performance was found in comparison to results in temperate environments (18°C [64°F]) (Watson et al., 2005). In 2011 a group of scientists found tyrosine improved cycling time to exhaustion by 11% under warm conditions (30°C [86°F]) (Tumilty et al., 2011). Although performance was improved, no differences in core temperature, heart rate, or rating of perceived exertion were noted. More research is needed to confirm these results; however, it appears that tyrosine supplementation may be capable of enhancing cognition under stressful conditions or improving performance during prolonged exercise in warm conditions.

Common usage: Tyrosine can be found in a variety of forms, pill and powder being most common. It's difficult to recommend an optimal usage strategy as more research is needed to confirm best-use procedures. A 2011 study of cyclists used a 150 mg/kg dose provided 1 hour before exercise. This would be equivalent to 9.5 g for a 64 kg (140 lb) athlete and up to 15 g for a 100 kg (220 lb) athlete (Tumilty et al., 2011). Tyrosine is sometimes recommended for treatment of depression, in which case 500 to 1,000 mg consumed 3 times/day is recommended. As noted, it has also been added to preworkout formulas, in part due to potential effects on epinephrine and norepinephrine secretion.

Health concerns: The use of tyrosine is safe for most people when consumed within recommended levels. Tyrosine supplementation may cause an increase in blood pressure in people taking antidepressant medications known as monoamine oxidase inhibitors (MAOIs), and those taking thyroid medication or levodopa should avoid tyrosine before consulting a physician. For comparison, in rats, which are not dosed the same as humans, the no-observed-adverse-effect level (NOAEL) of L-tyrosine was considered to be 600 mg/kg each day for males and 200 mg/kg each day for females (Shibui et al., 2016).

Ubidecarenone, Ubiquinone

(see *coenzyme Q10*)

Uncaria Guianensis, Uncaria Tomentosa

(see *cat's claw*)

Undenatured Type II Collagen (UC-II) 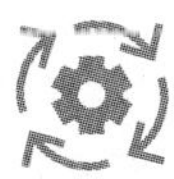 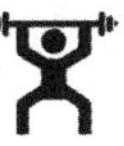

What it is: Glycosylated undenatured type II collagen (UC-II) is a dietary supplement that is produced from the sternum of chickens and is speculated to benefit arthritic joints and conditions such as osteoarthritis (OA) and rheumatoid arthritis. It is produced using a low-temperature procedure that prevents the proteins from being broken down, which is important for its effectiveness (Gupta, 2010).

Function: The exact mechanisms of UC-II are unknown; however, initial research suggests that stomach acids partially digest UC-II upon consumption, leaving chains of soluble collagen that can actively induce an immune response within the small intestine. In the case of rheumatoid arthritis, these proteins can downregulate autoimmune inflammatory responses—essentially, UC-II stops the immune system from attacking its own joint cartilage. In addition, UC-II has been shown to deactivate killer T cells, which also can induce an inflammatory response (Crowley et al., 2009).

Performance benefit: Because the physical demands of sport and daily training place a significant amount of stress on joints, many athletes experience chronic joint pain, reduced mobility, and decreased function. In addition, many athletes suffer injuries to joints that require surgery or joint reconstruction. UC-II may provide relief for athletes suffering from chronic joint pain or aid in recovery from injury.

Research: Current human data evaluating benefits of UC-II is limited but shows some promise as it relates to pain mitigation and improved functionality of joints affected by OA. Crowley and colleagues (2009) examined the effects of 40 mg of UC-II on subjects with OA of the knee. UC-II was found to be twice as effective as 1,500 mg of glucosamine and 1,200 mg of chondroitin in promoting joint health after 90 days. Improvements in physical function, stiffness, and pain were observed. Similarly, Lugo and colleagues (2013) found, in comparison to a control group, daily supplementation with 40 mg of UC-II over 120 days significantly improved knee joint extension while also significantly extending exercise time before pain arose in healthy subjects. Though early findings are positive, more research is needed before clear conclusions can be made relative to the effectiveness and mechanisms involved in the use of UC-II for treatment of joint pain and dysfunction in athletes.

Common usage: A supplementation protocol of 40 mg/day and consumed over at least 90 to 120 days is the current research-supported dose to mitigate pain and improve the functionality of joints inflicted with OA (Kumar et al., 2023).

Health concerns: The use of UC-II appears to be safe and well tolerated. A 2010 toxicological study concluded a broad spectrum of safety existed related to its use (Marone et al., 2010).

Valerian

aka *Valeriana officinalis*

What it is: *Valeriana officinalis* is a perennial herb found in North America, Europe, and Asia. More than 2,000 years ago Greeks used the herb as a treatment for anxiety, stress, insomnia, and other sleep disorders. It was used to relieve the stress of air raids in England during World War II. The use of valerian for treatment of anxiety, stress, and sleep disorders is still common today. Supplements are made from the roots, rhizomes, and stems of the plant, and extracts are often put into capsules.

Function: The exact mechanisms of valerian are unknown; however, a variety of constituents may be responsible for its biological effects. These include volatile oils, such as valeric acid, iridoids, alkaloids, and amino acids, including gamma-aminobutyric acid (GABA), tyrosine, arginine, and glutamine (Hadley & Petry, 2003).

Performance benefit: Athletes may benefit from improved quality, length, and onset of sleep. These benefits could produce improved recovery from training and subsequent performance. In addition, valerian can be used during extensive travel and time zone changes, assisting jet-lagged athletes in adapting circadian rhythms to new time zones.

Research: In one meta-analysis related to valerian, a total of 29 controlled studies were included; most found no significant differences between valerian and a placebo in healthy individuals suffering from general sleep disturbances or insomnia. As a result, it was concluded that, though the use of valerian is safe, it is not effective (Taibi et al., 2007). This review was in contrast to another review in 2006, which concluded that valerian might improve sleep quality; however, more research was recommended. It was noted that many studies included in the 2006 review had methodological flaws (Bent et al., 2006). A 2011 study conducted with oncology patients found valerian ineffective in relieving sleep disturbance in cancer patients (Barton et al., 2011). These results are similar to other recent studies, which were better controlled and less methodologically flawed. In conclusion, though early research suggested a potential benefit, more recent scientific studies have failed to show benefits. No known studies have been conducted with athlete-specific populations and the impact of improved sleep through valerian supplementation on recovery and performance.

Common usage: The potentially effective dosage of valerian used in scientific trials ranges from 300 to 600 mg and should be ingested between 30 minutes and 2 hours before bedtime.

Health concerns: No adverse side effects of valerian are known, nor are there contraindications to its use. Unlike some sleep aids, valerian use does not result in dependence.

Valine

(see *branched-chain amino acids*)

Vanadium (V) 

aka *Amanita muscaria, amavadin, sodium metavanadate, sodium orthovanadate, vanadyl sulfate*

What it is: Vanadium is considered a trace element. Vanadium is found in foods such as mushrooms, shellfish, black pepper, parsley, dill seed, and grains. *Amanita muscaria,* a species of mushroom, contains amavadin, which is a natural vanadium-containing compound (Vanadium/Vanadyl Sulfate, 2009).

Function: Vanadium is not considered an essential nutrient in the diets of humans; however, it is an essential nutrient for some animals such as chickens, which develop adverse effects in bones, feathers, and blood as a result of deficiency. Vanadium plays a role as a cofactor in a variety of enzymes, and some studies have shown it to mimic the actions of insulin. This effect is believed to produce a variety of beneficial effects on blood glucose control and possibly body composition. Various forms of vanadium are commonly added to dietary supplements marketed for weight loss and improvement of body composition.

Performance benefit: Athletes wanting to improve body composition or enhance muscle carbohydrate (glycogen) deposition may use vanadyl sulfate or vanadium.

Research: Research in support of vanadium for sports-related purposes remains scarce. Little work has been done in recent decades. A 12-week study completed in 1996 is the only known study related to vanadyl sulfate supplementation and athletes. The study on 31 weight-training athletes found no significant effects of supplementation on body composition (Fawcett et al., 1996). Another study in 2002 found that vanadyl sulfate supplementation did not affect insulin sensitivity in healthy active individuals (Jentijens & Jeukendrup, 2002). Although vanadium appears to have a role in insulin sensitivity, it does not improve body composition and is not recommended for use in athletes.

Common usage: There is no RDA for vanadium; however, a daily intake of 10 to 100 mcg is considered adequate. The average diet contains 6 to 18 mcg of vanadium/day. In scientific trials related to diabetes, a therapeutic dose of 100 to 300 mcg is often used. Another supplemental strategy often used in clinical trials is 50 mcg consumed 2 times/day.

Health concerns: Vanadium does not appear to be toxic; however, some mild effects such as abdominal cramps and diarrhea have been reported with higher doses (50 to 100 mcg). The vanadate form of vanadium can increase the effects of anticoagulants such as heparin (Vanadium/Vanadyl Sulfate, 2009).

Vanadyl Sulfate

(see *vanadium*)

Vinis Vinifera
(see *grape seed*)

Vinpocetine 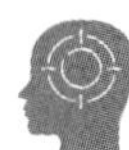 

aka *Cavinton (brand name), lesser periwinkle extract*

What it is: Vinpocetine is a synthetic derivative of a compound found in the periwinkle plant (*Vinca minor*). It has a history as a pharmaceutical drug in Europe and other regions, but in the United States, it is a dietary supplement. Lawsuits and Federal Trade Commission (FTC) actions against companies marketing vinpocetine have plagued its sale.

Function: Enhanced blood flow to the brain and neuroprotection are potential mechanisms in which people seeking memory enhancement have interest. These effects may be achieved by alterations in cellular sodium and calcium exchange or antioxidant effects.

Performance benefit: Enhanced cognition appears to be the primary candidate for affecting sport performance.

Research: In a Mayo Clinic Proceedings letter to the editor, physician Pieter Cohen (2015) raised concerns that vinpocetine, a pharmaceutical in Germany, Russia, and China, among other countries, is sold domestically as a dietary supplement despite never having been approved by the FDA for use in the United States; he also cited a 2008 Cochrane review suggesting it has no benefit for neuroprotection. In contrast, Zhang and colleagues (2018) stated that "Due to its excellent safety profile, increasing efforts have been put into exploring the novel therapeutic effects and mechanism of actions of vinpocetine in various cell types and disease models." More recently, Jędrejko and colleagues (2023) reported that "Many popular nootropics are unauthorized food or dietary supplement ingredients according to the European Commission including huperzine A, yohimbine, and dimethylaminoethanol; unapproved pharmaceuticals like phenibut or emoxypine (mexidol); previously registered drugs like meclofenoxate or reserpine; EU authorized pharmaceuticals like piracetam or vinpocetine." Pertinent to sport, these authors also point out that the World Anti-Doping Agency (WADA) does not define many nootropics as doping agents, although some may qualify as nonapproved substances or related substances according to the WADA Prohibited List.

Common usage: Vinpocetine has been used by adults in doses of 10 to 30 mg, 1 to 3 times/day. According to an older Cochrane review (Szatmari & Whitehouse, 2003), doses varied between 15 and 60 mg/day with a length of treatment from 12 weeks to 1 year.

Health concerns: The FDA issued a warning against vinpocetine in 2019 for consumers who are pregnant or may become pregnant. According to Cohen (2015), vinpocetine can lead to flushing, headaches, and decreased blood pressure. Vinpocetine may also interact with anticoagulant medications; consult a health care professional regarding this and other interactions.

Virgin Coconut Oil

(see *coconut*)

Vitamin B$_1$

(see *thiamine*)

Vitamin B$_2$

(see *riboflavin*)

Vitamin B$_5$

(see *pantothenic acid*)

Vitamin B$_9$

(see *folic acid*)

Vitamin B$_{12}$ 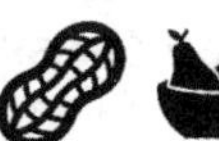

aka *cobalamin, cyanocobalamin, hydroxocobalamin, methylcobalamin*

What it is: Often considered nature's most beautiful vitamin due to the striking red color of its crystals, vitamin B$_{12}$ is a water-soluble vitamin that belongs to a family of chemically complex compounds containing the mineral cobalt—thus its secondary name, cobalamin. Naturally found in foods of animal origin such as organ meats, egg yolks, clams, crab, and salmon, vitamin B$_{12}$ plays an integral role in the formation of red blood cells, energy metabolism, normal nerve cell activity, and proper brain function.

Function: Because of its role alongside folic acid in the creation of red blood cells—important for oxygen transport throughout the body—as well as DNA synthesis, a deficiency in vitamin B$_{12}$ can result in such anemia-based symptoms as fatigue, poor energy levels, nausea and diarrhea, decreased appetite, weakening of the muscles, headaches, and tingling sensations. Vitamin B$_{12}$ also protects the outer covering of nerves, called the myelin sheath, which helps facilitate optimal conduction of energy throughout the nervous system. Suboptimal vitamin B$_{12}$ levels thus may compromise an athlete's ability to see, hear, think, and move. Although deficiencies are rare thanks to the body's ability to maintain stores for several years, the added stress of intense exercise on the body's energy-producing pathways and tissues may leave an athlete at elevated risk for diminished stores.

Performance benefit: Deficient athletes who supplement with vitamin B$_{12}$ may benefit from enhanced energy levels and better endurance through reversal of anemia symptoms.

Research: Limited research has been conducted to examine whether exercise increases the need for vitamin B$_{12}$. It has been confirmed that severe deficiency of B$_{12}$, especially in combination with folate, results in anemia and reduced endurance performance (Lukaski, 2004). More recently, Krzywański and colleagues (2020) evaluated the impact vitamin B$_{12}$ status has on red blood cell parameters in a group of elite track and field athletes. On average, vitamin B$_{12}$ levels were 739 ± 13 pg/mL, with no cases of deficiency being present. However, a small but significant relationship was found between vitamin B$_{12}$ and hemoglobin concentrations. With very low vitamin B$_{12}$ concentration (<400 pg/mL) there was a significant increase in hemoglobin, which was not seen with B_{12} levels above 700 pg/mL. Study investigators concluded that athletes should regularly monitor their blood vitamin B_{12} concentration and, if necessary, adjust dietary intake or supplement orally to optimize red blood cell parameters (400-700 pg/mL).

Common usage: The most common and recommended supplement form of vitamin B_{12} is cyanocobalamin. Delivery can be sublingual (under the tongue), in pill form, as part of a beverage, or by injection. According to the current Dietary Reference Intake (DRI), those age 14 and older should aim for 2.4 mcg daily; pregnancy and lactation warrant increased daily intake of 2.4 and 2.6 mcg, respectively. For reference, 1 oz (28 g) of salmon meets the 2 mcg/day recommendation. Supplementation of 25 to 100 mcg daily has been used to maintain vitamin B_{12} levels in at-risk populations, and therapeutic doses to correct deficiencies are often prescribed at doses of 125 to 2,000 mcg daily under the supervision of a doctor. Vitamin B_{12} shots (injectable B_{12}) are often marketed to boost metabolism, enhance energy, and speed weight loss; however, unless a deficiency is present, none of these claims carry any scientific merit.

Health concerns: Athletes who compete at the master's level, follow strict vegetarian or restrictive diets, or have undergone gastric bypass surgery are at greatest risk for deficiencies due to poor dietary intake or absorption. Severe deficiency cases, which are extremely rare even within an at-risk athletic population, can lead to anemia, gastrointestinal lesions, and neurological damage. Due to the body's ability to store vitamin B_{12}, it is generally considered nontoxic even in large doses. However, there have been a small number of anaphylactic reactions reported.

Vitamin C  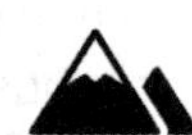

aka *antiscorbutic vitamin, ascorbate, ascorbic acid, calcium ascorbate, cevitamic acid, sodium ascorbate*

What it is: A water-soluble vitamin with powerful antioxidant qualities, vitamin C is an essential vitamin found naturally in abundance within fresh fruits and vegetables such as broccoli, peppers, brussels sprouts, strawberries, and kiwifruit.

Function: Vitamin C enhances wound healing and aids the growth and repair of injured tissue by facilitating the production of collagen. It also raises concentrations of key antibodies (IgA, IgM, IgG), helping to strengthen immune function. As an antioxidant, it hinders lipid peroxidation and reduces oxidative DNA and protein damage. Additionally, vitamin C serves as an enzyme cofactor for carnitine, important for the transport of fat into mitochondria for energy production, and aids the synthesis of peptide hormones, which are key factors for enhancing muscle size and strength.

Performance benefit: Playing a key role in the growth and repair of many tissues and supporting immune function, vitamin C may help enhance both short- and long-term recovery from intense exercise.

Research: Major reviews of vitamin C confirm that supplementation with the vitamin only aids physical performance in times of deficiency. In fact, a 2008 double-blind, randomized study of 14 trained men and 24 rats actually demonstrated a decline in physical performance with an oral dose of 1 g of vitamin C (dose altered in accordance to body mass in rats) taken over 6 weeks (Gomez-Cabrera et al., 2008). Specifically, vitamin C supplementation hindered important training adaptations such as increases in cytochrome C (a marker of mitochondrial content) and the powerful antioxidants superoxide dismutase and glutathione peroxidase, which limited improvements in aerobic capacity and time to exhaustion in supplemented subjects. Indeed, the current consensus is that, outside of cases of deficiency, caution is needed when supplementing with vitamin C, particularly at high doses (>1 g/day), as there is an increasing body of evidence showing no improvement or a deterioration of physical performance as well as undesirable metabolic changes and a decline in antioxidant activity (Higgins et al., 2020; Otocka-Kmiecik & Król, 2020).

Common usage: Available in capsule, tablet, and powder form as well as in multivitamin and antioxidant formulations, vitamin C is a commonly supplemented vitamin. The RDA for vitamin C is 90 mg for adult males and 75 mg for adult females; during pregnancy and lactation, RDA increases to 85 mg and 120 mg, respectively.

Health concerns: Severe vitamin C deficiency can lead to the onset of scurvy, a potentially fatal disease marked by fatigue, bleeding gums, joint pain and swelling, and hair and tooth loss. Although rare in developed countries, it has been reported in children and older adults on highly restricted diets. On the other hand, intake of vitamin C at levels upward of 3 g/day (well above the RDA) are generally well tolerated, although some experience stomach distress and diarrhea with high doses. Chronic supplementation at or above the threshold dose of 3 g/day also increases the risk for kidney stones.

Vitamin D

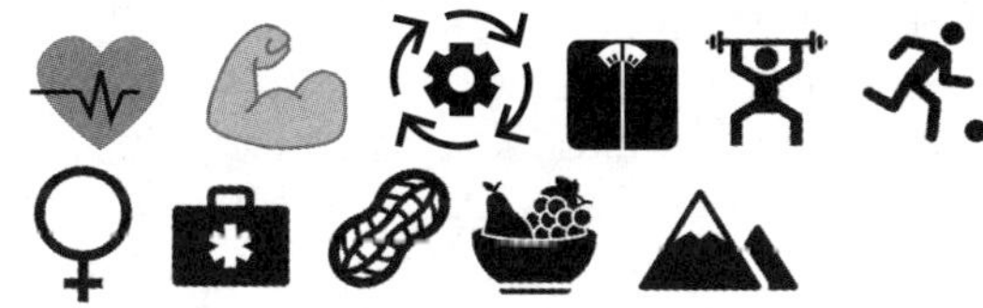

aka calcidiol, calcifediol, calcitriol, 1,25-dihydroxyvitamin D [1,25(OH)$_2$D], 25-hydroxyvitamin D [25(OH)D], vitamin D$_2$, vitamin D$_3$

What it is: Vitamin D is commonly referred to as the sunshine vitamin because it is produced in the skin from exposure to ultraviolet B (UVB) radiation. Vitamin D is classified as a fat-soluble vitamin (even though it is technically a prohormone, or any substance that can be converted to a hormone); its hormonally active form, calcitriol, plays a key role in calcium metabolism and bone health. Vitamin D levels are generally determined by measuring serum 25(OH)D concentrations; 30 ng/mL has been indicated as the cutoff to distinguish vitamin D deficiency, though there still is some uncertainty as whether this threshold should be higher for athletes (Amrein et al., 2020; Larsen-Meyer, 2013; de la Puente Yagüe et al., 2020; Thomas et al., 2016) .

Function: The discovery of vitamin D receptors within skeletal muscle initiated interest from sport scientists with respect to the possible role vitamin D plays in the world of sport performance and recovery from athletic injury. The active form of vitamin D works in conjunction with the parathyroid hormone and the hormone calcitonin to regulate serum calcium and phosphorus concentrations, generally by enhancing intestinal absorption of these minerals, facilitating normal bone mineralization, and protecting against debilitating osteoporotic and stress-related fractures. Vitamin D, which is obtained from sun exposure, food, and sometimes supplements, must undergo two chemical reactions within the body before it's available for use. Initially, vitamin D is converted to 25-hydroxyvitamin D [25(OH)D], also known as calcidiol or calcifediol, within the liver and then forms physiologically active 1,25-dihydroxyvitamin D [1,25(OH)$_2$D], also known as calcitriol. As a steroid hormone, calcitriol also regulates more than 50 genes in tissues throughout the body, including muscle and nerve tissue, a mechanism of action thought to have a positive impact on athletic performance, especially as it relates to the neuromuscular system. By reducing the production of proinflammatory cytokines and increasing the production of anti-inflammatory cytokines, vitamin D may also help speed the recovery process between hard workouts.

Performance benefit: Vitamin D–deficient athletes may benefit from improved muscle strength, power, and endurance; lower risk of stress fractures and other musculoskeletal injuries; and enhanced recovery from acute muscle injuries and inflammation following exhaustive exercise by increasing vitamin D stores through whole food intake, supplementation, and sun exposure.

Research: Vitamin D deficiency (30-40 ng/mL) is prevalent among all types of athletes and particularly those with limited exposure to sunlight (e.g., indoor athletes, athletes training in winter months) (Bârsan et al., 2023). One study revealed 84% of 342 professional soccer players competing in Qatar to have a vitamin D deficiency, with another 12% being severely deficient (<10 ng/mL) (Hamilton et al., 2014); another study revealed 41.2% of professional basketball players to present with vitamin D deficiency (Grieshober et al., 2018). These numbers fall in line with previous reports of vitamin D deficiency in athletes (Constatini et al., 2010) and presents a major cause for concern—an increase in morbidities and the onset of osteomalacia and osteoporosis, among a plethora of other health and performance detriments, is associated with this deficiency (Bikle, 2014; Farrokhyar et al., 2017; Koundourakis et al., 2016; Todd et al., 2015). Carswell and colleagues (2018) indeed found a correlation between vitamin D deficiency and compromised endurance performance, though, interestingly, restoration of optimal serum 25(OH)D levels through sun exposure and 1,000 IU/day of vitamin D supplementation did not translate to improved endurance performance in a study of 967 young, healthy men and women. Żebrowska and colleagues (2020) demonstrated a significant improvement in the serum 25(OH)D levels of nondeficient highly trained male ultrarunners (compared to a control group) with supplementation with 2,000 IU vitamin D over 3 weeks leading up to running a national championship ultramarathon race. Serum 25(OH)D levels in the supplemented group increased from baseline by 5.4 ± 2.8 ng/mL (to 40.3 ± 4.9 ng/mL) but decreased in the control group by -2.2 ± 3.6 ng/mL (to 31.8 ± 4.2 ng/mL). Implications for recovery and injury prevention were seen in the supplemented group with a significant decrease in postexercise biomarkers of muscle damage compared to the control group. Thus, achieving higher baseline levels of serum 25(OH)D via sun exposure, dietary intake, and supplementation might be warranted to offset the risk of musculoskeletal injuries in highly trained athletes competing in long distance running. Similarly, Bauer and colleagues (2019) demonstrated a correlation between vitamin D deficiency and musculoskeletal injuries as well as infection risk in elite handball athletes; Rakovac and Sajković (2023) revealed the same in a systemic review evaluating the relationship of serum 25(OH)D levels or vitamin D supplementation on reduced injury occurrence and enhanced muscular function in adolescent and elite professional ballet dancers. Indeed, previous data showed serum 25(OH)D concentrations of less than

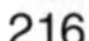

20 ng/mL to double the risk for stress fractures of the tibia and fibula as compared to concentrations of greater than 40 ng/mL in a group of young Navy recruits (Burgi et al., 2011). It has also been previously established that as serum 25(OH)D concentrations rise, increases in intracellular levels of calcitriol within muscle and nerve tissue and consequent improvements in the size and number of type II (fast-twitch) muscle fibers occur (Larson-Meyer & Willis, 2010). This may help explain why muscle strength has been shown to be significantly higher in male swimmers with sufficient vitamin D status (Geiker et al., 2017). A 2012 study also found a supplementation protocol incorporating 5,000 IU of vitamin D_3 over 8 weeks to significantly increase serum 25(OH)D concentrations in athletes and consequent performance in 10 m sprint time and in a vertical jump test (Close et al., 2012). Future research should continue to explore how supplementation with vitamin D can help achieve optimal 25(OH)D serum levels to yield favorable health and performance outcomes in athletes.

Common usage: Vitamin D is found naturally in such food sources as cod liver oil (1 tbsp = 1,360 IU), salmon (3.5 oz [99 g] = 360 IU), and egg yolk (1 = 20 IU); fortified in several products such as milk (1 cup = 98 IU); and as a supplement. The Institute of Medicine currently recommends an adequate intake, rather than a specific daily amount of vitamin D. This ranges from 600 IU (15 mcg) for adults up to age 70 to 800 IU (20 mcg) for adults age 71 and older. Athletes with serum 25(OH)D levels below 30 ng/mL, as revealed by a simple blood test, are encouraged to discuss ways to increase vitamin D via whole food intake, sun exposure, or supplementation with a doctor or a registered dietitian. A serum 25(OH)D concentration of 40 ng/mL or greater has been shown to be achievable with a daily supplementation protocol that incorporates 4,000 IU of vitamin D_3.

Health concerns: Chronically low serum 25(OH)D concentrations (<10 ng/dL) can lead to rickets in children and osteomalacia in adults, both characterized by soft bones and increased susceptibility to fracture. At the other end of the spectrum, toxicity symptoms, indicated at serum 25(OH)D levels ranging from 200 to 240 ng/mL or supplementation doses of 10,000 to 40,000 IU/day, include weakness, muscle pain, bone pain, loss of appetite, nausea, intestinal cramps, headache, metallic taste, and in the most severe cases renal impairment. Athletic performance has shown to decline with a supplementation protocol of 5,000 IU or more.

Vitamin E    

aka *alpha-tocopherol, alpha-tocotrienol, beta-tocopherol, beta-tocotrienol, delta-tocopherol, delta-tocotrienol, gamma-tocopherol, gamma-tocotrienol*

What it is: Found naturally in such foods as wheat germ, sunflower seeds, almonds, and vegetable oils, vitamin E, which collectively represents eight fat-soluble compounds, is a powerful and essential antioxidant that protects cell membranes and other fat-soluble parts of the body from free radical damage that can negatively affect both health and performance. Of its eight compounds, alpha-tocopherol is the only form actively maintained within blood and tissues and recognized to meet the human requirements for vitamin E.

Function: In response to strenuous or unaccustomed physical activity, the human body produces highly reactive oxygen species (ROS) known as free radicals that oxidize DNA, proteins, and lipids within cells, increasing the risk for cellular damage as well as cellular death. Such free radical production has been positively correlated with loss of muscle function, release of muscle enzymes, and histological evidence of damage and muscle soreness. Dietary antioxidants such as vitamin E serve as scavengers, repairing the damage free radicals leave behind and providing added protection against oxidative stress, thereby aiding the integrity of a multitude of physiological functions important to both health and performance.

Performance benefits: Athletes engaged in intense or prolonged endurance training may be able to better adapt to elevated levels of oxidative stress, therefore facilitating quicker recovery times. Athletes training or competing at altitudes above 6,000 feet (~1,800 m) may benefit from enhanced oxygen usage with increased vitamin E intake (Higgins et al., 2020). In addition, an acute intake of 250 mg of vitamin E taken 1 hour before moderate exercise in hypoxia simulating an altitude of 4,200 m has been shown to decrease postexercise cell damage markers and reduce the concentration of inflammatory cytokines, making it a possible recovery nutrient for athletes training and competing at altitude (Santos et al., 2016).

Research: Research has demonstrated a nearly 2-fold increase in markers of oxidative stress and a consequent rise in rate of vitamin E usage during a 50 km ultramarathon on rugged terrain (Mastaloudis et al., 2001), with a follow-up study showing a combined supplementation protocol of 400 IU of vitamin E and 1,000 mg of vitamin C over 6 weeks to elicit significant protection against oxidative stress compared to a control group, whose blood markers rivaled those of heart attack victims (Mastaloudis et al., 2004). A more recent meta-analysis of randomized control trials revealed similar outcomes, with a supplementation protocol consisting of 500 IU of vitamin E being shown to significantly reduce exercise-induced muscle damage in athletes (Kim et al., 2022). Although some research demonstrated an attenuation of exercise-induced oxidative stress with enhanced vitamin E intake and consequent storage, the translation to postexercise recovery and other parameters of sport performance is inconsistent, with some data showing antioxidant supplements, including vitamin E, to have no impact on performance or actually hinder positive cellular adaptations to training (Higgins et al., 2020; Martínez-Ferrán et al., 2020, 2022; Merry & Ristow, 2016; de Oliveira et al., 2019; Paulson et al., 2014). Interestingly, increasing daily whole food intake of antioxidants—specifically 50 g of dried berries and fruits; a 750 mL fruit, vegetable, and berry smoothie; 40 g walnuts; and 40 g dark chocolate (>70% cocoa content) over a 3-week altitude training camp—did not yield any negative impact on $\dot{V}O_2$max, erythropoietin, or hemoglobin mass compared to a placebo group of national team endurance athletes (Koivisto et al., 2018). In a follow-up to this study, investigators found the same daily intake of antioxidant-rich foods over a 3-week altitude training camp to significantly improve antioxidant capacity and decrease some of the altitude-induced inflammatory biomarkers compared to a control group of elite athletes (Koivisto et al., 2019). In another evaluation of whole food intake of antioxidants, Yi and colleagues (2014) found a single daily consumption of 75 g of almonds, which is a good source of vitamin E, taken before exercise over 4 weeks to improve the performance (measured as cycling distance traveled) of trained cyclists and triathletes compared to the control group. Similarly, an acute dose of 60 g almonds taken 2 hours before exercise was shown to enhance endurance performance in trained subjects (Esquius et al., 2020). Because of the potential hindrance vitamin E supplements may have on favorable adaptations to exercise training that do not seem to occur with whole food intake, the focus should remain on improving dietary intake of vitamin E from such rich sources as nuts, seeds, fish, avocado, wheat germ, and spinach.

Common usage: The RDA for adults over age 14 is 15 mg (22.4 IU). Because vitamin E is found in limited amounts in foods that generally are high in fat (e.g., vegetable oil), some may find it difficult meet recommendations from food alone without increasing fat intake above recommended levels. Thus, many foods are fortified with a synthetic form of vitamin E known as all-rac-alpha-tocopherol or DL-alpha-tocopherol, though it is not well absorbed by the body. The highest quality vitamin E supplements are naturally derived, containing only RRR-alpha-tocopherol (also labeled as d-alpha-tocopherol); a supplementation dose of 200 to 500 IU/day is indicated to help protect against exercise-induced oxidative damage.

Health concerns: Both deficiency and toxicity have rarely been reported in humans, although older athletes as well as those with celiac or muscle-wasting diseases are thought to be at greater risk for deficiency. Symptoms of deficiency include neurological damage, muscle weakness, loss of appetite, and anemia. The Food Institute of Medicine has established an upper tolerable intake level of 1,500 IU/day (1,000 mg/day for the natural form of alpha-tocopherol or 1,100 IU for the synthetic form of alpha-tocopherol). Doses above this level may cause bleeding problems.

Whey Protein

aka *whey protein concentrate (WPC), whey protein hydrolysate (WPH), whey protein isolate (WPI)*

What it is: Whey, a type of protein derived from the liquid portion of milk that separates from the curds when making cheese, makes up about 20% of the total protein found in cow's milk, with the other 80% coming from casein. It is a complete protein, meaning it contains all nine essential amino acids. The main components of whey protein include beta-lactoglobulin, alpha-lactalbumin, bovine serum albumin, and immunoglobulins. The three most common types of whey protein supplements, either as standalone products or added to pre- and postworkout supplements, are whey protein concentrate (WPC), whey protein isolate (WPI), and whey protein hydrolysate (WPH).

Function: With its rapid rate of digestion, whey protein offers the muscles a quick source of amino acids to aid in muscle protein synthesis as well as postexercise recovery of muscle function. The high leucine content (50%-75% more than other protein sources) is a key to the whey protein's anabolic qualities. The biological components of whey protein and its isolates have also been shown to provide antioxidant benefits and help regulate lipid metabolism.

Performance benefit: Because of its role in building new tissues in the body, whey protein can increase gains in lean body mass, which can also lead to improved strength and power, improved recovery from training, and less muscle soreness. Whey can also be used to maintain muscle mass in energy- or calorie-restricted states during weight loss. Finally, the amino acids found in whey are also believed to enhance and strengthen the immune system

Research: Much research has centered on the use of whey protein before and after workouts. Positive results have been seen related to mitigating protein breakdown and improving protein balance, decreasing markers of muscle damage, and promoting protein synthesis while also aiding muscle glycogen repletion when consumed in conjunction with carbohydrate (Morifuji et al., 2010). Schoenfeld and colleagues (2017) demonstrated favorable impacts on muscular adaptations to resistance training, including significant increases in maximal squat strength, when resistance-trained males consumed 25 g of WPI either before or after workout. In another study, administration of 0.9g/kg/day of whey protein divided into three 0.3g/kg daily doses over 5 days (a total of 13 doses or 3.9g/kg protein) after completing an exhaustive eccentric exercise protocol significantly reduced postexercise biomarkers of muscle damage compared to the water-only control group, with large effect sizes for creatine kinase and myoglobin demonstrated during the fourth and fifth days of recovery (Nieman et al., 2020). Kim and colleagues (2023) found supplementation with 60 g/day of WPI split into three doses (AM, postexercise, PM) over 4 weeks of a resistance-training program to significantly increase muscle mass and overall muscular strength and endurance, independent of dietary influence, compared to the placebo group of healthy men. For female athletes, both pre- and postexercise protein intakes of 0.32 to 0.38 g/kg have demonstrated beneficial physiological responses after completing resistance and intermittent exercise (Mercer et al., 2020). Of special relevance to athletes training or competing in the evening, consumption of 45 g (0.6 g/kg) of WPI after 60 minutes of endurance cycling (60% of maximal workload) and prior to sleep has shown to increase both mitochondrial and myofibrillar protein synthesis rates during overnight recovery compared to the placebo group of healthy men consuming a total daily protein intake of 1.2 g/kg (Trommelen et al., 2023). Overall, current evidence supports the notion that an athlete's total daily protein intake needs to remain adequate to support favorable adaptations to training. Both pre- and postworkout consumption of protein, via whole food or whey protein supplements, can be a valuable tool to support performance and promote optimal recovery.

Common usage: Target daily protein intake for athletes to support metabolic adaptation, repair, remodeling, and protein turnover generally ranges from 1.2 to 2.0 g/kg/day (Thomas et al., 2016). Higher intakes may be warranted over short periods when training is intensified or energy intake is restricted. Consuming 0.25 to 0.3 g/kg body mass or 15 to 25 g of whey protein in the 2 hours before and after exercise can help achieve daily protein needs as well as promote favorable adaptations to training (Thomas et al., 2016). Data are still limited in terms of which type of whey protein is best; however, there is little current evidence to suggest that any type of whey (WPC, WPI, or WPH) is superior to another (Hulmi et al., 2010).

Health concerns: High-protein diets do not appear to pose any health concerns; however, athletes need to understand that excessive protein intake could mean they are underconsuming other important macronutrients such as carbohydrate and healthy fats as well as vitamin-rich fruits and vegetables.

Willow Bark  

aka *salicin, salicylates, salix, Salix daphnoides, Salix fragilis, Salix purpurea*

What it is: Since ancient times the leaves and bark of willow trees, including the species *Salix purpurea, Salix daphnoides,* and *Salix fragilis,* have been used to treat pain, fever, and inflammation. Willow bark contains compounds known as salicylates, of which salicin is most common and believed to produce beneficial effects. Salicin is a precursor of salicylic acid, which is used to produce acetyl salicylic acid, the chemical name of aspirin. As a result, willow bark is often considered a natural form of aspirin and is used to treat similar conditions for which aspirin is prescribed. Willow bark is often found in dietary supplements used in the treatment of joint pain. In the late 1980s and early 1990s it was often used in combination with ephedrine and caffeine to produce supplements marketed as preworkouts, anorectics, or fat burners.

Function: Although many of the beneficial effects of willow bark are believed to result from salicin, other compounds such as polyphenols and flavonoids are speculated to contribute. Although the exact mechanism is unknown, willow bark's components are believed to inhibit inflammatory cytokines and inflammatory enzymes such as COX-2 (Nahrstedt et al., 2007; Shakibaei et al., 2012). Some experts believe that the additional

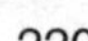

benefits of polyphenols and flavonoids found within willow bark make it superior to aspirin (Vlachojannis, Magora, & Chrubasik, 2011). This remains controversial, however, as work by Antoniadou and colleagues (2021) suggests that polyphenols are not relevant for the bioactivity of willow bark.

Performance benefit: Athletes suffering from muscle and joint pain resulting from training, competition, or injury may benefit from the pain-reducing and anti-inflammatory effects of willow bark.

Research: One study on the use of willow bark found that a dose equivalent to 240 mg of salicin significantly improved pain experienced by patients with osteoarthritis (Schmid et al., 2001). A 2009 meta-analysis of willow bark for musculoskeletal pain concluded that moderate evidence exists for the effectiveness of willow bark extract (Vlachojannis, Cameron, & Chrubasik, 2009). Willow bark is approved by the German Federal Health Agency for use in the treatment of fever, joint pain, and headaches. Willow bark appears to be effective; however, more research is needed to provide insight into the potential mechanisms beyond inhibition of prostaglandin E2 (PGE2) and confirm optimal doses needed to provide benefit.

Common usage: Currently, a dose of willow bark equivalent to 240 mg of salicin is recommended for treatment of inflammation, muscle soreness, and joint pain.

Health concerns: Use of willow bark is contraindicated in individuals with known aspirin allergy. Willow bark can also interact with anticoagulants and blood thinners. Products containing willow bark seldom contain warnings related to aspirin sensitivity and potential drug interactions, so consumers should proceed with caution.

Winter Cherry

(see *Withania somnifera*)

Withania Somnifera (WS) 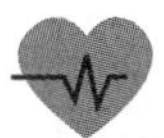 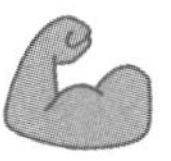 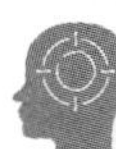 

aka *ashwagandha, Indian ginseng, winter cherry*

What it is: *Withania somnifera* (WS) or ashwagandha is a green shrub found in drier parts of the Middle East. WS is commonly used in Ayurvedic medicine, a traditional medical system of India, for treatment of a wide range of ailments.

Function: WS contains 12 alkaloids, 35 withanolides, and several sitoindosides, which are believed to be the active constituents of the plant. The diverse number of constituents is believed to be responsible for the multiple medicinal properties of WS (Kulkarni & Dhir, 2008).

Performance benefit: The suggested benefits of WS for athletes include anti-inflammatory, adaptogenic, anabolic, antioxidant, and immunomodulatory effects.

Research: Multiple studies on mice have reported WS to have an antistress effect on chronic fatigue induced by forced swimming (Archana & Namasivayam, 1999; Dhuley, 2000). WS has also been shown to improve activity of antioxidant defense enzymes such as superoxide dismutase, catalase, and glutathione peroxidase, especially in stress-induced conditions. In another study, WS provided a significant protective effect against foot strike–induced stress in mice (Bhattacharya & Muruganandam, 2003). Sumantran and colleagues (2008) also found WS to produce anti-inflammatory effects in osteoarthritic cartilage. More specific to human athletes, a 2021 systematic review by Bonilla and colleagues examined 12 studies with a low-to-moderate risk of bias and concluded that ashwagandha (*Withania somnifera*) "was more efficacious than placebo for improving variables related to physical performance" in healthy men and women. Earlier work from Sandhu and colleagues (2010) found that WS at a dose of 500 mg/day for 8 weeks with no training program implemented increased velocity, power, and $\dot{V}O_2$max, although sample sizes were relatively low. Another study of humans found 5 g/day of WS to improve resting cortisol and enzymatic antioxidant activity in cigarette-smoking men and psychologically stressed men.

Common usage: According to Bonilla and colleagues (2021), taking 300 to 500 mg 2 times/day (in the morning and at bedtime) might be a safe and effective supplementation protocol for those undertaking strenuous resistance or endurance training, but more research is needed. Supplementation used in human trials is 20 to 50 mg/kg used once daily. Research studies with mice have used higher dosages of 50 to 1,000 mg/kg without any known toxic effects, although rodent dosing differs from human dosing.

Health concerns: Extensive toxicological studies have demonstrated the plant to be nontoxic in a wide range of reasonable doses, and no adverse herbal or drug interactions have been reported (Kulkarni & Dhir, 2008).

Wood Spider

(see *devil's claw*)

Wu-Chu-Yu

(see *rutaecarpine*)

Yeast-Derived Beta-Glucan

(see *beta-glucan*)

Yohimbe  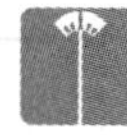

aka *Corynanthe johimbe, Pausinystalia johimbe*

What it is: Yohimbine is a pure alkaloid that can be isolated from the bark of the African yohimbe tree (*Corynanthe johimbe*). The bark of the yohimbe tree provides other indole alkaloids as well.

Function: Yohimbine works at least in part by blocking a subtype of adrenaline receptor in the body. Yohimbe (and similarly, the drug yohimbine hydrochloride) blocks alpha adrenaline receptors but also interacts with serotonin and dopamine receptors in the body. This can lead to vasodilation or lack of vasoconstriction (dizziness upon standing). Yohimbe can also increase the amount of epinephrine and norepinephrine in the bloodstream (Escalante et al., 2019).

Performance benefit: Yohimbe could potentially increase blood flow or fat loss, although its use is controversial.

Research: Although there is considerable literature on the drug yohimbine, there is less data on less-refined yohimbe supplements. A paper by McCarty (2002) on the use of yohimbine before exercise suggested that "it boosts lipolysis and serum FFA levels both during and following exercise; blockade of adipocyte alpha-2 adrenoreceptors makes at least a modest contribution to this pro-lipolytic activity." However, yohimbe supplements may contain unregulated amounts of yohimbine and therefore may not work like the prescription medication. The National Center for Complementary and Integrative

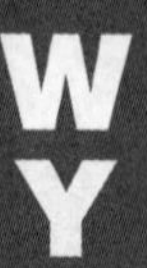

Yohimbe

Health (NCCIH) has concluded that there is limited evidence for many of yohimbe's purported uses.

Common usage: Yohimbe has been stacked with stimulant ingredients in preworkout supplements and energy drinks, as well as sold by itself for erectile dysfunction, fat loss, athletic performance, and other purported benefits. It has even been included in topical preparations (lotions) for spot-reduction of body fat. Yohimbine products are sold online at the time of this writing at 2 to 10 mg and yohimbe bark labels at 50 to 500 mg. Note that related labels have a history of controversy.

Health concerns: Largely through its effects on alpha-2 adrenoceptors, side effects could include feelings of anxiety or nervousness, dizziness, changes in blood pressure, and rapid heart rate (tachycardia), among other issues. The NCCIH cautions not to use yohimbe if you are taking a monoamine oxidase inhibitor (MAOI) antidepressant. Other drug contraindications include opioids and blood pressure medications. Pregnant or breastfeeding women should also avoid it. Consumers should consult their physician.

Zeaxanthin 

aka *macular pigment* (see also *lutein*)

What it is: A common carotenoid and antioxidant, zeaxanthin is the pigment that gives corn and paprika—among many other plants—their characteristic color. Foods rich in zeaxanthin also include green leafy vegetables like spinach and kale. Zeaxanthin and lutein are two xanthophyll carotenoids in the retina of the eye. Thus, zeaxanthin supplements are commonly supplemented to support eye health.

Function: Zeaxanthin may potentially contribute to enhanced vision, such as in conditions of high ultraviolet light or glare. It may also contribute to slowed progression of age-related macular degeneration and cataracts. Further, some of level of skin protection from UV light may be conferred.

Performance benefit: Athletes may benefit from potentially enhanced vision in sports involving bright and glaring conditions, especially outdoors.

Research: Studies and products often combine zeaxanthin with lutein, which could enhance the overall effect on eye health. Little research has been done specific to zeaxanthin and exercise.

Common usage: A mixture of lutein and zeaxanthin is common, with 10 mg/day of lutein and 2 mg/day of zeaxanthin. Americans do not typically consume this much from foods. According to Wilson and colleagues (2021), estimated intake among American adults is 1 to 2 mg/day of lutein and zeaxanthin from dietary sources.

Health concerns: There are few concerns in the common usage range listed. In a study of zeaxanthin concentrate, Ravi and colleagues (2014) reported "The findings of this sub-chronic toxicity and mutagenicity studies support safety of zeaxanthin concentrate." This conclusion was echoed by Johra and colleagues (2020): "Preclinical study results . . . have established the safety profile of several carotenoids [including zeaxanthin]. . . . Eight in vivo studies were mentioned in this review, and none of these studies observed any significant adverse effect or toxicity. Xu et al. (2013) suggested a daily intake of 3 mg/kg/day meso-zeaxanthin for humans." Note: meso-zeaxanthin is a stereoisomer of zeaxanthin.

Zinc (Zn)  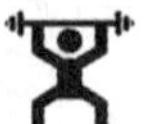 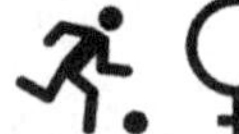    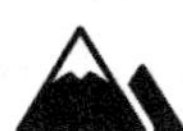

aka *zinc acetate, zinc aspartate, zinc gluconate, zinc methionine, zinc monomethionine, zinc oxide, zinc sulfate* (see also *zinc magnesium aspartate*)

What it is: An essential mineral derived naturally from such dietary sources as oysters, meat, seafood, and eggs as well as from fortified foods and supplements, zinc plays a key role in several aspects of cellular metabolism, aiding the functioning of over 300 enzymes in the body. Although zinc is found in virtually all cells of the body and is especially abundant in muscle tissue, there is no specialized storage system for the mineral, making daily intake necessary to avoid deficiencies. Athletes may need to consume more zinc than the general population to help offset mineral losses via sweat during physical training. Zinc is often combined with magnesium and vitamin B_6 to form a supplement cocktail known as zinc magnesium aspartate (ZMA).

Function: Zinc plays a key role in a wide range of biological functions important to sport performance, including muscle energy production and protein synthesis. Many scientists believe zinc's involvement in energy metabolism to be an important determinant of an athlete's endurance capacity, with suboptimal levels triggering premature fatigue during exercise. Additionally, because blood testosterone levels are in part regulated by zinc, a deficiency may hinder gains in muscle mass and strength. The antioxidant qualities of zinc may also help reduce postexercise free radical activity, thereby promoting recovery and supporting immune functionality.

Performance benefit: Zinc may help enhance recovery by aiding tissue repair postworkout and protecting immune functionality, especially in deficient athletes.

Research: It is known that acute endurance and muscular strength exercise decrease serum zinc levels while increasing urinary zinc, particularly in the case of exhaustive exercise (Chu et al., 2017; Maynar et al., 2018). Combined with dietary zinc intakes that fall below the RDA, negative outcomes on health and performance would be expected (Bakaloudi et al., 2021; England & Cheng, 2024; Garner et al., 2021; Wan & Zhang, 2022). Lukaski (2005) confirmed this, finding that poor dietary intake of zinc over 9 weeks (3.8 mg/day, or <50% of the current RDA for adults) compromised zinc status, impaired metabolic responses to exercise, and significantly reduced peak oxygen uptake; this culminated in an 11% decline in total work capacity during submaximal exercise when compared to a supplemental zinc protocol that incorporated 18.8 mg/day over 9 weeks. The performance effects on a nondeficient population have not been confirmed, although some scientists believe zinc supplementation aids the short- and long-term health of an athlete by enhancing antioxidant activity. A supplementation protocol of 22 mg of zinc/day over 12 weeks in football players (de Oliveira et al., 2009) and a shorter protocol of 8 weeks for elite wrestlers (Kara et al., 2010, 2011) have been shown to do just that, decreasing markers of oxidative stress and consequent free radical damage to cells important to immune functionality postworkout. Yet, the overall available evidence fails to support performance benefits of zinc supplementation beyond the RDA, which, for most athletes, can be obtained through a balanced diet (Davison et al., 2016; Hernández-Camacho et al., 2020; McClung, 2019). Future research should continue to explore the impact zinc supplementation may have on those athletes at greatest risk for low intake and deficiency.

Common usage: The current RDA for zinc in adult men and women (ages 19 and up) is 11 mg and 8 mg, respectively, with pregnancy and lactation increasing needs to 11 mg and 12 mg, respectively. Many experts believe intense sport training to warrant an increase in intake to 25 to 30 mg/day. Deficiencies are generally corrected at doses of 30 to 40 mg/day. Zinc should not be taken with high-fiber or dairy foods, which can impair absorption. Due to malabsorption and excretion issues, athletes at heightened risk for a zinc deficiency and thus most likely to benefit from supplementation include strict vegetarians and vegans, energy-restricted athletes, master athletes (age 60+), those carrying the sickle cell trait, pregnant and lactating athletes, and those having undergone gastrointestinal surgery (e.g., gastric bypass) or experiencing digestive disorders such as Crohn's disease, ulcerative colitis, or irritable bowel syndrome.

Health concerns: Consuming large doses of zinc, especially above the current upper limit of 40 mg/day, increases risk for copper deficiencies and altered iron status as well as such symptoms as nausea, vomiting, fatigue, neuropathy, and metallic taste.

Zinc Magnesium Aspartate (ZMA)

What it is: Zinc magnesium aspartate (ZMA) is a nutritional supplement that was popular for a number of years. Its main ingredients are the minerals zinc and magnesium; however, various proprietary blends can be found that include additional B-vitamins, herbs, and plant sterols. ZMA is still marketed to athletes wanting to increase lean body mass, improve sleep and recovery, and enhance testosterone levels.

Function: Effects depend in part on baseline zinc and magnesium status. Research has identified that zinc deficiency results in low testosterone levels, and magnesium intake affects the secretion of insulin-like growth factor 1 (IGF1) and increases testosterone bioactivity. However, its relationship with anabolic hormones such as testosterone in men needs further study.

Performance benefit: Athletes may benefit from the enhanced levels of testosterone promoting gains in muscle strength, size, and power. It's also possible that ZMA may positively affect rest, sleep, and recovery. In addition, athletes may benefit from the immune-enhancing effects of zinc and its role in the function of superoxide dismutase, a powerful cellular antioxidant.

Research: Data on ZMA are mixed, in part depending on which potential benefit is tested. After documenting that zinc and magnesium may play a role in sleep via interactions with gamma-aminobutyric acid (GABA), Gallagher and colleagues (2024) tested whether supplementation of ZMA (30 mg zinc, 450 mg magnesium, 10.5 mg vitamin B_6) during partial sleep deprivation affected sleep quality and subsequent morning resistance exercise, concluding that supplementation of ZMA for 2 nights of partial sleep deprivation (4 hours sleep) had no effect on submaximal (40%-80% 1RM) bench press and squat performance in 16 trained males. Earlier research created a lot of initial excitement related to ZMA as it was found that supplementation resulted in an increase in plasma testosterone of approximately 30% and significantly improved muscle strength in semiprofessional athletes (Brilla & Conte, 2000). However, another study on weightlifters in 2004 found ZMA was not effective and did not produce any significant differences in anabolic or catabolic hormones, body composition, strength, or anaerobic capacity (Wilborn et al., 2004). Similar results were found in a 2009 study specifically evaluating the effectiveness of ZMA on increasing testosterone levels. No other studies have found zinc, ZMA, or similar supplements to produce any significant benefits (Koehler et al., 2009). ZMA supplementation shows promise only if zinc and magnesium deficiencies exist.

Common usage: Research studies have evaluated supplements containing approximately 30 mg of zinc and 450 mg of magnesium. The RDA for zinc is roughly 11 mg for men and 8 mg for women. The RDA for magnesium is 420 mg for men and 320 mg for women.

Health concerns: Because minerals can compete with each other for absorption and transport in the body, consuming large doses of zinc (>40 mg/day) increases risk for copper deficiency and altered iron status as well as symptoms of nausea, vomiting, fatigue, neuropathy, and metallic taste. Side effects associated with magnesium include diarrhea, abdominal pain, and nausea.

Zinc Magnesium Aspartate (ZMA)

Supplements for Special Groups and Environments

In a simple world, there would be a one-size-fits-all strategy for nutrition, but the human body is an intricate machine, and every athlete has different genetics, habits, and needs with different nutritional requirements. Some may have food sensitivities and intolerances that create extra performance obstacles unless nutritionally tended to. Others may have metabolic disorders, such as diabetes, that require close monitoring for success in sport. Dramatic differences can exist just based on sex. Furthermore, some athletes make lifestyle choices, such as vegetarianism, that affect nutritional needs. Additionally, every sport has physiological demands that affect an athlete's nutritional requirements, and if injury occurs, a specialized nutrition approach may be needed to enhance recovery. Even Mother Nature can dictate that a nutrition plan be adjusted for environmental conditions. Thus, not unlike clear trends in individualized, precision medicine, a customized approach to nutrition and dietary supplementation is essential. In this chapter, we discuss specialized nutrition and dietary supplement recommendations for athletes across the age spectrum and for female athletes, athletes recovering from injury, athletes with diabetes, athletes with food allergies and intolerances, athletes with plant-based diets, athletes competing in heat and humidity, and athletes competing at altitude.

ATHLETES WITH SPECIALIZED CONCERNS

Athletes with specialized concerns are encouraged to work closely with a registered sport dietitian and exercise physiologist or certified strength and conditioning specialist (CSCS) as well as their doctor to develop both nutritional and supplemental plans best suited for their needs. A list of qualified dietitians can be found at www.eatright.org, a list of qualified exercise physiologists can be found at www.asep.org, and a list of reputable strength and conditioning professionals can be found at https://directory.nsca.com. Consumers should ask about any nutritionist's or trainer's university education.

Master Athletes

Older athletes must be aware of the physiological changes that result from aging in order to maintain high levels of performance. For the endurance athlete, peak performance is typically maintained until age 35. Performance in strength and power sports is similar, with athletes who stay injury free often increasing in strength through middle age. Master athletes commonly experience fat gain, slowed recovery time, nagging injuries, and diminished performance. Even so, many master athletes continue to conquer the physiological changes of aging: Jenny Hitchings, a female American distance runner, broke the 60+ womens world record mark for the marathon at the 2023 Chicago Marathon. Oksana Chusovitina, gymnast from Uzbekistan, received a standing ovation from her fellow Olympians as she concluded her record-setting eighth Olympic appearance at the 2020 Tokyo Games at age 46. Female Brazilian soccer legend Formiga, at age 43, became the oldest soccer player to ever compete at the Olympics in the 2020 Tokyo Games. Two NFL quarterbacks, Tom Brady and Brett Favre, led their teams to the playoffs while in their 40s, with Brady being the oldest quarterback in history to win a Super Bowl with a win in Super Bowl LIII against the Rams—his sixth Super Bowl win. As simple as it may sound, peak performance for all ages across all sports relies heavily on two key controllable factors: smart training and proper nutrition. Athletes who optimize these factors will continue to defy odds and break records as well as extend quality of longevity.

Performance Obstacles for Master Athletes

A number of physiological changes are responsible for decreases in performance with age. Impacts on endurance performance are caused by significant declines in maximal aerobic capacity ($\dot{V}O_2$max)—although anaerobic threshold and exercise economy are well maintained, $\dot{V}O_2$max declines roughly 5% to 10% per decade after age 30. These changes are the result of reduced cardiac output, a product of maximum heart rate and stroke volume. Maximum heart rate declines at a rate of 0.7 beats per year starting in early adulthood. Mild decreases in stroke volume are observed in older endurance athletes, who typically have stroke volumes that are roughly 80% to 90% of the volume typical of younger trained counterparts.

There is still considerable debate about whether performance declines are a natural result of aging or a reduction in the intensity and amount of training typically practiced by older athletes. It has been found that drops in total weekly running distance of approximately 15 mi (24 km) may cause $\dot{V}O_2$max to drop by 2.4%. The loss of muscle mass and mitochondrial efficiency that occurs with aging can also affect $\dot{V}O_2$max. A loss of 3 kg (6.6 lb) of lean body mass can drop $\dot{V}O_2$max by 4.5%.

Unfortunately, the impact of aging on strength and power athletes is less understood. Most significantly for these types of athletes, aging is associated with losses in muscle mass and a decline in the number of fast-twitch muscle fibers, resulting in reductions in speed, strength, and power. Metabolic changes within the muscle such as enzyme activity and alterations in the ATP-PC energy system can also negatively affect anaerobic exercise. Further, tendonitis and tendinosis can weaken musculoskeletal connection and force transfer, even leading to evulsion injury, which can set back training many months. However, master athletes should take heart in knowing that although several physiological systems begin to decline with age, these systems are still very adaptable and responsive to training. Both strength and power and endurance master athletes can achieve significant improvements in performance through training.

Other important changes associated with aging include declines in resting metabolic rate (RMR), which can result in increased body fat and weight gain. RMR decreases by about 10% from early childhood to adulthood and another 10% from adulthood to the 60s. Several factors have been shown to directly influence RMR: thyroid hormones; genetics, body or environmental temperature; and stress. Other factors related to RMR are body surface area, total body weight, lean body mass, sex, age, and aerobic fitness. Of these factors, there seems to be the strongest correlation between lean body mass and RMR. When metabolically active muscle tissue is lost and replaced with less metabolically active adipose or fat tissue, RMR inevitably declines. Fortunately, RMR can be kept elevated by master athletes who continue to train at high levels while meeting individual nutritional needs.

AGING AND BONE HEALTH

A progressive decline in calcium content in the bones begins around age 30, increasing risk for stress fractures and development of osteoporosis. Declines in sex hormones worsen this loss. Other risk factors that exacerbate the aging effect on bone include smoking, alcohol intake, inactivity, and poor nutrition. More than 25 million people in the United States alone are affected by osteoporosis, leading to as many as 1.5 million bone fractures per year. According to the National Health and Nutrition Examination Survey (NHANES) data, prevalence of osteoporosis is on the rise for those over 50, increasing from 9.4% in 2007-2008 to 12.6% in 2017-2018 (Sarafrazi et al., 2021). Indeed, in the United States, the incidence of the disease has been projected to grow by 32% between 2010 and 2030 (Li et al., 2024).

Women tend to be more affected by osteoporosis, especially after menopause when levels of estrogen, a bone-protecting hormone, are significantly reduced. According to NHANES data, the most significant rise in osteoporosis rates among those over 50 occurred in women, with rates increasing by 5.6% from 2007-2008 to 2017-2018 (Sarafrazi et al., 2021). It has previously been estimated that one-third of all women will experience osteoporosis-related fractures in their lifetimes, but with increasing rates of osteoporosis, these numbers will also likely rise (Riggs & Melton, 1992).

Mortality has been shown to increase 2.8 to 4 times during the first 3 months after a hip fracture (Moyer, 2013). Thus, it is critical to address measures that help prevent and treat osteoporosis. Fortunately, bone health can be maintained with a healthy lifestyle, including proper training, particularly weight-bearing exercise, and a well-balanced, energy-sufficient diet rich in key bone-building nutrients like calcium and vitamin D.

Aging also affects the immune system. Decreased resistance to infections, increased inflammation, autoimmune activation, lower immune surveillance, and lower vaccination efficiency are all recognized immunological changes. Proper nutrition and certain supplements addressed in this book may assist in preventing some of these changes.

Finally, changes to joint structures and connective tissues can result in pain, dysfunction, and higher rates of inactivity in master athletes. Cartilage, a flexible connective tissue found in many joints, often degenerates over time, a change often responsible for pain and dysfunction. Certain dietary supplements may protect against this degeneration.

Nutritional Recommendations for Master Athletes

Nutrition can have a significant impact in delaying changes associated with aging. Although calorie needs of master athletes are often lower due to drops in resting metabolic rate and lower intensities and volumes of training, preservation of available energy has been shown to be a critical factor in maintaining sufficient physical activity levels with age and reaping the benefits of an active lifestyle (Gibala et al., 2012; Schrager et al., 2014). The ability of older adults to accurately regulate energy intake, however, is often impaired. A number of possible causes include delayed rate of absorption of macronutrients, reductions in taste and smell acuity, changes in numerous hormonal and metabolic mediators of energy regulation, changes in patterns of dietary intake, and a reduction in the variety of foods consumed in older age that may further reduce energy intake (Roberts & Rosenburg, 2006). Furthermore, among adults aged 40 and above, it has been reported that anywhere from 2% to 7.7% of women and approximately 1% of men meet the diagnostic criteria for an eating disorder, with rates being higher for those experiencing disordered eating and body images without meeting the full diagnostic criteria for an eating disorder (Mangweth-Matzek et al., 2013). Prevalence of low energy availability associated with disordered eating and eating disorders are likely to be higher in master athletes given statistics across all ages demonstrating elevated risk in an athletic population, particularly in those competing in sport where weight or body image and size is emphasized for performance (Bratland-Sanda & Sundgot-Borgen, 2013). Recommended intake for maintaining energy balance and consequently supporting optimal physical activity levels, health, and performance of older athletes is approximately 45 kcal/kg of FFM (fat-free mass) per day (Thomas et al., 2016).

Because musculoskeletal deterioration and consequent declines in strength and functionality is common with aging, it is recommended that baseline protein intake increase from 0.8 g/kg/day to 1.2 g/kg/day after age 40. Exercise training, like that with younger athletes, further increases this demand, with intakes of 1.6 to 2.0 g/kg/day being warranted for master-level athletes age 40 and older, and even greater intakes of 2.2 g/kg/day being supported for senior-level athletes (age 80+) to optimally support muscle protein synthesis, recovery, and long-term adaptations to training (Doering et al., 2016). Pre-, peri-, and postmenopausal athletes are also recommended to target the high end of these protein guidelines (Sims et al., 2023). Ideally, daily protein demands will be met by consuming smaller, more frequent (4-5) meals consisting of 0.3 to 0.4 g/kg protein (e.g., chicken, whey, casein, egg, perhaps soy), including a protein-rich snack before bedtime. Master athletes focused on soy protein should note that, at least acutely, it has been compared unfavorably to similar-dose whey protein, with a typical 20 g scoop not being statistically better than 0 g regarding muscle protein synthesis (Yang, Churchward-Venne, et al., 2012). Increasing the dose of soy does help somewhat, however.

Research has shown that even with the same type of protein, master athletes may need double postworkout protein intake (40 g) compared to their younger, trained counterparts (20 g) to maximize muscle protein synthesis and promote recovery, particularly when in a detrained state (Yang, Breen, et al., 2012). To optimize the anabolic response of resistance exercise and muscle protein synthesis postworkout, athletes are encouraged to consume a protein source providing a total of 0.03 to 0.045 g/kg of leucine taken pre- or postworkout or in a split dose manner both pre- and postworkout. Researchers have stated that for an adult to consume 2.7 g of leucine, or 10.9 g essential amino acids, they would have to ingest ~32 g of whey protein, ~48 g of pea protein, or ~55 g of soy protein

(Putra et al., 2021). Athletes who struggle to achieve these guidelines may benefit from supplemental protein intake.

Fat and carbohydrate intake are also important, though recommendations for older athletic populations have not been shown to differ from those of younger athletes. Note that for some master athletes to maintain energy balance while achieving elevated protein needs, overall energy intake from carbohydrate and especially fat may need to be reduced. It is difficult to make specific macronutrient recommendations as demands vary significantly between individuals and often need to be manipulated to achieve specific athletic goals. Therefore, it is best to consult a registered dietitian to devise a specific macronutrient and overall nutrition plan for optimal health and performance.

The need for certain vitamins and minerals also increases with age. Vitamin D is essential for the prevention of osteoporosis and many chronic diseases as well as for immune system and muscle function. Most of it is produced from exposure to sunlight; however, the body's ability to produce vitamin D from this exposure decreases with age and makes supplementation more important. A 25(OH)D value of less than 75.8 nmol/L has been shown to elevate risk for a stress fracture (Knechtle et al., 2021), which not only inhibits the athlete's ability to train but also has been shown to increase risk of morbidity. Adequate calcium intake is also important in preventing the loss of calcium from bone and the development of osteoporosis and fracture.

Vitamin B_{12} also has a variety of functions that are vital for optimal muscle function and performance, including red blood cell production, DNA synthesis, and nerve function. B_{12} requires a special protein produced in the GI tract, known as intrinsic factor, in order to be absorbed, but production of intrinsic factor decreases with age, limiting the ability of the body to absorb B_{12} and increasing requirements. The need for the antioxidant vitamins C and E can also increase with age; research supports the added supplementation of these vitamins for providing protection against free radicals and preventing some of the declines in immune system function associated with aging. Athletes should note, however, that muscle adaptations to exercise may be hampered by high doses of vitamins C and E, so it is important to consider lower doses (e.g. 250 mg vitamin C and 200 IU natural vitamin E). Iron, thiamin, riboflavin, folate, niacin, and vitamin A are also noted as commonly being consumed in inadequate amounts. A daily multivitamin and multimineral supplement with additional antioxidants will serve as a nutrition insurance agent. Research results for any added benefit of nutritional supplementation remain controversial.

Supplement Options for Master Athletes

In cases of deficiency, certain dietary supplements can be of particular importance to maintain the health and performance of older populations. Addressing some of the physiological changes associated with aging through nutrition and dietary supplements can assist in preventing declines in function and performance. Following is a list of physiological changes important for older athletes to consider.

- Preservation of lean body mass
- Immune support
- Joint support
- Antioxidant defense
- Skeletal health

Potential supplements to address these changes are discussed in table 4.1.

TABLE 4.1 Highlighted Supplement Options for Master Athletes

Supplement	Potential benefit	Recommended dose
Protein (whey, casein, egg, soy)	Builds and preserves muscle mass	Baseline daily total protein intake: 1.2 g/kg When training: 1.6-2.2 g/kg, including 0.25 g/kg or ~40 g (>40 g soy) consumed after exercise To promote muscle protein synthesis during sleep, 20-40 g casein can be supplemented before bed
Leucine	Builds and preserves muscle mass	0.03-0.045 g/kg prior to and after exercise
Branched-chain amino acids (BCAAs)	Preserves muscle mass	6-14 g/day (ratio of leucine, valine, isoleucine: 2-3:1:1); note that leucine alone is also an option
Arginine	Preserves muscle mass and supports blood flow	2-9 g/day spread over multiple doses
Undenatured type II collagen (UC-II)	Supports joint health	40 mg/day over 90-120+ days
Glutamine	Supports immune system and may preserve muscle mass	1.5-4.5 g/day split into pre-, during, and postworkout doses or throughout the day, particularly during periods of potential overtraining
Omega-3 fatty acids	Supports immune system, brain health, and mood; preserves muscle mass	1-2 g EPA and DHA/day
Vitamin D	Supports bone health, immune system, and potentially mood; preserves muscle mass and strength	4,000 IU/day to increase serum 25(OH)D >40 ng/mL
Vitamin B_{12}	Prevents deficiency	To maintain optimal blood levels: 25-100 mcg/day To correct deficiency: 125-2,000 mcg/day
Fiber	Supports immune system	3-5 g fermentable fibers like inulin and other fructooligosaccharides to feed existing healthy bacteria; 250 million to 20 billion organisms; 2.5-20 CFU/day
Curcumin	Provides immune system, gut, and joint support	3 mg/kg/day

Supplement	Potential benefit	Recommended dose
Ginger	Provides immune system and joint support	1 g/day
Avocado soybean unsaponifiables (ASU)	Supports joints	300 mg/day
Glucosamine	Supports joints	1,500 mg/day (500 mg 3×/day)
Chondroitin	Supports joints	800-1,200 mg/day (those with melanoma risk, consult a physician)
Zinc (Zn)	Supports immune system	10-20 mg/day
Calcium (Ca)	Supports skeletal health	1,200 mg/day
Creatine	Fights muscle loss, improves cognition, reduces inflammation	4-6 g/day for 1 month (loading phase)
Tart cherry	Improves recovery	Extract/pill: Equivalent of 40-270 mg/day of anthocyanins Fruit: 45-100 Montmorency cherries Concentrate: 240 mL (12 oz) tart cherry juice 1-2×/day
Hyaluronic acid	Supports joint health	Oral: 225 mg/day
Fenugreek	Improves muscle strength and endurance	500-900 mg/day
Coenzyme Q10 (CoQ10)	Provides antioxidant defense, improves aerobic performance, enhances recovery	60-300 mg 2-3×/day for 3+ weeks
Thiamine (Vitamin B1)	Higher intakes of thiamine have been shown to lower risk of early-onset sarcopenia, particularly in men	Men: 2.09-12.05 mg/day Women: 1.55-7.33 mg/day

Youth Athletes

Throughout late childhood and early adolescence, nutrition plays a formative role in the timing and pattern of puberty, with consequences for adult height, body composition, and health in later life (Norris et al., 2022). An average bone mass increase of 45% has been noted during growth spurts throughout adolescence, with peak bone formation and skeletal maturity typically being achieved by the time the young athlete reaches their early 20s. Soft tissues, organs, and red blood cells also grow in size during adolescence. Peak muscle mass is typically reached between the ages of 16 and 20 in females and 18 and 25 in males.

To support these changes, nutritional demands peak during adolescence. Adolescence is also a pivotal time for young athletes to establish a healthy relationship with food, a positive body image, and a basic understanding of fueling for sport. With the added metabolic demand of sport training, it is not uncommon for energy deficits, also known as relative energy deficiency in sport (RED-S), and consequent macronutrient and micronutrient deficiencies to arise. Furthermore, many young athletes struggle balancing school, training, work, and social commitments, and may be influenced by their peers' eating habits, making meeting nutritional demands even more challenging. Young athletes also often have unrealistic expectations based on portrayals of recreational and professional athletes on social media and as a result adopt unhealthy behaviors, both in training and nutrition, to try to achieve similar success. Dietary supplement abuse, adoption of extreme dietary behaviors (e.g., cutting out major food groups), and nutritional deficits driven by poor nutritional choices not only can compromise growth and delay sexual maturation but can have a negative impact on an athlete's overall health and longevity in the sport (Savarino et al., 2021). Thus, sport nutrition education with principles that support sound physical, physiological, and psychosocial development of the young athlete should be integrated into any youth sport program.

Understanding how to best support the nutritional journey of a young athlete, including the safety and efficacy of dietary supplements in this population, can be challenging for coaches, parents, and trainers. Helping the young athlete adopt a positive body image while educating them on how to meet elevated daily nutrition needs to support growth and development through consistent and balanced whole food consumption should always be the first line of defense. In addition, it is important that young athletes practice recommended fueling and hydration strategies before, during, and after workouts to support the additional nutritional demands associated with general physical activity, training, and competition and maximize favorable adaptations to their training. Dietary supplements may be used to help fill voids that may be hindering the young athlete's performance and possibly provide an added boost to overall health and performance.

Nutritional Recommendations for Youth Athletes

Throughout adolescence, adequate energy intake is required to meet both the growth and development needs of the young athlete, as well as individual macronutrient demands associated with general physical activity, exercise training, and competition. Optimizing energy availability (EA) is key, with data suggesting a minimum of 45 kcal/kg fat-free mass (FFM) and 40 kcal/kg FFM needed in female and male athletes, respectively to support health and performance.

To compute energy availability, simply take the athlete's intake (in kcal), subtract what is spent in exercise (kcal), and divide by their fat-free mass (in kg), as follows:

Energy availability (EA) = [Energy intake (EI) – Exercise energy expenditure (EEE)] / Fat-free mass (FFM)

Youth athletes with low EA, defined as less than 30 kcal/kg fat-free mass (FFM)/day, have been shown to be more likely to have negative performance effects, including decreases in coordination, concentration, endurance, and training response (Ackerman et al., 2019; Desbrow, 2021; Rogers et al., 2021). Furthermore, low EA may lead to serious health consequences, including delayed puberty, menstrual irregularities, poor bone health, short stature, the development of disordered eating behaviors, and increased risk of injury (Desbrow et al., 2019). To help estimate energy demands, a new equation was created to predict the resting metabolic rate (RMR) of young developing athletes (Reale et al, 2020):

$$RMR\ (kcal/day) = RMR = 11.1 \times body\ mass\ (kg) + 8.4 \times height\ (cm)$$
$$- (340\ male\ or\ 537\ female)$$

This equation does not account for energy deposited in growing tissues, estimated as approximately 2 kcal/g of daily weight gain, nor the energy that the young athlete expends during exercise training and competition. Because these numbers can be highly variable from day to day, it is important that the young athlete pays attention to (and actively addresses) hunger cues and that the athlete's supporting crew be aware of and address any symptoms associated with low EA the athlete may be displaying. The bulk, if not all, of the energy burned in training should be replaced to help maintain optimal energy availability. Supplemental nutrition in the form of energy gels, energy bars, sports chews, sports drinks, and protein powders can serve as a convenient means to help fuel the young athlete during workouts as well as maximize favorable adaptations to their training.

Protein Needs of Youth Athletes

Daily protein requirement rises from 0.86 g/kg for ages 4 to 7 years to 0.92 g/kg and 1.0-1.4 g/kg from 7-12 years in prepubertal ages to support the increase in muscle mass, erythrocytes, and myoglobin and to support hormonal changes (EFSA, 2017; Savarino et al., 2021). During peak growth, which generally occurs within 2 years of reaching puberty, increases in lean body mass nearly triple compared to the prepubertal period. To support growth periods during puberty as well as the metabolic demands of exercise, youth athletes—particularly those competing in more than one sport or training and competing in both club and school sports—require additional protein, with total intake guidelines increasing to 1.5 g/kg/day (e.g., 0.3 g/kg protein spread across five meals). This is in line with the American College of Sports Medicine and Academy of Nutrition and Dietetics protein intake guidelines for adult athletes, which lie at 1.2 to 1.8 g/kg body mass. Additionally, research has shown the ingestion of 20 g of protein following exercise helps maintain positive protein balance in youth athletes. For reference, a pint of low-fat flavored milk will provide just under 20 g of protein. Coaches and parents of youth athletes should recognize that insufficient protein intake, often seen in athletes with low EA, can delay growth and sexual maturation, reduce muscle mass, depress immune function, and hinder athletic performance (Lassi et al., 2017). On the flipside, however, it is also important to note that young athletes often believe that more is better when it comes to protein, although science does not necessarily support this notion in practice.

Of course, the context of an age-appropriate, balanced diet must be considered as well. With practicality in mind, consumption of quality protein from whole foods should be encouraged at each meal and snack. Youth athletes who struggle to meet adequate protein intake through whole food consumption during the day or need a convenient option for after practice or competition when they are away from home may benefit from supplementation with protein powder such as egg, whey, casein, and perhaps to a lesser extent soy. There are also recovery nutrition products that generally offer a combination of carbohydrate and protein in powder or bar form. Amino acid supplements are not warranted for young athletes, particularly when dietary protein intake is sufficient.

Carbohydrate Needs of Youth Athletes

The availability of carbohydrate plays a large role in exercise-driven training adaptations, making dietary intake of carbohydrate key to overall health and performance. It has been demonstrated that young athletes not only have a reduced capacity to store carbohydrate but also rely more on exogenous carbohydrates for energy compared to adults, making optimal daily carbohydrate intake and carbohydrate supplementation during and around training increasingly important to support maintenance of performance in this population.

To support optimal glycogen storage and availability, it is recommended that the youth athlete consume between 3 and 8 g of carbohydrate/kg/day, depending on exercise intensity and total exercise volume (Bonci, 2010; Nisevich, 2008). To help support these guidelines, the youth athlete should be encouraged to incorporate carbohydrate-rich snacks and meals over 4 to 6 smaller meals throughout the day so that at least 50% of their daily energy intake encompasses carbohydrate. In addition, proper fueling with carbohydrate before, during, and after training sessions will help enhance overall performance, support recovery, and maximize favorable adaptations to training. For each hour prior to completing a workout, a youth athlete should aim to consume approximately 1 g of easy-to-digest carbohydrate/kg. For example, a 45 kg (100 lb) athlete should aim to consume around 45 g of carbohydrate for each hour prior to starting a workout, which would equate to consuming a medium banana and one graham cracker sheet.

If the youth athlete is unable to eat prior to a shorter (<1 hour) workout, consuming small amounts of carbohydrate (e.g., sipping on a sports drink versus plain water) during the workout can benefit performance. For example, Dougherty and colleagues (2006) demonstrated significant performance improvements in both shooting and on-court sprinting ability in male basketball players aged 12 to 15 when they sipped on 6% carbohydrate solution, such as that seen in the popular sports drink Gatorade, rather than water. During prolonged training sessions (60-90+ minutes) of moderate to high intensity, young athletes can oxidize up to 0.6 g/kg/hour of a single carbohydrate source (e.g., glucose)—a lower rate than that of adult athletes—and beyond 0.6 g/kg/hour with multiple transportable forms of carbohydrate (e.g., glucose plus fructose) with benefits to their overall endurance, performance, and recovery (Burke et al., 2011). For example, Batatinha and colleagues (2013) found that gymnasts aged 11 to 14, whose daily practices were 4 hours in duration, fell less often on their balance beam routines when a 20% maltodextrin solution was provided during practice versus a sugar-free control. In the sport of gymnastics, falls not only represent a significant reduction in overall points scored but also put the young athlete at risk for sidelining injuries. Supplemental carbohydrates such as energy chews, energy gels, and sport drinks offer quick and convenient ways for youth athletes to meet these needs.

To support posttraining recovery, young athletes are encouraged to consume 1.0 to 1.5 g of carbohydrate/kg within 30 minutes of finishing exhaustive training. For example, a 45 kg (100 lb) athlete should aim for approximately 45 g of carbohydrate as soon as possible after a workout, which could be accommodated by drinking a pint (600 mL) of low-fat chocolate milk or 12 oz (360 mL) of 100% fruit juice.

Fat Needs of Youth Athletes

Because a long-term high-fat diet has been linked to increased risk of several chronic diseases, particularly cardiovascular disease, guidelines for intake are no different for youth athletes compared to their adult counterparts. Current guidelines state that dietary fat intake should comprise 20% to 35% of daily energy intake, with no more than 10% of total energy intake coming from saturated fat. Adequate intake of calorie-dense fat (9 kcal/g) helps support elevated energy demands during puberty—when nearly 50% of adult body mass and skeletal mass is achieved—as well as aids the synthesis of hormones and promotes healthy growth and maturation. Dietary fat sources also help athletes meet the requirements for the fat-soluble vitamins A, D, E, and K as well as essential fatty acids.

Some youth athletes may be allured by commercial marketing stating that lipid-based dietary supplements such as fish oil may enhance fat metabolism, thereby providing a boost to endurance performance, and reduce inflammatory damage, thereby aiding recovery. Increased intake of two underconsumed fatty acids found in fish oil—eicosapentaenoic acid (EPA) and docosahexaenoic acid (DHA)—have indeed been associated with decreased prevalence of cardiovascular diseases, as well as reduced markers of inflammation, and a review by Tomczyk and colleagues (2023) determined that EPA and DHA can benefit athletes, including young adults. Their effects on youth athletes still need investigation, however. Another lipid-based dietary supplement that has been marketed to boost performance and body composition is conjugated linoleic acid (CLA)—actually a series of isomers—which is found naturally in beef and dairy foods. A combination of CLA and fish oil supplementation was previously reported to promote an anabolic response from exercise, potentially as a result of increased testosterone synthesis. There are also indications in the literature that CLA may enhance strength and decrease inflammatory markers, but data are mixed and modest for adults and lacking in youth sports settings. At the time of this writing, CLA lacks the evidence for a recommendation for those under 18 years of age, and intentional manipulation of hormone levels during puberty is not advised.

Micronutrient Needs of Youth Athletes

A balanced whole food intake is crucial to support both the macronutrient as well as micronutrient needs of the young athlete. All types of food provide a variety of nutrients essential for athletes (see chapter 3 for discussions of many of these nutrients). Whole grains and their three main components—the bran, germ, and endosperm—house health-promoting nutrients, including carbohydrate, dietary fiber, B-vitamins, vitamin E, iron, copper, zinc, magnesium, antioxidants, and phytochemicals. The Dietary Guidelines for Americans recommend that one-quarter of a meal plate comprise whole grains to support optimal health. Eating a rainbow of colors from fruits and vegetables provides an array of many vitamins and minerals, including vitamin C, beta-carotene (provitamin A), and potassium; they also provide dietary fiber and are sources of many phytochemicals, like quercetin and resveratrol, that function as antioxidants, phytoestrogens, and natural anti-inflammatory agents. The Dietary Guidelines for Americans recommend that one-half of a meal plate comprise fruits and vegetables to support optimal health.

Dairy foods provide a valuable source of protein and are the main source of calcium and vitamin D in many diets, all nutrients key to optimal bone formation in the youth athlete. Foods in the dairy group also provide potassium, phosphorous, vitamin A, vitamin B_{12}, riboflavin, zinc, choline, magnesium, and selenium. Such dairy foods as yogurt and kefir offer a natural source of probiotics.

Lean meats and plant-based proteins offer protein and amino acids (glutamine, arginine, branched-chain amino acids) as well as a variety of vitamins and minerals including iron, zinc, vitamin B_{12}, and vitamin B_6. The Dietary Guidelines for Americans recommend that one-quarter of a meal plate comprise a protein source (plant or animal) for optimal health. Finally, healthy fats such as olive oil, fish oil, nuts (almonds, walnuts, peanuts), coconut milk, flaxseed, and borage oil contain fatty acids that can benefit health and function of cells. A sprinkling of healthy fat should be present at each meal. By consuming a balanced and varied diet, athletes will ensure they are consuming adequate amounts of vitamins and minerals.

Youth athletes who are picky eaters, have poor appetites, have food allergies, or who are intentionally or unintentionally restricting energy intake often have low energy availability that puts them at greater risk for nutrient deficiencies. Additionally, the daily time constraints of youth athletes, particularly those competing in more than one sport or bouncing from school to club sport practices after a full day of school, can make achieving a balanced diet challenging, thus elevating risk for micronutrient deficiencies.

Iron, vitamin D, and calcium are the most common nutritional deficiencies reported in children and adolescents; however, deficiencies in magnesium, phosphorus, and vitamins A, C, and E have also been noted. Increases in hemoglobin production, blood volume, and muscle mass account for the majority of increased iron needs in young athletes. For the young female athlete, iron requirements become even greater at the onset of menstruation. As a result, iron deficiency and anemia are commonly seen in this population (WHO, 2005), with negative impacts on sport performance as well as health (Solberg et al., 2023). From ages 9 to 13, the RDA for iron for boys and girls is 18 mg per day; for ages 14 to 18, the RDA is 11 mg/day for boys and 15 mg/day for girls. Achieving optimal iron status should be encouraged through consumption of iron-rich foods such as red meat, chicken, beans, peanuts, and green vegetables, though supplementation with iron, as overseen by a health professional, may be necessary to correct anemia or low levels of ferritin in some young athletes.

Prior to achieving peak skeletal maturity, the availability of calcium and vitamin D, which aids calcium absorption, is important for bone development, support for enhanced bone loading during exercise, and protection against bone fractures and osteoporosis later in life (Bonjour & Chevalley, 2014). Requirements for calcium peak during adolescence at 1,300 mg/day for both girls and boys ages 12 to 18, yet average calcium intake for this age group in the United States falls short of these guidelines (Ross et al., 2011). Youth athletes are encouraged to include calcium-rich sources at each meal and snack (e.g., milk in cereal at breakfast, yogurt as a snack, cheese on a sandwich at lunch, almonds as a snack, broccoli as a side at dinnertime) to help accommodate increased needs. Dairy foods fortified with vitamin D will help accommodate needs for both nutrients. Those athletes who struggle to consume adequate calcium and vitamin D through whole foods may benefit from calcium supplements fortified with vitamin D.

Fluid Needs of Youth Athletes

Consuming adequate amounts of fluids throughout the day and during exercise is important for a young athlete's health and overall performance. Although sweat rates for preadolescent children tend to be lower than those of adolescent and adult athletes, losses are similar when adjusted for size and body mass. Just a 1% loss of body mass from fluid has been shown to have adverse effects of the performance of young athletes; adult athletes experience a similar drop in performance at 2% loss. Dehydration in youth athletes decreases endurance and overall performance by negatively affecting the cardiovascular system, thermoregulation, and central fatigue or perceived exhaustion. Signs and symptoms that a youth athlete may be suffering from dehydration include acute weight loss, headache and lightheadedness, noticeable thirst, irritability, nausea, muscle cramping, dark yellow urine, difficulty paying attention, weakness, and fatigue.

Dehydration increases a young athlete's risk for exertional heat illness, including heatstroke, especially when competing in hot and humid conditions. Youth athletes face unique challenges when they exert themselves in the heat. Because smaller athletes absorb more heat than adults as a result of their greater ratio of surface area to body mass, youth athletes are more prone to overheat (Falk and Dotan, 2008; Cheng et al, 2020). The smaller the athlete, the faster the heat absorption, making children aged 10 and under particularly vulnerable. Children and adolescent athletes also have a reduced ability to dissipate heat through sweating. Because young athletes also frequently lack the physiological drive to drink enough fluids to replenish sweat losses, particularly during longer exertional sessions, and are more likely to be distracted when occasions allow them to rest and rehydrate, it is important that coaches and parents implement strategies to combat dehydration on hot days, such as more frequent hydration breaks and reminders to drink, increased rotation of players on a competitive field, and cooling misters and shaded rest areas.

To help maintain optimal hydration, young athletes should meet daily fluid guidelines shown in table 4.2. Additionally, youth athletes should aim to consume 6 mL/lb (13.2 mL/kg) of body weight for each hour of exercise. For a 60 lb (27 kg) athlete, this would equate to 360 mL (0.35 L)/hour or 90 mL (0.09 L) every 15 minutes; for a 100 lb (45 kg) athlete, the comparable amount would be 600 mL (0.59 L)/hour or 150 mL/oz (0.15 L) every 15 minutes. These guidelines are likely to increase when intensity of exertion is high and the young athlete is competing in heat. Youth athletes can be encouraged to keep track of urine color as means to monitor hydration status, with a pale yellow urine (like lemonade) indicating good hydration and darker yellow to brown (like apple juice) being an indication of dehydration and a need to drink more.

TABLE 4.2 Daily Fluid Goals for Youth Athletes

Ages 4-8	
All children	1.7 L/day
Ages 9-13	
Boys	2.4 L/day
Girls	2.1 L/day
Ages 14-18	
Boys	3.3 L/day
Girls	2.3 L/day

Note: Based on Dietary Reference Intakes.

Electrolytes—namely sodium and potassium and in smaller amounts magnesium and calcium—are also important in assisting in fluid absorption and aiding hydration status. The concentration of sodium in sweat can vary widely, but it typically ranges from 460 to 1840 mg/L; potassium ranges from 160 to 320 mg/L; and magnesium and calcium are far lower at 4 to 15 mg/L and 0 to 40 mg/L (Barnes et al., 2019).

A combination of water and carbohydrate-electrolyte drinks should be used during exercise to help prevent dehydration and replace some of these losses. Sports drinks that contain an optimal ratio of carbohydrate, water, and electrolytes for hydration are encouraged when total exercise exceeds 1 hour or the youth athlete is competing in hot and humid conditions where both fluid and electrolyte losses are greater. Water is sufficient when total exercise is less than an hour and in cooler conditions. Water is also an acceptable hydration beverage when consumed in combination with food containing sodium and other electrolytes while exerting in hot and humid conditions. Electrolyte supplements are available in effervescent tablets, powders, chews, and capsules for young athletes who prefer to consume carbohydrate sources that are low in sodium (e.g., orange slices during a soccer game).

It is important to observe the youth athlete's hydration behaviors to see if there are fluid options that encourage the athlete to drink more throughout practice and competition. For many youth athletes, total fluid intake, hydration status, and consequent performance is enhanced when they drink something with flavor versus plain water. Ultimately, maintaining a healthy hydration status in the youth athlete should be the first priority when putting a performance plan in place.

Supplementation Options for Youth Athletes

If a youth athlete wants to begin taking a dietary supplement, parents and coaches may explore providing their athlete vitamins (vitamin D, multi); minerals (calcium, iron, multi); calorie replacements; energy gels, chews, and bars; sports drinks; electrolytes (sodium, potassium); protein powders; and fish oils. These supplements can assist youth athletes in meeting some of the nutritional guidelines mentioned previously. However, if the youth athlete is looking at more advanced supplements containing creatine, beta-alanine, amino acids, herbs, caffeine, prohormones, or other ingredients, more caution—and education—is warranted. Table 4.3 lists some supplement options.

TABLE 4.3 Highlighted Supplement Options for Youth Athletes

Supplement	Potential benefit	Recommended dose (ages 4 to 8)	Recommended dose (ages 9 to 13)	Recommended dose (ages 14 to 18)
Calorie-replacement shakes and bars	Assists in meeting energy needs, promotes weight gain	Varied depending on diet and calorie needs	Varied depending on diet and calorie needs	Varied depending on diet and calorie needs
Protein (whey, casein, egg, soy)	Assists in meeting protein needs and with nutrient timing	0.86 g/kg/day, including 15 g consumed prior to and after exercise	0.92-1.5 g/kg/day, including 15-20 g consumed prior to and after exercise	1.5 g/kg/day, including 20-25 g consumed prior to and after exercise
Folic acid	Supports red blood cell formation, DNA synthesis, and protein metabolism	200 mcg/day	300 mcg/day	400 mcg/day
Pantothenic acid	Enhances energy metabolism	3 mg/day	4 mg/day	5 mg/day
Riboflavin	Enhances energy metabolism	0.6 mg/day	0.9 mg/day	Girls: 1.0 mg/day Boys: 1.3 mg/day

Supplement	Potential benefit	Recommended dose (ages 4 to 8)	Recommended dose (ages 9 to 13)	Recommended dose (ages 14 to 18)
Thiamine	Enhances energy metabolism and supports nervous system function	0.6 mg/day	0.9 mg/day	Girls: 1.0 mg/day Boys: 1.2 mg/day
Vitamin B_{12}	Supports red blood cell formation, DNA synthesis, and neurological function	1.2 mcg/day	1.8 mcg/day	2.4 mcg/day
Vitamin C	Provides antioxidant and immune support, enhances collagen formation, improves absorption of iron	25 mg/day	45 mg/day	Girls: 65 mg/day Boys: 75 mg/day
Vitamin D	Assists in protein synthesis, provides immune support, promotes bone health	600 IU/day (15 mcg/day)	600 IU/day (15 mcg/day)	600 IU/day (15 mcg/day)
Vitamin E	Provides antioxidant support	10.5 IU/day (7 mg/day)	16.5 IU/day (11 mg/day)	22.4 IU/day (15 mg/day)
Calcium (Ca)	Supports skeletal health and muscle contraction	1,000 mg/day	1,300 mg/day	1,300 mg/day
Chromium (Cr)	Enhances insulin sensitivity	15 mcg/day	Girls: 21 mcg/day Boys: 25 mcg/day	Girls: 24 mcg/day Boys: 35 mcg/day
Copper (Cu)	Supports health of bones, muscle, and blood vessels	440 mcg/day	700 mcg/day	890 mcg/day
Iron (Fe)	Supports red blood cell function	10 mg/day	8 mg/day	Girls: 15 mg/day Boys: 11 mg/day

(continued)

TABLE 4.3 *(continued)*

Supplement	Potential benefit	Recommended dose (ages 4 to 8)	Recommended dose (ages 9 to 13)	Recommended dose (ages 14 to 18)
Magnesium (Mg)	Assists in bone formation, nerve transmission, enzyme homeostasis, and muscle contraction	130 mg/day	240 mg/day	Girls: 360 mg/day Boys: 410 mg/day
Potassium (K)	Controls electrolyte and fluid balance	2,300 mg/day	Girls: 2,300 mg/day Boys: 2,500 mg/day	Girls: 2,300 mg/day Boys: 3,000 mg/day
Selenium (Se)	Provides antioxidant and immune function support	30 mcg/day	40 mcg/day	55 mcg/day
Sodium chloride (aka salt)	Controls electrolyte and fluid balance	<1,900 mg/day*	<2,200 mg/day*	<2,300 mg/day
Zinc	Supports growth, provides immune system and antioxidant support	5 mg/day	8 mg/day	Girls: 9 mg/day Boys: 11 mg/day
Choline	Assists in neurotransmitter synthesis and cell signaling	250 mg/day	375 mg/day	Girls: 400 mg/day Boys: 550 mg/day
Omega-3 fatty acids	Supports brain and neuromuscular development and immune function	0.9 g/day ALA, 0.5-1 g/day EPA, 0.5-1 g/day DHA	Girls: 1 g/day ALA, 1-3 g/day EPA, 1-3 g/day DHA Boys: 1.2 g/day ALA, 1-3 g/day EPA, 1-3 g/day DHA	Girls: 1.1 g/day ALA, 1-3 g/day EPA, 1-3 g/day DHA Boys: 1.6 g/day ALA, 1-3 g/day EPA, 1-3 g/day DHA

Note: Correcting a deficiency typically brings greater benefits than hypersupplementation in a healthy, replete athlete. Some B-vitamins, for example, are inherently common in the U.S. food supply: Enriched flour must contain particular levels of thiamin, riboflavin, niacin, folic acid, and iron (21 CFR 137.165).

*Additional sodium may be warranted to offset losses when sweating during exercise.

It may be advisable for parents and coaches to consult with team of experts rather than turn to dietary supplements; this may include a registered dietitian (preferably a board-certified specialist in sport dietetics) who can provide guidance on daily nutrition as well as workout demands and a strength and conditioning specialist or sport-specific coach who can help develop an integrated training program. Most dietary supplements can provide only mild benefits ranging from 3% to 15% improvement; the majority result in only a 3% to 5% improvement. Furthermore, all athletes have a genetic ceiling above which further improvement cannot be achieved. This genetic ceiling takes years (10-15+) to achieve, and improvements in performance get smaller the more well trained the athlete becomes. As a result, athletes might benefit most from using dietary supplements once they have seen the greatest improvements from training along with following recommended principles of nutrition, and improvements in performance have become smaller and more difficult to achieve.

CREATINE AND YOUTH ATHLETES

According to the International Society of Sports Nutrition position stand on creatine use, which includes evidence on youth athletes, supplementation with creatine monohydrate may provide a safer nutritional alternative to potentially dangerous anabolic androgenic steroids.

Creatine supplementation only should only be considered for use by youth athletes who are involved in serious or competitive supervised training, are consuming a well-balanced and performance-enhancing diet, are knowledgeable about appropriate use of creatine, and do not exceed recommended dosages.

The current body of evidence demonstrates that doses ranging from 0.3 to 0.8 g/kg/day of creatine for up to 5 years across all ages poses no adverse health risks while possibly providing a number of health and performance benefits.

Kreider et al., 2017

The following criteria might assist parents, coaches, and younger athletes in understanding when it would be appropriate to begin supplementing with some of these more advanced products.

1. The athlete has a solid food foundation and is consistently practicing sport nutrition principles of adequate calorie intake, nutrient timing, consumption of a balanced and varied diet, adequate fluid and electrolyte intake, and consistent fueling.
2. The athlete has reached full maturity and is nearing the end of adolescence.
3. The athlete has consistently practiced a resistance-training program or structured endurance-training program for 2 consecutive years.

The A-to-Z guide in chapter 3 can provide athletes with added information on effective and high-quality supplements to consider for various performance variables.

Female Athletes

Since the passage of Title IX—the law that expanded opportunities for females in sports over 50 years ago—the number of girls and women participating in various sport activities has skyrocketed. According to data from the National Federation of State High School Associations and presented within a 2022 Women's Sports Foundation report, from 1971-1972 to 2018-2019, the number of girls participating in high school varsity sports increased from 294,015 to 3.4 million (Staurowsky et al, 2022). Similar trends have been observed at the collegiate level. According to the Women's Sports Foundation (Staurowsky et al., 2022), the percentage of female athletes competing on college teams has risen from 15% in 1972 to 44% during the 2020-2021 academic year. Such milestones are a cause for celebration. However, in order to truly embrace the benefits of sport participation, it is essential that athletes and coaches alike understand the unique nutritional demands that female athletes face during sport training and competition.

Nutritional Recommendations for Female Athletes

Dissimilar male and female chromosomes and sex hormones, including estrogen, progesterone, and androgens, drive the unique nutritional demands of the female athlete. Furthermore, significant differences exist between the structure and function of other organ systems in boys and girls, which are highlighted during puberty and very much driven by dietary and lifestyle choices. Notable sex differences have been observed across a variety of parameters, including mitochondrial function (Miotto et al., 2018; Silaidos et al., 2018), substrate utilization and insulin sensitivity (Hevener et al., 2018, 2020; Montero et al., 2018), immune responses (Gupta et al., 2020; Klein & Flanagan, 2016), muscle morphology and body composition (Haizlip et al., 2015; Landen et al., 2021), iron metabolism (Badenhorst et al., 2021; McKay et al., 2020), thermoregulation (Baker et al., 2020; Yanovich et al., 2020), hydration (Giersch et al., 2021; Wickham et al., 2021), appetite control (Hagobian & Braun, 2010; Hirschberg, 2012), and energy availability and endocrine function (Fahrenholtz et al., 2018; Heikura et al., 2018). Thus, nutritional guidelines, including recommendations for dietary supplement use, need to consider the unique needs of the female athlete.

Perhaps the most important nutritional consideration for women engaged in sport is fulfilling the elevated energy demands of training, particularly from carbohydrate and protein, and thereby achieving an optimal energy availability (EA) to support overall health as well as maximize favorable adaptations to physical training. Well-controlled laboratory studies have revealed that an EA of 45 kcal/kg of fat-free mass (FFM) per day is necessary to support physiological functions and body mass maintenance in female athletes. For female athletes seeking weight gain and muscle hypertrophy, an EA greater than 45 kcal/kg FFM is needed. These thresholds are likely to increase more than 300 kcal/day during the luteal phase of the menstrual cycle as a result of enhanced energy needs (Slater et al., 2017); conversely, when progesterone levels are low during the late follicular phase of the menstrual cycle, resting metabolic rate (RMR) is at its lowest and thus the EA threshold is likely to decrease. Similarly, in aging women, these EA thresholds are thought to be lower as a result of changing ratios of estrogen and progesterone, which contribute to decreases in metabolic rate and changes in body composition (Hodson et al., 2014).

For female athletes looking to optimize body composition through intentional restriction of calories, it is important to note that even modest reductions in EA over as little as 5 days, with the threshold being indicated at 30 kcal/kg FFM, have been shown to suppress metabolic hormones. Such reductions can also decrease luteinizing hormone (LH) pulse frequency, which, in turn, initiates menstrual disturbances and inhibits reproductive function (Koltan et al., 2020; Melin et al., 2019; Reed et al., 2015). Thus, EA should remain well above the threshold amount of 30 kcal/kg FFM, though likely below 45 kcal/kg FFM to promote healthy body fat loss. Furthermore, female athletes restricting energy should focus on nutrient timing (pre-, during, and postworkout nutrition) to reduce time spent in a catabolic state, thereby improving favorable adaptations to training and in turn facilitating optimal health and performance.

A major consequence of low EA and consequent hormonal aberration is low bone mineral density, impaired bone geometry and structure, and reduced bone strength, all of which is associated with an elevated risk of fractures that can sideline an athlete for weeks if not months—or, in severe cases, end an athletic career altogether. The combination of low EA, menstrual dysfunction, and low bone mineral density was initially coined the female athlete triad. Later, this condition was subsumed under a broader umbrella of symptoms named relative energy deficiency in sport (RED-S). With RED-S, energy deficiency is identified as the key to the disruption of a wide range of physiological functions, including reproduction, bone, endocrine, metabolic, hematological, growth and development, physiological, cardiovascular, gastrointestinal, and immunological systems, with consequences for the performance and health of the athlete regardless of sex (Mountjoy et al., 2018). Further medical problems arise when energy and weight-control behaviors become recognized diagnoses of eating disorders, including anorexia nervosa (severe energy restriction) and bulimia nervosa (binge and purge disorder).

Low EA has been reported to be moderate to high in female athletes, with one study demonstrating a range of 11% to 55% of female athletes, with athletes who were engaged in sports where leanness is emphasized (e.g., gymnastics, dance, diving, distance running) trending in the higher risk category. In this same cohort of 112 female athletes, 80% were experiencing at least one symptom consistent with RED-S and 37% were experiencing two to three symptoms. Impaired immune function, blood abnormalities, and gastrointestinal distress were the most common symptoms reported (Rogers et al., 2021). Although details are beyond the scope of this section, it should also be noted that male athletes who participate in sports emphasizing leanness, including endurance sports such as cycling and running, also appear to have a greater prevalence of low EA and disordered eating (Cupka & Sedliak, 2023).

Female athletes struggling with low EA can benefit from working with a registered dietitian (RD) who can provide guidance on increasing caloric intake to meet the needs

RISK FACTORS FOR LOW EA

1. Prolonged periods of dieting or weight fluctuations
2. Traumatic events such as illness or injury, new coach, leaving home (college), failure at school or work, family problems, relationship issues, loss
3. Large increase in training volume and significant weight loss associated with increase in training volume
4. Belief that menarche (first period) has been reached too early
5. Early start of sport-specific training
6. Large discrepancy between desired ideal weight and actual (healthy) ideal weight
7. Casual comments about weight; recommendation to lose weight without guidance
8. Social influences for thinness
9. Performance anxiety
10. Negative self-appraisal, generally as it relates to performance

of exercise energy expenditure, reducing exercise activity, or both to optimize energy availability. Additional medical intervention from a team of experts, including an RD and preferably an exercise physiologist, becomes necessary when eating disorders are suspected or formally diagnosed.

Carbohydrate Needs of Female Athlete

Alongside EA, carbohydrate availability is a limiting factor to performance, especially endurance performance, due to reduced muscle glycogen and lower levels of circulating carbohydrate contributing to fatigue and impaired cognition (aka hitting the wall or bonking). Female athletes oxidize more fat and less carbohydrate than male athletes given the same relative intensities of exercise. There are also significant sex differences and hormonal influences on carbohydrate metabolism, meaning carbohydrate needs may be affected by the different phases of an athlete's menstrual cycle.

During the follicular phase of the menstrual cycle (days 1-14), when levels of estrogen progressively increase and progesterone levels stabilize, the oxidation of carbohydrate increases, which, in turn, reduces glycogen storage, an environment that will tend to favor shorter high-intensity exercise sessions rather than prolonged endurance-focused training. However, as long as energy intake from carbohydrate is sufficient for exercise demands, this should not have a negative impact on performance of any duration or intensity. The ability to store glycogen improves as the athlete enters the midfollicular to midluteal phase of the menstrual cycle, which is a great time to increase carbohydrate intake. Research has shown a higher carbohydrate intake of 8.4 to 9 g/kg/day during the midfollicular phase to increase muscle glycogen stores 17% to 31% (James et al., 2001; Paul et al., 2001; Walker et al., 2000). Following carbohydrate-loading intake guidelines—which entails consuming 10 to 12 g/kg/day over 24 to 72 hours leading up to any training or competition that extends beyond 90 minutes—may provide further benefit to athletes entering the late follicular to midluteal phase of their menstrual cycle. During the luteal phase of the menstrual cycle (days 14-28), when estrogen and progesterone levels peak, there is a greater effect of sex hormone suppression on gluconeogenesis, making increased carbohydrate intake helpful to muscle glycogen storage and performance, particularly endurance performance. Similarly, increasing carbohydrate intake during the active pill weeks of oral contraceptive users can aid performance.

Current recommendations for fueling with carbohydrates are based on male-centric research. However, it is known that, regardless of sex, consuming adequate energy from carbohydrate to support general metabolic demands as well as the additional metabolic demands of exercise (see table 4.4) is essential to promote peak athletic performance. Proper timing of carbohydrate intake can also help support favorable adaptations to training as well as performance.

TABLE 4.4 Daily Carbohydrate Intake Goals for Female Athletes

Light activity (<1 hour of exercise per day)	3-5 g/kg BM/day
Moderate activity (1 hour of exercise per day)	5-7 g/kg BM/day
Endurance activity (1-3 hours of exercise per day)	6-10 g/kg BM/day
Extreme activity (>4 hours of exercise per day)	8-12 g/kg BM/day

To account for body composition differences between male and female athletes, it may be prudent to use fat-free mass rather than total body mass to calculate carbohydrate needs for female athletes. It is recommended to consume 1 g of carbohydrate/kg of body mass for each hour prior to exercise; the female athlete fueling 3 hours prior to exercise may therefore target 3 g of carbohydrate/kg of fat-free mass leading up to her workout. This guideline is particularly important to mitigate the performance detriments associated with impaired metabolism during the luteal phase of the menstrual cycle.

During exercise, carbohydrate recommendations stand at 30 to 60 g/hour for sessions lasting 1 to 2.5 hours and 60 to 90 g/hour for sessions lasting more than 2.5 hours. Compared to their male counterparts, however, female athletes have demonstrated slower rates of gastric emptying and gut mobility as well as a greater incidence of exercise-induced gastroparesis, particularly during the early follicular and late luteal phases of the menstrual cycle (Bernstein et al., 2014; Gonzalez et al., 2020; Mori et al., 2017). Thus, tapering back carbohydrate intake during exercise may be warranted if GI upset ensues, though the low end of these guidelines should still be met to support performance. Female athletes should be encouraged to work on training their gut to meet carbohydrate guidelines during training and monitor their overall tolerance so they know the best fueling approach for competition regardless of where it may fall in relation to their menstrual cycle.

Postexercise carbohydrate intake aids restoration of muscle and hepatic glycogen stores; guidelines recommend 1.2 g/kg/hour for 4 to 6 hours after completing a glycogen-depleting workout. Adding protein in a ratio of 1 g of protein for every 4 g of carbohydrate consumed can further enhance recovery. These guidelines are particularly favorable when muscle glycogen repletion is reduced during the follicular phase of the menstrual cycle. Because insulin sensitivity is significantly greater in a 30 to 40 minute window after exercise, peri- and postmenopausal athletes, who experience heightened levels of insulin resistance, are encouraged to follow the same recommendations with special attention to timing of nutrition (Yu et al., 2022).

SUPPLEMENT TIP

Carbohydrate supplements, available as sports drinks, chews, powders, and gels, are easy to digest and can serve as a convenient means for the female athlete to support fueling needs before, during, and after training and competition.

Protein Needs of Female Athletes

Adequate dietary protein is necessary to support optimal physiological adaptations to exercise, regardless of sex. Sex differences, hormonal status, types of exercise, and training status are all variables that play into how *adequate* is quantified for female athletes. Current sports nutrition guidelines for daily protein intake fall between 1.4 and 2.0 g/kg, which, based on a review by Mercer and colleagues (2020), closely matches the protein intake seen in eumenorrheic (regularly menstruating) recreationally active and competitive female athletes who perform endurance exercise (1.28-1.63 g/kg), resistance exercise (1.49 g/kg) and intermittent exercise (1.41 g/kg) (Jäger et al., 2017; Thomas et al., 2016). Female athletes with low EA, whether intentional or unintentional, may benefit from protein intakes on the upper end of these guidelines and possibly higher (Carbone et al., 2019; Houlthan & Rowlands, 2014). Due to the catabolic nature of progesterone, eumenorrheic athletes in the luteal phase should also target closer to 2.0 g/kg BM/day. With declining estradiol levels and consequent insulin and anabolic resistance, perimenopausal and postmenopausal athletes should aim for 1.8 to 2.0 g/kg BM/day (Agostini et al., 2018; Gould et al., 2022; Phillips et al., 2016). Female athletes seeking skeletal muscle hypertrophy are likely to respond favorably to protein intakes above 2.0 g/kg BM/day (Bosse & Dixon, 2012).

Alongside meeting daily protein requirements, timing protein intake so that 0.32 to 0.38 g/kg BM is consumed both prior to and immediately after exercise can help reduce exercise-induced amino acid oxidative losses and initiate muscle protein remodeling and repair, thereby maximizing favorable adaptations to training in both premenopausal and eumenorrheic athletes as well as those using oral contraceptives (Jäger et al., 2017). Peri- and postmenopausal athletes may also benefit from a more favorable anabolic response, with muscle protein synthesis rates increasing in the 4-hour postexercise window, with the inclusion of a single dose of 6 to 10 g of essential amino acids from whole foods or supplements taken after completion of resistance-focused exercise (Bukhari et al., 2015; Ispoglou et al., 2017).

Female athletes who struggle meeting daily protein guidelines or need a convenient on-the-go option may benefit from supplementing with protein powders, with the gold standard being considered whey and amino acids.

Fat Needs of Female Athletes

Recommendations for fat intake do not differ based on sex, with guidelines targeting a range of 20% to 30% of calories being derived from a variety of fat sources, preferably plant- and fish-based, to ensure adequate energy intake as well as intake of essential fatty acids and fat-soluble vitamins (A, D, E, and K) (Thomas et al., 2016). Adequate fat intake is also essential for sex hormone concentrations. For female athletes seeking body fat and weight loss, further guidelines for fat intake have been indicated at 0.5 to 1.0 g/kg BM/day (Kerksick et al., 2018).

The American Heart Association, along with the American College of Cardiology, encourage keeping intake of saturated fat intake to less than 7% of total energy intake and trans fat intake to no more than 1% of energy intake to help reduce the risk of cardiovascular events and all-cause mortality (Eckel et al., 2014). Heart disease remains the number one cause of death in women, claiming the lives of one in five women every year. The most powerful risk factor for heart disease in women is elevated blood pressure, which omega-3 fatty acids—specifically eicosapentanoic acid (EPA) and docosahexanoic acid (DHA), found in fish oil—have been shown to help reduce, thereby helping to improve overall cardiovascular health. Omega-3 fatty acids are a popular supplement choice among athletes as well as the general public, with some research also demonstrating a protective impact against bone catabolism and inflammation, which can aid recovery and lower risk for injury and illness in athletes. The Institute of Medicine recommends women consume 1.1 to 1.4 g/day of omega-3 (alpha-linoleic acid), though research-supported doses related to various sport performance parameters range from 1.5 to 2.0 g/day (Thielecke & Brannin, 2020).

Female athletes should be encouraged to include small amounts of healthy fat at each meal (e.g., small handful of nuts in oatmeal, sliced avocado added to a sandwich or olives in a salad, baked salmon). Fat intake, however, should be limited in the 2 to 3 hours before moderate- to high-intensity exercise as fat takes longer to clear the gut and can elevate risk for gastrointestinal distress. The overall composition of any preworkout meal should be low fat, meaning less than 3 g of fat per 100 calories consumed.

Micronutrient Needs of Female Athletes

Beyond a heightened risk for altered hormonal status and diminished bone health, female athletes, especially those following restrictive diets with low EA, are vulnerable to micronutrient deficiencies that can result in fatigue, stunted growth (for adolescent athletes), poor immune function, loss of motivation, inability to concentrate, and significant declines in both strength and endurance. Deficiencies in iron, vitamin D, and calcium are commonly reported in female athletes; thus, nutritional strategies to help correct deficiency and prevent symptoms from arising should be taught and implemented.

Iron is one of the most prevalent micronutrient deficiencies found in female athletes, partially due to restrictive energy intake that may include elimination of such iron-rich foods as red meat and dark meat (poultry) or adoption of a vegan diet, which is more common in this population. In addition, blood loss during menstruation along with a phenomenon known as exercise-induced hemolysis can cause hemoglobin (the protein that carries iron) levels to drop and increase the risk for iron deficiency (Castell et al., 2019; Pedlar et al., 2018). Declines in both physical and cognitive performance have been demonstrated in female athletes with poor dietary intake of iron, especially those with iron-deficiency anemia (DellaValle & Haas, 2011; McClung, 2012). Athletes who have low EA, whose lifestyle choices may make adequate consumption of iron difficult (e.g., plant-focused diets), or who may be displaying symptoms consistent with iron deficiency should consult with their doctor and a sports dietitian to evaluate iron status and optimize their daily nutrition plans for iron intake, which may include supplementation.

Female athletes are also at increased risk for calcium and vitamin D deficiencies; these nutrients play a role in building bone and muscle as well as supporting immune function and protecting against injury (Gabel, 2006; Thomas et al., 2016). Because calcium levels are difficult to measure in a clinically meaningful manner for athletes, a valid means to estimate calcium intake in the female athlete is through a dietary recall. Those with low EA or who are avoiding dairy or fortified dairy alternatives like soy milk should target 1,500 mg of calcium per day to optimize bone health and protect against stress fracture (Mountjoy et al., 2014). To improve the intestinal absorption of calcium and ultimately optimize bone health, it is integral to establish adequate serum vitamin D levels, which have been indicated at >50 ng/mL for female athletes (Thomas et al., 2016). Those with suboptimal vitamin D levels may benefit from improved vitamin D status with a daily maintenance supplementation of 1,000 to 2,000 IU/day vitamin D_3.

As a general rule, female athletes should aim to consume four to six closely calorie-matched meals throughout the day. The three staple meals (breakfast, lunch, and dinner) should include a balance that incorporates 25% protein (e.g., edamame, Greek yogurt, cottage cheese, eggs, lean beef, skinless poultry, fish), 25% starch (e.g., sweet potato, oats, quinoa, brown rice, corn, peas, legumes, 100% whole grain breads), and 50% color (fruits and vegetables) along with small doses of healthy fat (e.g., avocado, olives, nuts, seeds, fatty fish, vegetable oils). Avoidance of major food groups is highly discouraged as deficiency risks, including those common among female athletes (e.g., iron, calcium, vitamin D, zinc), tend to be heightened with food restriction. To improve iron intake, female athletes should include more animal protein such as beef in the diet. Plant sources of iron such as whole grains, fortified cereals, and legumes should be combined with foods rich in vitamin C (e.g., oranges) to aid iron absorption. To boost intake of calcium and vitamin D, female athletes should aim to consume three to four servings of dairy or fortified dairy alternatives such as soy or almond milk (1 serving = 1 cup [0.24 L] milk, three-fourths cup [170 g] yogurt, 1 ounce [28 g] cheese, 0.5 cup [113 g] cottage cheese). It is also desirable to consume prepared foods with short, recognizable ingredient lists (e.g., "clean label" foods): Those failing to meet these criteria tend to be highly processed and generally score low on the nutrition grading scale.

Fluid Needs of Female Athletes

Although female sex hormones alter certain aspects of fluid dynamics and electrolyte balance, the current data—albeit limited in nature, with less than 30% of recent studies using female subjects—have shown minimal effects of the menstrual cycle phase on whole body sweat rate, fluid balance, or the physiological and performance impact of dehydration (Casanova et al., 2019; Gifford et al., 2019; Nuccio et al., 2017). Rather, variables such as body size, overall workload, fitness status, and whether an athlete is environmentally acclimated play a more significant role in determination of sweat loss and fluid balance. Thus, it is currently recommended that hydration strategies be personalized based on individual sweat losses, exercise type, and environmental conditions, with the overall goal of preventing any significant fluid and electrolyte imbalances that could compromise health and performance (ACSM et al., 2007). The United States Institute of Medicine's (IOM) adequate intake for total water, based on the median total water intake from the U.S. National Health and Nutrition Examination Survey data, is 2.7 L/day for women, with 2.2 L consumed as liquids and the remainder coming from food (Erdman, 2005). Note that these guidelines do not account for sweat output during exercise, making overall daily fluid demands higher on training days.

Drinking excessive amounts of any type of fluid, especially water, can cause hyponatremia (low blood sodium); symptoms include clear urine, muscle fatigue, pressure headache, dizziness, confusion, nausea, and vomiting. Female athletes, especially those new to endurance sports who may be on a race course for a longer duration than usual, seem to be at greatest risk for hyponatremia and associated symptoms (Hew-Butler et al., 2015; Rosner & Kirven, 2007). Vulnerability may be further heightened during menstruation because both estrogen and progesterone hinder the function of the sodium-potassium pump, which helps maintain sodium levels and protect against hyponatremia. Due to a slower rate of water excretion, female athletes entering perimenopause and menopause are also at heightened risk for hyponatremia (Hew-Butler et al., 2015).

Female athletes may choose to work with a sports dietitian, who can help with the development of customized hydration plan beneficial for preventing fluid and electrolyte imbalances and optimizing performance.

Supplement Options for Female Athletes

Because there is no research suggesting that supplementation with vitamins and minerals is beneficial to performance (except when an athlete has a documented deficiency), the first line of defense for the female athlete—and any athlete for that matter—should always be via whole food intake. If a deficiency is detected by a doctor, therapeutic levels of specific vitamins and minerals in supplement form may help blood levels normalize and allow the athlete to regain optimal health and peak performance (see table 4.5). Female athletes whose bloodwork tests are healthy yet consistently struggle to meet the recommended daily intake amounts of key nutrients through whole food intake, especially with iron, zinc, calcium, and vitamin D, may benefit from supplementation with a once-a-day multivitamin and multimineral supplement to help bridge the gap and protect against deficiency Multivitamin and multimineral supplements generally provide lower doses (up to 100% of the current RDA) of nutrients and can serve as nutritional insurance for concerned athletes.

Evidence for sex-specific supplementation is lacking due to the paucity of female-specific research and any differential effects in women. To foster and promote high-quality research investigations involving female athletes, researchers are first encouraged to stop excluding women unless the primary endpoints are directly influenced by sex-specific mechanisms. In all investigative scenarios, researchers across the globe are encouraged to inquire and report on more detailed information surrounding the athlete's hormonal status, including menstrual status (days since menses, length of period, duration of cycle, etc.), hormonal contraceptive details, and menopausal status. Caffeine, iron, and creatine have the most evidence for use in female athletes, with both iron and creatine being highly efficacious.

TABLE 4.5 Highlighted Supplement Options for Female Athletes

Supplement	Potential benefit	Recommended dose
Avocado soybean unsaponifiables (ASU)	Natural alternative for hormone replacement therapy for menopausal women	300 mg/day
Beta-alanine	Helps protect against muscle acidosis and consequent fatigue during intense training	3.2-6.4 g/day
Caffeine	Reduces perceived effort of exertion, improves mental focus, enhances endurance	3-6 mg/kg 60 minutes prior to exercise
Calcium (Ca)	Supports bone health, may help reduce cramping associated with PMS	Premenopausal: 1,000-1,200 mg/day Postmenopausal, adolescents: 1,500 mg/day
Carbohydrate	Enhances endurance	30-90 g/hour during prolonged training
Cinnamon	Relieves menstrual cramping	3-6 g/day
Copper (Cu)	Supports bone health	2.5-3 mg/day
Creatine	Preserves muscle protein dynamics	3-5 g/day; postmenopausal females may benefit from higher doses (0.3 g/kg/day) (Smith-Ryan et al, 2021).
Beetroot	Decreases oxygen cost of submaximal exercise	500 mL of juiced beetroot (or 3,000-4,000 mg) taken 2.5 hours before a short, high-intensity period of exercise
Fenugreek	Reduced symptoms associated with perimenopause and menopause	500-900 mg/kg
Fiber	Supports general health	25 g/day
Flaxseed	Supports general health	1-3 tbsp ground or whole flaxseed/day

(continued)

TABLE 4.5 *(continued)*

Supplement	Potential benefit	Recommended dose
Folic acid	Supports pregnancy and lactation health Carrier of MTHFR gene mutation, high homocysteine levels (Dai et al, 2021)	600-800 mcg/day
Iron (Fe)	Offsets losses seen with menstruation, facilitates oxygen delivery to working muscles and ATP production	RDA: 18 mg/day Therapeutic dose for anemia: 50-100 mg 3×/day
Magnesium (Mg)	May help reduce cramping associated with PMS	100-350 mg/day
Omega-3 fatty acids	Supports general health, reduces inflammation	1-2 g of EPA and DHA/day
Probiotics	Supports immune health	1×10^9 to 1×10^{11} CFU
Tart cherry juice	Helps fight inflammation, aids recovery, improves sleep efficiency	12 oz (0.35 L) taken 1-2×/day
Vitamin B$_{12}$	Carrier of MTHFR gene mutation (Dai et al, 2021)	2.4-2.6 mcg/day
Vitamin D	Supports bone health	1,000-2,000 IU/day
Protein (whey, casein, egg, soy)	Promotes nitrogen balance and recovery; protects against muscle breakdown when restricting calorie intake	1.4-2.0 g/kg/day, including 0.32-0.38 g/kg consumed prior to and immediately after exercise

Injured Athletes

Injuries are common to athletes in all sports. Some injuries are much more serious than others; however, recovery from all types of injury can be improved with appropriate nutritional strategies. Any type of tissue damage—muscle, tendon, ligament, cartilage, or bone—goes through distinct stages of repair. Immediately following injury, an important inflammatory response is initiated that can last from a few hours to several days. This is a vital step toward optimal recovery, and trying to prevent this response may be counterproductive. Following this phase is a period of repair and regeneration for the damaged tissue; it begins with the formation of scar tissue, which is later broken down and replaced by type II collagen. Over time, new tissue is formed, and repair is complete. Providing the body with essential nutrients to assist in these steps is essential.

Performance Obstacles for Injured Athletes

Some injuries require immobilization of muscles, joints, or bones for extended time to allow appropriate healing. This will result in significant losses to the muscle mass surrounding the immobilized joints. Other muscles not affected by injury will also be affected because the athlete's training program will be significantly altered as a result of injury. Preventing these losses in lean body mass is a key component to speeding recovery. In addition, athletes must provide the proper stimulation for muscle recovery. Tension and stress placed on the injured joint or muscle during rehabilitation will affect the formation and repair of new tissue. Initiating blood flow to the injured area will also assist in providing the adequate nutrients needed to speed healing.

Nutritional Recommendations for Injured Athletes

Adequate protein intake is also important. Proteins can assist in preventing the loss of muscle mass as well as initiate and provide the building blocks for repair and rebuilding of new tissue. While needs are elevated, an intake of 0.75 to 0.9 g/lb (1.6-2.0 g/kg) of body mass/day is sufficient. A balanced intake of macronutrients (fat, carbohydrate, protein) is important. As the intensity and duration of training activity significantly decrease, the need for carbohydrate is slightly reduced. Injured athletes should aim to consume 20% to 25% of their calories from protein, 40% to 45% from carbohydrates, and 30% to 35% from healthy sources of fat. Healthy fats, including olive oil, mixed nuts (e.g., walnuts, almonds, pecans), avocados, coconut oil or milk, and flaxseeds or oil, can provide powerful fatty acids that limit inflammation and may decrease pain in injured tissues. Injured athletes should also emphasize fruit and vegetable intake. Consuming a variety of naturally colored (i.e., polyphenol-rich) fruits and vegetables will provide an array of nutrients with antioxidant and anti-inflammatory benefits.

The benefits of nutrient timing experienced by uninjured athletes also apply during injury and rehabilitative workouts. Rehabilitative exercise facilitates the use of injured muscles and joints, resulting in increased blood flow and delivery of nutrients. Providing important nutrients during these types of exercise will assist in delivering important nutrients to the injured site. Protein and carbohydrates should be consumed both before and after rehabilitative exercise. Due to the lowered intensity of this form of exercise, carbohydrate needs are decreased relative to those of uninjured athletes; a 1:1 or 2:1 ratio of carbohydrates to protein may be used depending on the duration and intensity of rehabilitative exercise. It is important that injured athletes not eliminate carbohydrates from the diet, especially during these nutrient-timing windows. Carbohydrates both before and after exercise can limit stress and immune suppression during training and increase levels of the powerful anabolic hormone insulin.

Adequate intakes of vitamins and minerals are also needed. A clear relationship between zinc, vitamin C, vitamin A, and wound healing has been found (Tipton, 2010). In addition, intakes of calcium and vitamin D are also important. Injured athletes should focus on a balanced diet, emphasizing whole foods such as fresh fruits, vegetables, whole grains, dairy, lean protein, and healthy sources of fat. These are the best sources of a wide array of nutrients needed for proper recovery. Athletes restricting certain food groups or consuming inadequate quantities of these food groups will not recover as optimally as those who eat a variety of whole foods.

Supplement Options for Injured Athletes

Dietary supplements can assist athletes in meeting additional nutritional needs during periods of injury. Following is a list of areas dietary supplements might target and benefit (see table 4.6 for specific guidelines).

TABLE 4.6 Highlighted Supplement Options for Injured Athletes

Supplement	Potential benefit*	Recommended dose**
Protein (whey, casein, egg, and possibly soy, collagen)	Prevents muscle atrophy and may support wound repair	1.2-2 g/kg/day, including 15-25 g consumed prior to and after exercise Collagen: 15-30 g, co-supplemented with vitamin C, 1 hour prior to exercise
Leucine	Prevents muscle atrophy	0.015-0.022 g/lb consumed prior to and after exercise
Branched-chain amino acids (BCAAs)	Prevent muscle atrophy	6-14 g/day (ratio of leucine, valine, isoleucine: 3:1:1)
Arginine	Prevents muscle atrophy and may support wound repair	Acute supplementation: 0.15 g/kg consumed between 60 and 90 before exercise Chronic supplementation: 1.5 to 2 g/day for 4 to 7 weeks for improved aerobic performance; 10 to 12 g/day for 8 weeks for enhanced anaerobic performance
Hydroxy-beta-methylbutyrate (HMB)	Prevents muscle atrophy in some populations and conditions	3 g/day (1.5 g, 2×/day)
Glutamine	Provides immune support and may support wound repair; preserves muscle mass; decreases tissue losses	Up to 7.5g one to two times daily
Omega-3 fatty acids	Preserves muscle mass; provides immune and joint support	1-3 g/day of EPA and DHA
Vitamin D	Preserves muscle mass; provides immune and joint support	2,000-4,000 IU/day
Calcium (Ca)	Supports skeletal repair	1,200 mg/day
Copper (Cu)	Supports repair and regeneration	100 mg/day
Vitamin C	Supports repair and regeneration	250-1,000 mg/day
Zinc (Zn)	Supports repair and regeneration	10-30 mg/day
Garlic	Anti-inflammatory	2-4 g/day (600-1,200 mg of aged garlic extract)
Boswellia serrata (BS)	Anti-inflammatory	600-3,000 mg/day
Bromelain	Anti-inflammatory	200-2,000 mg/day

Supplement	Potential benefit*	Recommended dose**
Curcumin	Anti-inflammatory	0.5-3 g/day
Ginger	Anti-inflammatory	0.5-2 g/day
Tart cherry juice	Anti-inflammatory; aids in recovery	12 oz (350 mL) 1-2×/day
Quercetin	Anti-inflammatory; aids in recovery	200-400 mg 2-3×/day
Glucosamine	Provides joint support	1,500 mg/day
Chondroitin	Provides joint support	800-1,200 mg/day (those with melanoma risk, consult a physician)
Avocado soybean unsaponifiables (ASU)	Provides joint support	300 mg/day
Methylsulfonyl-methane (MSM)	Provides joint support	1,500-3,000 mg/day (500-1,000 mg 3×/day)
S-adenosyl methionine (SAMe)	Provides joint support	1,200 mg/day (400 mg 3×/day)

* Potential benefits have been suggested by some literature.

** Recommended dosage should take individual tolerance; consult with a medical professional for more information.

- ***Preservation of lean body mass.*** Protein supplements, including calorie- or meal-replacement shakes and bars, can assist injured athletes in meeting elevated calorie and protein needs. Consuming them can also help ensure proper nutrient timing in relation to exercise. Branched-chain amino acids (BCAAs), particularly leucine, the leucine metabolite hydroxy-beta-methylbutyrate (HMB), vitamin D, and fish oils, also have evidence to suggest benefits in preventing losses in muscle mass.

- ***Joint support.*** Glucosamine, chondroitin, methylsulfonylmethane (MSM), avocado soybean unsaponifiables, collagen, EPA and DHA from fish oils, hyaluronic acid, and S-adenosyl methionine (SAMe) are all thought to provide benefits in the preservation of joints and prevention of pain. Mechanically, all promote the synthesis and limit the degradation of cartilage. There is little evidence to suggest these types of supplements would provide benefit to inflammation-related joint conditions such as tendonitis, with the exception of SAMe and avocado soybean unsaponifiables.

- ***Anti-inflammatory effects.*** Although preventing inflammation within the first 48 to 72 hours appears counterproductive to injury repair, it is beneficial for speeding long-term recovery. Dietary supplements can often provide natural anti-inflammatory protection.

Athletes With Diabetes

Speaking broadly, diabetes is a metabolic disorder in which the body either fails to produce insulin (type 1) or is unable to use what is produced (type 2). According to a position statement from the American Diabetes Association (Colberg et al., 2016):

Type 1 diabetes (5%–10% of cases) results from cellular-mediated autoimmune destruction of the pancreatic b-cells, producing insulin deficiency. Although it can occur at any age, b-cell destruction rates vary, typically occurring more rapidly in youth than in adults. Type 2 diabetes (90%–95% of cases) results from a progressive loss of insulin secretion, usually also with insulin resistance.

Secreted by the pancreas, insulin influences the metabolism of all body fuels and regulates blood glucose (sugar), helping to facilitate muscle development, growth, and fuel storage for energy use. Without insulin, sugar from food could not reach cells, causing muscle and fat stores to shrink, energy levels to plummet, and performance to suffer. People with type 1 diabetes are insulin dependent, meaning injection through a syringe or pump is necessary; those with type 2 diabetes, in many cases, can manage the disease with changes to diet and exercise. Because of the correlation between greater body fat and type 2 diabetes, athletes who have diabetes, especially those at the competitive or professional level where body fat levels tend to be low, are more likely to have type 1; for this reason, this condition gets more focus in this section. By 2050, projections show that 1 in 8 (approximately 853 million) adults will be living with diabetes worldwide. This number is an increase of 46%, making education regarding all treatment options, including potentially beneficial dietary supplements, essential. Even athletes who are more likely to have the less-common type 1 can benefit from such education.

Performance Obstacles for Athletes With Diabetes

The primary goal of diabetes management is maintenance of optimal blood glucose levels, which is not always an easy feat for athletes with diabetes due to the combined challenges of diminished or nonexistent insulin activity and the physical demands of training and competition. Both exercise-induced hypoglycemia (low blood sugar) and hyperglycemia (high blood sugar) are serious issues that athletes with diabetes face. Athletes should monitor and log their blood glucose before, during, and after exercise. According to the American Diabetes Association (Colberg et al., 2016), blood glucose responses to physical activity in persons with type 1 diabetes are highly variable based on activity type and timing, thus requiring different adjustments. For example, added carbohydrate or insulin reductions are typically required to maintain glycemia during and after physical activity. Frequent blood glucose checks—again, including before exercise—are required to implement these dosing adjustments.

DRUG TESTING WARNING

Insulin is on the current World Anti-Doping Association (WADA) List of Prohibited Substances and Methods. Therefore, in order to compete legally, athletes with diabetes who take insulin and are exposed to drug testing must complete a Therapeutic Use Exemption (TUE) form, found on the WADA website, before competition. See the WADA banned substances list from the References and Resources file at \bb\.

The mere stress associated with sporting competition, including pre-event jitters and any trauma or injury during the event, can trigger a fight-or-flight hormonal response that may cause blood glucose levels to rise. For athletes with diabetes, hyperglycemia can further ensue during exercise; this is due to inadequate insulin being available for transport coupled with increased glucose release from the liver. Outside of training, a high dietary intake of refined carbohydrates and sugar can also promote a deleterious blood sugar response. Left untreated, hyperglycemia can lead to a dangerous metabolic disturbance called ketoacidosis, where, in the absence of insulin, fatty acids are broken down to create ketones for energy production. This causes the pH of the blood to drop and the kidneys to work overtime trying to achieve homeostasis, which causes a plethora of problems detrimental to health and performance. Among these problems are dehydration, falling blood pressure (often coupled with passing out), kidney failure, tachycardia (rapid heartbeat), blindness, poor wound healing, and damage to nerve endings. Thus, it is critical that athletes with diabetes make note of precompetition blood glucose levels to ensure personal safety. If blood glucose levels rise above 250 mg/dL, especially in the presence of ketosis, athletic participation is discouraged.

On the opposite end of the blood sugar spectrum, hypoglycemia ensues when uptake of blood glucose by the muscles during exercise exceeds that released by the liver or supplied from carbohydrate sources (e.g., sport drinks). Inadequate energy intake to support training demands may also trigger or exacerbate an episode. Furthermore, nearly all people with diabetes who use insulin will experience a hypoglycemic episode at some point. Mild cases elicit hunger, fatigue, and dizziness, hardly a prescription for athletic success. In moderate or severe cases, these symptoms intensify and are often joined by poor concentration, shaking, cold skin, blurred vision, seizures, or loss of consciousness. Consequently, athletes with diabetes are encouraged to always carry emergency sources of sugar such as juice, glucose tablets, sport drinks, energy gels, energy chews, or raisins to combat hypoglycemia should such a situation arise during training or competition. An athlete with these symptoms should not return to competition until blood glucose rises to normal levels. For more information on glucose management and exercise, athletes may wish to consult joint guidelines such as those published by Moser, et al. (2020).

Nutritional Recommendations for Athletes With Diabetes

Success in sport for any athlete, including those with diabetes, requires consuming adequate amounts of macronutrient energy (calories) to support daily training demands. Both acute and chronic intake must be considered. Considerations immediately before and after exercise can be even more important to diabetic athletes, whereas chronic recommendations are sometimes less diabetes specific. Due to the highly variable glycemic responses known to occur in response to acute exercise, diabetic athletes need to work with their physician.

The aforementioned position statement from the American Diabetes Association (Colberg et al., 2016) suggests additional carbohydrate intake and/or reductions in insulin are typically required during prolonged (>30 minutes), predominantly aerobic exercise. For low- to moderate-intensity aerobic activities lasting 30 to 60 minutes, performed when circulating insulin concentrations are low (fasting or basal conditions), 10 to 15 g of carbohydrate may prevent hypoglycemia. For activities performed with relative hyperinsulinemia (after bolus insulin), 30 to 60 g of carbohydrate/hour of exercise may be needed—not unlike the carbohydrate recommendations for nondiabetic athletes.

For athletes with chronic conditions (not diabetic athletes, per se), a joint position statement issued by the ACSM, the American Dietetic Association, and the Dietitians of Canada (Rodriguez et al., 2009) offered general nutrient requirements:

1. Although daily energy requirements are highly variable based on daily training as well as activity levels outside of training, recommendations range from 16 to 18 kcal/

lb (35.2-39.6 kcal/kg) for endurance athletes and 20 to 22+ kcal/lb (44-48+ kcal/kg) for strength-trained athletes.

2. As a means to maintain optimal blood glucose levels and replenish depleted muscle glycogen stores during training, daily carbohydrate consumption should be 2.7 to 4.5 g/lb (5.9-9.9 g/kg), with variations being dependent on the athlete's daily total energy expenditure, sport type, sex, and environmental circumstances. Low-glycemic and nutrient-dense carbohydrate sources such as whole grains, legumes, and whole fruits and vegetables are recommended for optimal blood sugar control (see table 4.7).

TABLE 4.7 Carbohydrate Recommendations for Athletes With Diabetes

Type of activity	Blood glucose level	Carbohydrate intake recommendations	Example of snack
Short duration, low- to moderate-intensity exercise (e.g., walk 0.5 mi [800 m], leisurely bike ride <30 minutes)	<80 mg/dL	30 g	Medium banana
	>80 mg/dL	10-15 g	One-half cup (0.12 L) juice
Moderate-intensity exercise (e.g., swim, jog, cycle for 1 hour)	<80 mg/dL	30 g + small amount of protein	One-half peanut butter sandwich
	80-180 mg/dL	10-15 g	1-2 figs
	180-300 mg/dL	No extra food	N/A
	>300 mg/dL	Exercise not recommended	N/A
High-intensity, strenuous exercise (e.g., racing, interval workout, scrimmaging)	<80 mg/dL	~50 g + some protein	Blend 0.75 cup (0.18 L) nonfat milk with 2 tbsp nonfat Greek yogurt, 1 banana, 0.5 cup (113 g) mango
	80-180 mg/dL	~30 g + some protein	1 banana sliced into 0.5 cup (113 g) nonfat Greek yogurt
	180-300 mg/dL	10-15 g + some protein	One-third energy bar (e.g., PowerBar)
	>300 mg/dL	Exercise not recommended	N/A

In addition to consuming the right quantity and balance of overall macronutrient energy, a key component of sport success for athletes with diabetes is proper supplementation with carbohydrate energy before, during, and after competition to help protect against exercise-induced hypoglycemia, sustain peak levels of performance, and promote recovery. Because blood sugars can be affected by such factors as exercise intensity, exercise duration, time of day, environmental conditions, emotional stress or excitement, and absorption of insulin and dietary supplements, there is not a standard recommendation

TYPE 2 DIABETES: A CONSENSUS STATEMENT

A consensus statement from the ACSM further states that individuals with type 2 diabetes "should focus on sustainable eating plans that consider the amount and timing of carbohydrate intake in combination with an active lifestyle to manage glycemia, insulin sensitivity, body weight, and CVD risk" (Kanaley et al., 2022). This consensus statement largely relied on the 2020-2025 U.S. Dietary Guidelines for Americans. Similar to the 2009 joint position paper noted above (Rodriguez et al., 2009), a healthy eating plan provides appropriate daily calories from fruits, vegetables, and whole grains as well as reduced or nonfat dairy products, lean meats, poultry, fish, beans, eggs, and nuts. It is also one that is low in saturated and trans fats, cholesterol, salt, and added sugar. Whole foods are a focus because they are dense in micronutrients, rich in antioxidants, and beneficial in preventing and managing type 2 diabetes. The consensus statement covers popular diets as well, including low carbohydrate, Mediterranean, and vegan diets, which are frequently followed for management of type 2 diabetes. These should be discussed with a physician. Various types of intermittent fasting and ketogenic diets are cautioned against due to limited data on type 2 diabetic persons.

for athletes with diabetes. Therefore, frequent self-monitoring of blood glucose levels and maintaining logs of such data are important for determining an optimal dietary management plan for safe participation in sport. Until a dietary management plan is created, general guidelines can be followed.

1. *Preworkout.* For pre-exercise nutrient intake, see acute nutritional recommendations noted previously, based on American Diabetes Association (ADA) general information. Diabetic athletes should work with a physician to tailor those suggestions.

2. *During workout.* Although supplementation with carbohydrate exerts the greatest benefit during prolonged exercise sessions (>60 minutes), athletes with diabetes whose blood sugars run low preworkout or whose insulin levels are too high may need to eat small amounts of carbohydrate during competition to avoid a hypoglycemic episode. In fact, diabetes-specific nutritional shakes with specific carbohydrate blends and micronutrients that help control blood sugar fluctuations also exist and can be discussed with a health care professional.

3. *Postworkout.* Consuming carbohydrate with small amounts of protein immediately after workout has been shown to significantly increase glucose uptake by the muscles of nondiabetic individuals as well as reduce postworkout muscle damage, thereby enhancing recovery. Athletes with diabetes may further benefit from prevention of late-onset hypoglycemia, which can occur up to 24 hours after exercise. As noted, those with diabetes may have to adjust their insulin accordingly depending on blood glucose level. Because glycogen repletion occurs at a rate of only 5% to 7% per hour in nondiabetic persons, those with diabetes should work with their physician to devise a plan to continue consuming additional carbohydrate-focused meals throughout the day until energy stores are replenished.

Supplement Options for Athletes With Diabetes

The power that blood sugar control can have on the performance and health of athletes with diabetes cannot be emphasized enough. Premature fatigue and sluggishness brought on by a swing in blood sugars are detriments to several aspects of performance, including recovery, as well as to overall health. Chronically elevated blood sugars can also cause permanent damage to nerves, triggering a burning sensation, numbness, tingling, and pain, most commonly in the legs and feet. Several dietary supplements are purported to help protect against such blood sugar swings and the consequent detriments associated with the stress of poor glycemic control. These should be reviewed individually in chapter 3 and discussed with a physician, particularly regarding potential drug interactions.

Supplements That May Increase Blood Sugar

- Caffeine
- DHEA
- Fish oil (high doses)
- *Ginkgo biloba*
- Glucosamine sulfate
- Melatonin
- Niacin
- Vitamin C (high doses)

Supplements That May Decrease Blood Sugar

- Alpha-lipoic acid
- Biotin
- Chlorogenic acid (coffee extract)
- Chromium
- Cinnamon
- CoQ10
- Fenugreek
- Fiber
- Garlic
- Ginseng, American
- *Gymnema sylvestre*
- Magnesium
- Quercetin
- Thiamine
- Vanadyl sulfate
- Zinc

A key area of research is the impact of antioxidant supplementation on ameliorating damage from unstable oxygen molecules called free radicals, which can increase to levels beyond the body's own defense capabilities during times of extreme stress (e.g., strenuous exercise), especially in the presence of uncontrolled blood sugars. According to health scientists from Duke University Medical Center, poor control of blood glucose in itself can deplete the body's stores of antioxidant nutrients (Opara et al., 1999; Opara, 2004). Add the stress of intense training and competition, and athletes with diabetes may find themselves recovering poorly, getting sick, and experiencing some of the serious complications of diabetes such as nerve damage. Supplementation with antioxidants—vitamins C and E, coenzyme Q10, pine bark extract, resveratrol, quercetin, and alpha-lipoic acid—may help protect against these complications, particularly during intense training cycles (Ansar et al., 2011; Brasnyo et al., 2011; Chao et al., 2009; Dakhale et al., 2011; Gupta et al., 2011; Brasnyo et al., 2011; Kobori et al., 2009; Koh et al., 2011; Porasuphatana et al., 2012; Sing & Jialal, 2008). Although there is evidence in recent literature that short-term vitamin C supplementation may improve glycemic control, megadoses of it are contraindicated because they may actually elevate blood sugars as well as be of detriment to both performance and health.

B-vitamins, which include thiamine, riboflavin, niacin, pantothenic acid, vitamin B_6, biotin, folic acid, and vitamin B_{12}, play in important role in production of enzymes that aid the conversion of glucose into energy. Furthermore, though not consistently supported in research, B-vitamins may help protect an athlete against nerve ending damage associated with poor blood sugar control. Some research has shown the blood levels of certain B-vitamins to be significantly lower in those with diabetes than in those without, making supplementation of possible benefit (Davis, Calder, & Curnow, 1976; Satyanarayana et al., 2011). For instance, blood levels of thiamine (B_1) have been shown to be significantly lower in those with diabetes due to increased clearance through the kidneys (Luong & Nguyen, 2012). Vascular health, regardless of glucose homeostasis, is ultimately hurt because of increased inflammation (Page, Laight, & Cummings, 2011). People with diabetes also seem to be at greater risk for deficiencies in pantothenic acid (B_5) (Tahiliani & Beinlich, 1991). Biotin (B_7) plays an especially important role in helping the body use glucose, its basic fuel. Administration of supplemental biotin has been shown to prevent the development of insulin resistance in skeletal muscles, thereby aiding the transport of glucose energy to muscle and fat cells (Sasaki et al., 2012). Of important note, high doses of niacin (B_3) may increase blood sugars, possibly making adjustment of insulin dosing necessary with supplementation.

Perhaps the most studied mineral as it relates to the treatment and maintenance of diabetes, especially type 2, is chromium, which facilitates the transportation of glucose into cells by enhancing the action of insulin. A chromium deficiency, thought to be more prevalent among people with diabetes, impairs the body's ability to use glucose, compromising energy levels and increasing the need for insulin. Therefore, supplementation is purported to help, particularly in diabetics who are chromium deficient (Singer & Geohas, 2006). Magnesium and zinc are two additional minerals of pronounced importance to diabetics. Levels of magnesium, one of the most abundant minerals in the body, are known to be depleted with insulin use (Rosner & Goefien, 1968). Lowered magnesium levels can negatively affect glucose homeostasis as well as increase risk for muscle cramping, making supplementation of potential merit for athletes with diabetes. Deficiencies in zinc, which plays an integral role in the regulation of insulin production and consequent glucose use by muscle and fat cells, are also more common among those with diabetes, likely due to a reduced rate of intestinal absorption (Chooi, Todd, & Boyd, 1976; Huber & Gershoff, 1973). For this reason, zinc supplementation may be of potential benefit. Finally, though evidence from well-controlled studies has not been conclusive, vanadium or vanadyl sulfate carries insulin-like properties that may help enhance the delivery of glucose energy to the muscles, making it another mineral of potential merit for athletes with diabetes (Crans, 2000; Willsky et al., 2011).

Several additional ingredients, including dietary fiber, American ginseng, cinnamon, flaxseed, fenugreek, taurine, garlic, and *Gymnema sylvestre,* have shown promise in promoting glucose homeostasis through improvements in insulin sensitivity and consequent decreases in blood sugars (Bartlett & Eperjesi, 2008; Benzie & Wachtel-Galor, 2011; Fabian et al., 2011; Lee & Dugoua, 2011; Moloney et al., 2010; Yeh et al., 2003). Because supplements are poorly regulated compared to pharmaceuticals, and because taking several may affect optimal glycemic control as well as interfere with kidney function, it is important that athletes with diabetes consult with a physician and registered dietitian (www.eatright.org) before implementing a supplementation protocol (see table 4.8). With an appropriate dietary management action plan, safe participation as well as achievement of personal performance goals are possibilities for athletes with diabetes.

TABLE 4.8 Highlighted Supplement Options for Athletes with Diabetes

Supplement	Potential benefit	Recommended dose
Alpha-lipoic acid	Lowers blood sugars, decreases nerve pain	150-200 mg 2-4×/day
B-complex with extra biotin	Improves metabolism of glucose	50 mg 3×/day
Carbohydrate	Prevents exercise-induced hypoglycemia (adjustment to insulin levels may be needed)	15-90 g/hour of exercise
Chromium picolinate	Lowers blood sugars, increases insulin sensitivity	150-200 mcg/day 3×/day with meals
Cinnamon	Lowers blood sugars	3-6 g/day
Coenzyme Q10 (CoQ10)	Lowers blood sugars, reduces oxidative stress associated with elevated blood sugars	60-80 mg/day
Fenugreek	Lowers blood sugars	5-30 g/meal
Fiber	Lowers blood sugars	Up to 50 g/day
Flaxseed	Lowers blood sugars	600 mg 3×/day of a flaxseed lignan extract
Garlic	Lowers blood sugars	300 mg 2× daily
Ginseng, American	Lowers blood sugars	1-3 g/day in capsule form or 3-5/mL 3×/day dissolved in liquid
Gymnema sylvestre	Lowers blood sugars, increases insulin sensitivity	200-250 mg 2×/day
Magnesium (Mg)	Lowers blood sugars	250-500 mg 1-2×/day
Pine bark extract	Reduces oxidative stress associated with elevated blood sugars	50-200 mg/day
Quercetin	Lowers blood sugars	100 mg 3×/day
Resveratrol	Increases insulin sensitivity, reduces oxidative stress associated with elevated blood sugars	10 mg/day
Taurine	Facilitates the release of insulin	500 mg 2×/day on an empty stomach
Vanadium (vanadyl sulfate)	Lowers blood sugars, increases insulin sensitivity	<1.8 mg/day
Vitamin C	Reduces oxidative stress associated with elevated blood sugars	1,000 mg/day
Vitamin E	Reduces oxidative stress associated with elevated blood sugars	200 mg/day
Zinc (Zn)	Increases insulin sensitivity	30 mg/day

Athletes With Food Allergies or Intolerances

The prevalence of food allergies has seemingly grown in the past several decades, with as many as 25% of adults believing that they or their children suffer from food allergies. Nevertheless, according to results from the National Health and Nutrition Examination Survey 2005-2006 (Liu et al., 2010), clinically proven diagnoses for true allergic reactions by an appropriate medical professional (board-certified allergist or immunologist) remain low, with only an estimated 2.5% of the U.S. population affected. Slightly higher incidence numbers were reported for Black subjects, male subjects, and children. Food intolerance, on the other hand, is much more common. Its associated gastrointestinal symptoms, including bloating, gas, diarrhea, and stomach cramping, present debilitating problems for many athletes. Thus, exploration of treatment options, including adjustments to whole food intake and possible introduction of dietary supplements, is important.

Performance Obstacles for Athletes With Food Allergies or Intolerances

When an allergy to a food or specific ingredient within a food product exists, an abnormal immune response occurs (see table 4.9). Initially, the food allergen triggers the production of immunoglobulin-E (IgE) antibodies, which cause particles found within large cells to release chemicals such as histamine that are responsible for the onset of inflammatory symptoms. These symptoms range in severity and generally arise within a couple minutes, although they can sometimes appear a few hours after consuming the allergen; the symptoms are thought to intensify after exercise. On the mild-to-moderate end of the symptom spectrum are hives (red, itchy skin), stuffy or itchy nose, sneezing, itchy or teary eyes, vomiting, stomach cramps, shortness of breath and asthma, diarrhea, and swelling of the tissue beneath the skin. On the severe end of the symptom spectrum, and indicative of a reaction known as anaphylaxis, are a tingling sensation in the mouth, swelling of the tongue and throat, wheezing, chest tightness, difficulty breathing, hoarseness, intense stomach cramping, vomiting, pale or red color to face and body, and loss of consciousness. If not treated immediately with an injection of adrenalin from an EpiPen, anaphylaxis can be fatal.

Unlike food allergy, which is immunity based and can be life threatening, food intolerance relates to the inability of the digestive system to properly process a food ingredient, generally as a result of deficiencies in digestive enzymes such as lactose in milk, an imbalance of bacteria and yeast in the intestines, sensitivities to food additives and dyes, or reactions to naturally occurring chemicals in foods (see table 4.10). This can cause

TABLE 4.9 Most Common Food Allergies

Child athletes	Adult athletes
Cow's milk	Fish
Eggs	Peanuts
Fish	Shellfish
Peanuts	Tree nuts
Shellfish	
Soy	
Tree nuts	
Wheat	

partially or undigested food to enter the bloodstream, which triggers the production of immunoglobulin-G (IgG) antibodies and onset of uncomfortable (but not life-threatening) gastrointestinal symptoms such as nausea, bloating, gas, stomach cramping, and diarrhea. These symptoms can linger as long as the food ingredient remains in the diet and certainly hinder an athlete's ability to perform at peak.

TABLE 4.10 Common Food Intolerances

Ingredient	Food sources
Lactose	Dairy foods
Gluten	Wheat, barley, rye
Monosodium glutamate (MSG)	Meat, fish, poultry, many vegetables, sauces, soups, marinades
Sulfites	Red wine
Nitrites	Processed meats
Salicylate	Several fruits and vegetables, some cheeses, tomato paste, soy sauce, vinegar, some nuts, coffee, wine, beer, rum, jams, jellies, mint
Amines	Fish, cheese, some meats, bananas, avocados, mushrooms, chocolate, sauerkraut, soy sauce

Athletes experiencing symptoms, especially gastrointestinal ones, may be at greater risk for energy imbalances and consequent nutrient deficiencies that can cause performance to plummet. If diarrhea ensues, dehydration and electrolyte imbalances also can present serious risks to the athlete's performance, recovery, and overall health. Those with multiple food allergies and intolerances are generally instructed to avoid all food triggers and may therefore struggle to put together a menu plan that includes enough calories and nutrients to support training demands.

Nutritional Recommendations for Athletes With Food Allergies or Intolerances

Treatment of a food allergy or intolerance is as simple as limiting intake or eliminating the culprit food. The first step in discovering a food allergy or intolerance is to develop a list of suspect foods over a period of a month that seem to trigger the onset of one or more unpleasant symptoms. Once this list is compiled, the suspect foods can be eliminated from the diet over the next month to see if the recorded symptoms disappear. After a month's period, one suspect food can be reintroduced into the diet to determine if symptoms reappear. A positive reaction will almost always manifest itself with one or more symptoms in coordination with a spike in heart rate. A board-certified immunologist, commonly referred to as an allergist, is the health professional most qualified to diagnose a food allergy and can confirm by running a series of tests that generally includes a skin test. Upon confirmation from a doctor, the athlete is encouraged to consult with a registered dietitian, preferably one board-certified in sport dietetics, to help create a custom training menu that is allergy friendly and incorporates the right balance of nutrition to support peak performance.

Supplement Options for Athletes With Food Allergies or Intolerances

The National Center for Complementary and Alternative Medicine (NCCAM), a branch of the National Institutes of Health, is responsible for investigating the effectiveness of alternative forms of allergy treatment, including dietary supplements. Although avoidance of the culprit food is currently the only proven effective nutritional treatment for food allergies, preliminary evidence suggests that certain dietary supplements may help alleviate specific allergy-driven symptoms, such as gastrointestinal distress, inflammation, and asthma, making them of potential benefit for the affected athlete (see table 4.11).

TABLE 4.11 Highlighted Supplement Options for Athletes With Food Allergies or Intolerances

Supplement	Potential benefit	Recommended dose
Boswellia serrata	Reduces inflammation; may reduce asthma symptoms	600-3,000 mg/day
Bromelain	Reduces inflammation, enhances action of quercetin	500 mg split into 3-4 doses and taken with meals
Folic acid	Lowers IgE antibodies, may reduce asthma symptoms	400 mcg/day
Ginger	Reduces inflammation	0.5-2 g/day
Omega-3 fatty acids	Reduces inflammation	EPA and DHA: 1-3 g/day (3:2 ratio) ALA: 3-5 g/day
Probiotics	Enhances immune function	Should contain >10 billion CFU of bifidobacteria and lactobacillus species
Quercetin	Reduces inflammation, may reduce asthma symptoms	200-400 mg 2-3\x\/day before meals
Curcumin	Reduces inflammation	500-3,000 mg/day
Vitamin D	Reduces inflammations, may reduce allergy symptoms	1,000-2,000 IU/day

Probiotics are one increasingly popular ingredient under investigation for the treatment of food-related allergies. Probiotics, microorganisms within the gut also known as friendly bacteria, are found in such foods as yogurt and kefir as well as in dietary supplement form; they seem to help enhance the immune response by introducing these beneficial bacteria into the gut. Although research is still in an infancy state, a probiotic supplement containing at least 10 billion CFU of bifidobacteria species and lactobacillus species may be helpful for athletes with food allergies (Fiocchi et al., 2012; Isolauri, Rautava, & Salminen, 2012; Isolauri & Salminen, 2008).

Spices such as turmeric and ginger, easily added into the diet through their use in cooking, have demonstrated potent anti-inflammatory properties that may help mute the inflammatory responses, including asthma, associated with allergic reaction (Ghayur,

Gilani, & Janssen, 2008; Maeda-Yamamoto, Ema, & Shibuichi, 2007; Zhou, Beevers, & Huang, 2011). It has also been postulated that the apparent rise in food allergy and intolerance is associated with the modern diet that emphasizes omega-6 fatty acids over omega-3 fatty acids, which is a recipe for inflammation. Research has found increased intake of omega-3 fatty acids from such sources as fish oil, flaxseed, and chia seed reduces symptoms associated with food allergies (de Matos et al., 2012).

Deficiencies in vitamin D, the sunshine vitamin, have recently been correlated with increased incidence of allergic diseases, including food allergy, asthma, and allergic rhinitis, with one study demonstrating a significantly higher prevalence of severe vitamin D deficiency in patients with allergic rhinitis than the normal population (30% versus 5.1%) (Arshi et al., 2012). Additional research is needed, however, to determine if supplementation is effective in alleviating symptoms. Folic acid, or vitamin B_9, is another vitamin that may help suppress allergic reactions and lessen the severity of allergy and asthma symptoms, according to researchers from Johns Hopkins. Specifically, investigators found that people with higher levels of folate (the naturally occurring form of folic acid) had fewer IgE antibodies, fewer reported allergies, less wheezing, and lower likelihood of asthma. People with the lowest folate levels (<8 ng/mL) had a 40% greater risk of wheezing than people with the highest folate levels (>18 ng/mL) (Matsui & Matsui, 2009).

Quercetin, a dietary flavonoid found naturally within apple skin, has been shown to ameliorate allergy-driven inflammation, especially that associated with asthma, by lowering levels of IgE antibodies (Chirumbolo, 2011; Lee, Ji, & Sung, 2010). Bromelain, an enzyme found naturally in pineapple, enhances this action and thus is commonly paired with quercetin in dietary supplements. *Boswellia serrata* is another ingredient that presents strong anti-inflammatory properties of particular promise for athletes with allergy-driven asthma (Ammon, 2006; Houssen et al., 2010).

Although preliminary evidence demonstrates potentially beneficial applications of supplement ingredients for alleviating food allergies and corresponding symptoms, continued research is needed to confirm their effectiveness as well as determine optimal dosing for therapeutic use.

Plant-Based Athletes

There are a variety of well-balanced plant-based diets, which vary from exclusion of all animal products and byproducts (vegan) to exclusion of select animal products (semivegetarian, lacto-vegetarian, lacto-ovo-vegetarian). The health and performance benefits of plant-based diets are potentially profound when they include higher intake of such cardioprotective nutrients as dietary fiber, folic acid, potassium, magnesium, and anti-inflammatory phytonutrients as well as a lower intake of proinflammatory saturated fat. Indeed, for well over 100 years, there have been cases of vegetarian athletes from all sports achieving as highly as—and even outperforming—their meat-eating counterparts. For example, Scott Jurek, an ultramarathoner and vegan athlete who has racked up wins in many of the sport's most prestigious races, set a new U.S. record in 2010 for distance run in 24 hours with 165.7 mi (266.7 km) at the 24-Hour World Championships in Brive-la-Gaillarde, France. The plant-focused eating habits of successful athletes like Jurek, who chronicles his journey as a vegan athlete in his book *Eat & Run,* has garnered the attention of other athletes, leading to an increased number taking on a plant-based approach to fueling performance.

PLANT-BASED EATING EXPLAINED

Consumers have a multitude of reasons for eliminating particular animal-derived products from their diets.

Semivegetarian: The term includes some but not all animal-derived products, including meat, poultry, fish, seafood, eggs, and dairy foods.

Lacto-vegetarian: Includes dairy foods but excludes eggs, fish, seafood, and meat.

Lacto-ovo-vegetarian: Includes only dairy foods and eggs.

Ovo-vegetarian: Includes only eggs.

Vegan: Excludes all animal products, including eggs, dairy, and foods that include animal byproducts.

Performance Obstacles for Plant-Based Athletes

A well-balanced diet containing adequate amounts of calories, protein, vitamins, and minerals is a proven component of an athlete's health and success in sport. Even so, many athletes struggle to strike the right nutritional balance to adequately meet the metabolic demands of training. This holds especially true for those following specialized dietary plans such as vegetarianism, where restriction of various foods can increase the risk for nutritional deficiencies and make nutritional planning more challenging. Numerous studies have demonstrated plant-based diets to be deficient in several nutrients, including protein, iron, zinc, calcium, and vitamin B_{12} (Craig, 2009, 2010). The greatest risk for deficiency is for athletes who practice vegetarianism for weight control, common among female athletes; athletes involved in sports where a perceived ideal body weight is thought to influence performance (e.g., running); and athletes who simply lack the knowledge to create a menu plan suitable to meet the demands of training and competition. The impact that a poorly implemented plant-based diet can have on athletic performance cannot be overstated. Risks include decreased metabolic efficiency, nutrient deficiencies, and altered hormonal status, all of which can significantly compromise the health and performance of an athlete.

Decreased Metabolic Efficiency

Athletes can expend extraordinary amounts of energy during training and competition. In fact, it has been estimated that athletes require anywhere from 16 to 30 kcal/lb (35.2-66 kcal/kg) of lean body weight to meet the high demands of competitive sport. Energy needs in plant-based athletes may be even higher, because resting energy expenditure has been shown to be approximately 11% higher in vegetarians compared to nonvegetarians (Toth & Poehlman, 1994). Because vegetarians typically eat lots of high-fiber, low-fat foods (e.g., whole grains, fruits, vegetables), it is not uncommon to discover inadequate energy intakes in plant-based endurance athletes, especially those expending greater than 1,000 kcal/day via exercise. When energy expenditure exceeds intake by over 1,000 calories, there is significant catabolism of lean body mass, leading to a drop in metabolic efficiency and athletic performance.

Nutrient Deficiencies

Beyond energy intake, adequate intakes of both macro- and micronutrients are critical to the health and performance of a plant-based athlete. Protein is perhaps the most recognized nutrient of concern for vegetarians due to the incomplete nature and reduced digestibility of most plant sources of protein. With the exception of soybeans, milk, and egg whites, other vegetarian food choices lack some of the essential amino acids necessary for maximal tissue growth and repair. Even soy, arguably the most heavily relied on protein source by strict vegans, has a lower protein quality score than dairy proteins based on the modern DIAAS. Most plant-based foods need to be combined to attain all the essential amino acids; for example, tortillas and beans, rice and lentils, peanuts and wheat bread. The concept of complementary proteins is controversial from a per-meal perspective because amino acids can linger in the bloodstream, but it does emphasize the fact the larger doses and a wider variety of plant proteins may be needed compared to animal proteins. Endurance-trained athletes require 0.5 to 0.6 g of protein/lb (1.1-1.3 g/kg) of body weight; strength-trained athletes require 0.7 to 0.8 g of protein/lb (1.5 to 1.8 g/kg) of body weight, which is approximately 150% to 200% the RDA for protein intake.

Additional amounts of protein are needed to replace the loss of amino acids during exercise and to help repair exercise-induced muscle damage that occurs during weight-bearing activities such as running. The World Health Organization (WHO) suggests that plant-based endurance athletes consume 110% of their calculated protein requirement because the high fiber content of plant foods reduces their protein digestibility. Plant-based diets providing adequate energy and a variety of proteins will supply all the essential amino acids needed for efficient protein metabolism, thereby enhancing recovery from exercise and helping to prevent muscle injury. A rule of thumb for vegetarians is to eat a higher total dose of protein, from a broader variety of sources.

Micronutrients of particular concern to plant-based athletes include calcium, vitamin D, vitamin B_{12}, iron, and zinc. Vegetarians who do not consume dairy products become especially vulnerable to low calcium and vitamin D intake. A chronically low calcium intake, especially when combined with an inadequate energy intake, is associated with decreased bone mineral density, leading to elevated risk for bone fracture (Myburgh et al., 1990; Talbott et al., 1998; Zanker & Swaine, 1998). In fact, over a period of just 1 year, an athlete with a restrictive eating pattern (often the case with vegetarians) may develop osteopenia, increasing the risk for stress fractures 8-fold (Bennel et al., 1995; Pettersson et al., 1999). Dietary restriction of calcium over a mere 9-week period has also been shown to elevate the rate of bone turnover and consequent loss of bone mass, leading to increased risk for stress fractures (Talbott, Rothkopf, & Shapses, 1998). In addition, a calcium deficiency may play a part in muscle cramping and weakness during exercise (Yu-Yahiro, 1994). Recommended intake of calcium ranges from 1,000 to 1,500 mg. In order to prevent loss of bone mass and consequent stress fracture, plant-based athletes are encouraged to consume an energy-sufficient diet that includes a variety of calcium-rich foods. Good nondairy sources of calcium include calcium-fortified foods, calcium-processed tofu (4 oz [113 g] = 145 mg), almonds (1 oz [28 g] = 332 mg), legumes (1 cup [227 g] = 90 mg), and collard greens (0.5 cup [113 g] = 179 mg). Because vitamin D enhances the intestinal absorption of calcium, low serum levels (<40 ng/mL) can also increase risk for fracture (McCabe, Smyth, & Richardson, 2012). Vitamin D is found in fortified dairy foods as well as fatty fish. Recommended intake of vitamin D ranges from 600 to 800 IU depending on the individual, although considerably more is recommended by many physicians, with a tolerable upper limit (UL) of 4,000 IU.

Vitamin B_{12}, which is naturally present only in animal products, is essential for maintaining healthy red blood cells and nerve fibers. Vegetarians who restrict calorie intake may be at elevated risk for a deficiency, leading to premature fatigue during exercise and potential nerve damage. Furthermore, a relationship between poor vitamin B_{12} status in vegetarians and increased bone turnover and risk for fracture has been demonstrated (Herrmann et al., 2009). Fortunately, the RDA (2.4 mcg) for vitamin B_{12} is very small and quite easy to attain through such fortified plant sources as soy milk, nutritional yeast, and breakfast cereals.

Iron, a trace mineral, is a major component of the body's red blood cells, or hemoglobin, whose role is to carry oxygen to various body tissues, including muscle, for use during aerobic activity. An iron deficiency may lead to premature fatigue during exercise due to lack of oxygen transport to working muscles. Indeed, greater fatigue can occur before anemia is present. Although iron is found extensively in several plant foods, the absorption is reduced by 20% compared to the iron found in animal products (Hurrell, 1997). Therefore, the risk for iron deficiency is increased in plant-based athletes even if total iron intake meets the RDA of 10 to 15 mg. For added absorption of plant-based iron sources, they should be consumed with foods rich in vitamin C, such as orange juice.

Along with iron, zinc deficiency tops the list of the most common dietary deficiencies among plant-based athletes. This is likely due in part to urinary and sweat losses during heavy training and the fact that plant sources of zinc (e.g., legumes, whole grains, wheat germ, fortified cereals, nuts, tofu, miso) are not absorbed as efficiently as animal sources of zinc (Lukaski, 1995). A study of female distance runners discovered that 50% fell below the recommended daily intake for zinc (12 mg/day), which may lead to an altered zinc status (Deuster et al., 1989). An altered zinc status will compromise immune function as well as basal metabolic rate and thyroid hormone levels, which can have a major impact on performance and health (Wada & King, 1986). Fortunately, data from the U.S. Department of Agriculture suggests that zinc status can be maintained within normal limits with a vegetarian (lacto-ovo) diet that includes such zinc-rich foods as beans, milk, yogurt, tofu, and peanut butter (Hunt, Matthys, & Hohnson, 1998).

Altered Hormonal Status

There has been some concern that plant-based athletes are at increased risk for altered hormonal status, especially for the sex hormones estrogen and testosterone. In a study of 8 male athletes, engagement in a lacto-ovo-vegetarian diet over a period of 6 weeks caused a slight decrease in total testosterone levels, although performance detriments were negligible (Raben et al., 1992). Similarly, female plant based athletes have reported lower circulating estrogen levels as compared to their meat-eating counterparts (Goldin et al., 1982). It is thought that the cessation of hormonal function is merely an energy-conserving adaptation to energy deficit, which can be caused by reduced energy intake; high energy expenditure from chronic, intense exercise; or a combination of the two. In addition, some studies have found that those eating plant-based diets with a high fiber content report greater loss of sex hormones in feces compared to non-plant-based diets (Gorbach & Goldin, 1987). However, it is unclear whether hormonal function diminishes as a result of the composition of the plant-based diet or simply because of a reduction in total energy intake. Regardless of the cause, altered hormonal status can lead to serious health and fitness implications. Symptoms of altered hormonal status include fatigue, weight loss, frequent infections, decreased physical performance, diminished bone health (including increased risk for stress fractures), and increased injury. In order to maintain normal hormonal status, vegetarians should follow a well-balanced diet that meets individual energy needs.

Nutritional Recommendations for Plant-Based Athletes

As the popularity of plant-based diets increases among athletes, the risk for poorly planned diets and consequent nutritional deficiencies also increases, which can have a profound negative effect on health and endurance performance. However, an athlete can reap many health and performance benefits from a well-planned vegetarian diet. The following tips offer a framework for achieving a healthy plant-based lifestyle:

• ***Achieve energy balance by consuming enough calories to meet training demands.*** The average endurance athlete requires anywhere from 16 to 30 kcal/lb (35-66 kcal/kg) to meet the high demands of endurance training; plant-based endurance athletes may need about 10% more. To meet the demands of endurance training, plant-based athletes are encouraged to eat six or more medium-sized meals or snacks containing such energy-dense plant foods as nuts, avocado, dried fruit, and dairy products.

• ***Keep in touch with your hormones.*** Despite popular belief, absence of hormones, specifically loss of a menstrual cycle for female athletes, does not mean that training is going well. For male athletes, low testosterone levels also can be problematic for bone density and performance. Listen to your body. If you are feeling tired, training is not going well, and illness becomes common, your hormones may be out of whack. Try reducing your training load or adding more energy-dense foods to your daily meal plan to see if normal hormone function returns.

• ***Include a variety of protein-containing plant foods throughout the day.*** The average athlete requires a daily protein intake of 0.5 to 0.8 g/lb (1.1-1.8 g/kg) to allow for efficient tissue growth and repair. Plant-based athletes benefit from at least a 10% greater amount due to the reduced digestibility of plant proteins. Also seek a variety of plant-based protein sources, or even consider the amino acid profiles of each.

• ***Don't skimp on bone-building nutrients.*** Vegetarians should include 3 to 4 servings of dairy to fulfill daily calcium needs—for example, 1 cup (0.24 L) skim, soy, or almond milk; 0.75 cup (170 g) Greek yogurt, or 0.5 cup (113 g) nonfat cottage cheese.

• ***Pump up the iron.*** Recommended daily allowances of iron can be fulfilled in one day by consuming 0.5 cup (113 g) firm tofu and 0.5 cup (113 g) lentils. Plant sources of iron are absorbed better when taken with vitamin C.

• ***Enhance dietary intake of vitamin B_{12}.*** Although additional amounts of B_{12} will not enhance oxygenation of blood, B_{12} is essential for maximal energy and normal nervous system function. Good vegetarian sources include fortified soy milks, meat analogs, and breakfast cereals.

• ***Zinc up.*** Help keep the bugs away: Consume a well-balanced vegetarian diet that includes lentils, beans, whole grains, nuts, and soy.

Supplement Options for Plant-Based Athletes

Although dietary supplements should never serve as a crutch to a poorly planned diet, there are several nutrients found primarily in animal-based foods that are often lacking in the diets of plant-based athletes; as a result, supplementation may be warranted to avoid deficiency and consequent declines in performance. As discussed earlier, protein, zinc, iron, calcium, vitamin D, and vitamin B_{12} are among these nutrients (see table 4.12).

Additional supplements of potential merit for the plant-based athlete include beta-alanine and creatine monohydrate. Studies have shown the plasma concentration of the

TABLE 4.12 Highlighted Supplement Options for Plant-Based Athletes

Supplement	Potential benefit	Recommended dose
Beta-alanine	Provides a boost to muscle carnosine levels, which helps reduce muscle fatigue associated with acidosis	3.2-6.4 g/day for 12 weeks
Calcium (Ca)	Supports bone health	1,000-1,500 mg/day
Creatine monohydrate	Promotes the resynthesis of ATP for use during explosive periods of activity, helps enhance speed and overall strength gains	5 g/day or 0.3 g/kg loading phase for 3-5 days followed by a maintenance dose of 3-5 g/day
Iron (Fe)	Supports oxygen delivery to muscles, particularly if deficient; increases ATP production	20-30 mg/day (higher doses may be warranted for deficiency)
Protein (soy, whey, casein, egg)	Promotes positive nitrogen balance, supports maintenance and growth of muscle, aids recovery	Typically 25 g per serving to help an athlete achieve recommended daily goal of 1.4-2.0 g/kg
Vitamin B_{12}	May enhance energy metabolism and endurance, if deficient	25-100 mcg/day
Vitamin D	Supports bone health	600-800 IU/day (higher levels may be warranted for deficiency)
Zinc (Zn)	Enhances recovery; supports immune function	25-30 mg/day

zoochemical creatine to be lower among vegetarian athletes (Lukaszuk et al., 2005); supplementation with oral creatine monohydrate therefore may be warranted. Similarly, muscle carnosine levels have been shown to be more than two times greater in meat eaters than vegetarians, making supplementation with beta-alanine—a key limiting factor in the storage of carnosine—of potential benefit.

Before using any dietary supplements, however, athletes who have concerns regarding nutritional status and supplemental ingredients of potential benefit to health and performance are encouraged to consult with a doctor as well as a registered dietitian, preferably one who is a board-certified specialist in sport dietetics or has exercise physiology education.

Athletes Competing in Hot and Humid Environments

Most athletes, whether in training or competition, have been forced to perform in hot and humid conditions. American football players typically begin training camps and two-a-day practices during some of the hottest and most humid times of the year. Some athletes can lose over a gallon (3.8 L) of fluid during one practice. Besides the obvious impact on sweat rates and fluid and electrolyte losses, the heat can produce other physiological effects that influence performance. The decision to hold the 1996 Olympic Games in Atlanta created a lot of interest in the impact of heat and humidity on performance and similar concerns were carried for the most recent Summer Olympics in Paris; many scientific experts believed it would be impossible for some athletes to reach performance norms under hot and humid conditions typical for summer in these locations. Scientists have determined that for the endurance athlete, a temperature of 10°C to 12°C (50°F-54°F) is optimal. Thus, athletic performance is likely to be affected once temperatures exceed these temperatures. Less scientific data is available for strength and power sports, but it's reasonable to assume these same optimal temperatures would apply.

Performance Obstacles for Athletes Competing in Hot and Humid Environments

Core temperature and fluid balance present the greatest concerns for athletes in the heat. Exertion during training and competition expend energy, which is dissipated in the form of heat. Dissipating heat from the body can take many forms, including convection (using a fan to blow heat away from the body), conduction (using cold water towels on the back of the neck or sitting in an ice bath), and most significantly, evaporation (sweating). Some of these forms of heat dissipation can be limited by equipment or gear worn by athletes (e.g., helmets, shoulder pads, pants). These types of equipment trap heat close to the body. As a result, many athletes rely heavily on sweating for thermoregulation. The loss of fluids results in drops in blood plasma and a subsequent drop in stroke volume, cardiac output, and maximal aerobic capacity, as well as a decline in blood flow to working muscles. A secondary concern is that warm environments increase an athlete's reliance on carbohydrates for fuel. Interestingly, although reliance on carbohydrates increases, it has not been shown to affect muscle glycogen levels at the point of fatigue, leaving scientists to conclude that decreased performance is not a result of fuel availability but thermoregulation.

Hot conditions can also affect the brain. Recently, a theory has been developed that elevation of core and brain temperature could be responsible for preventing the body from working harder or longer in hot conditions. Other mechanisms could be related to neurotransmitters, such as dopamine, which act on sites in the brain and affect fatigue (Roelands et al, 2015). Scientists have shown that the administration of bupropion may enhance performance in the heat by promoting the activity of dopamine, a powerful neurotransmitter, which positively influences motivation and perceptions of fatigue (Cordery et al, 2017). As a result, athletes tend to perform at higher intensities for longer in hot and humid conditions when taking bupropion. However, bupropion does not have beneficial effects in more temperate conditions (Watson et al, 2005). More research will further increase scientists' understanding of the brain's role in these conditions.

Nutritional Recommendations for Athletes Competing in Hot and Humid Environments

Athletes should focus on fueling strategies to improve thermoregulation and potentially affect mechanisms in the brain related to fatigue. Maintaining fluid balance and plasma volume during exercise are most vital. This is accomplished through proper fluid and electrolyte intake before, during, and after exercise. Current pre-exercise guidelines recommend consuming 16 to 24 oz (0.47-0.71 L) of fluid in combination with carbohydrates or electrolytes in the form of food or sport drinks in the 2 hours leading up to and another 7 to 12 oz (0.2-0.35 L) of fluid immediately prior to exercise in heat.

During exercise, typical fluid losses have been reported at 0.5 to 1.9 L/hour (16.9 to 64.2 ounces/hour, 507 to 1927 mL/hour) (Baker et al., 2016). American football players restricted in thermoregulation because of their equipment have been found to lose over 2 L/hour (67.6 oz/hour, 2029 mL/hour) during practices in hot environments; this is compared to average losses by runners of 1.75 L/hour (59.2 oz/hour, 1775 mL/hour) in hot temperatures, 1.6 L/hour (54.1 oz/hour, 1623 mL/hour) by basketball players training indoors, and 1.25 L/hour (42.3 oz, 1268 mL/hour) by soccer players (Godek, Bartolozzi, & Godek, 2005). Current guidelines for fluid intake encourage 4 to 8 oz (0.11-0.23 L, 120-240 mL) of fluid every 15 to 20 minutes of exercise. However, because sweat rates can be highly variable, calculation of sweat rate, which is highest in the heat for any given metabolic rate, is key to developing a sound hydration strategy for training and competition (Cheuvront & Kenefick, 2021). Sweat rate can be estimated by measuring body weight both immediately prior to and immediately after exertion while also monitoring volume of fluid consumed and urine output (see figure 2.2).

CALCULATING SWEAT RATE

1. Subtract postexercise weight (in pounds) from preexercise weight (in pounds).
2. Multiply by 16 to convert to ounces.
3. Add total fluid intake during exercise (in ounces).
4. Subtract any urine output (in ounces).
5. Divide by exercise duration (in hours).

Athletes can also monitor urine color, aiming to achieve a pale yellow color, and adjust fluid intake accordingly. If dehydration ensues after a workout in heat, particularly when losses are greater than 2% of body mass (as indicated by a sweat test or dark urine color), the American College of Sports Medicine Guidelines on Exercise and Fluid Replacement (2007) and the Position of the Academy of Nutrition and Dietetics on Nutrition and Athletic Performance (Thomas et al., 2016) recommend the athlete consume 1.25 to 1.50 L (42.3 to 50.7 oz, 1269 to 1522 mL) of fluid/kg of body mass lost to replenish body water content and a facilitate quicker recovery time.

Both carbohydrates and electrolytes assist in optimal fluid absorption, and both can be obtained from food sources or from the beverage itself. Intake of carbohydrate prior to and during exercise in hot environments has been shown to benefit exercise performance in heat, likely secondary to improvements in fluid uptake (Burke et al., 2019). However, concentration of carbohydrate consumed, particularly a single sugar type, should not exceed 8%; levels beyond this will lower the rate of fluid uptake in the body. When multiple types of sugars are consumed (e.g., glucose plus fructose), concentration of total carbohydrate consumed shouldn't exceed 10% to ensure optimal fluid uptake. For example, if an athlete is consuming 60 g of carbohydrate from multiple types of sugar, a fluid consumption of 20 to 30 oz (0.5 to 0.8 L) ideally will accompany it.

Loss of electrolytes, specifically sodium, ranges between 200 to 1,700 mg/L of sweat lost during exertion, with an average content being 1 g/L (Rodriguez et al., 2009). These numbers, however, can change significantly based on an athlete's state of heat acclimation as well as fitness level, with sweat sodium loss and consequent replacement needs decreasing at peak fitness and in an acclimated state. Endurance athletes also tend to have higher sweat sodium concentrations than more power-focused athletes (Veniamakis et al., 2022). Other electrolytes lost in sweat include potassium, calcium, and magnesium; the amounts of these nutrients lost in sweat are significantly less than those of sodium and chloride.

Co-ingestion of an osmotically active agent, such as sodium and glycerol, can increase voluntary water consumption and assist with retention of fluids, thereby resulting in pre-exercise hyperhydration and assisting thermoregulation and performance during prolonged exertion in heat (Morris et al., 2015). Acute salt loading (20 to 40 mg sodium/kg with 10 mL/kg fluid taken 1 to 2 hours prior to exercise) can expand blood volume, improve thermoregulation, and lower perceived effort during continuous exertion in the heat (Hamouti et al., 2014; Sims et al., 2007a, 2007b) and is equally or more effective than sodium loading over a more extended period (McCubbin et al., 2019a). Sodium loading before exercise has also been shown to exert a greater benefit to an athlete's performance than sodium intake during exercise.

Commercially prepared sports drinks as well as energy gels and chews contain varying levels sodium as well as other electrolytes to help replace sweat salt losses and to facilitate the transport of glucose across the intestinal wall. Electrolyte supplements, generally offered as a dissolvable tablet or powder to be mixed with water or a capsule to be swallowed, can also help an athlete replace sweat sodium and electrolyte losses. Broth, salted pretzels, salted boiled potatoes, and crackers are whole food options that can be consumed with water to meet individual sweat rate needs. An intake of 500 to 700 mg of sodium/L of fluid is advised by the ACSM, with endurance athletes competing in heat being advised to target at least 300 to 600 mg of sodium each hour (Veniamakis et al., 2022). Rapid restoration of hydration status after exercise can also be aided by increasing salt intake. This can either be achieved by consuming foods naturally rich in sodium along with water or using any of the electrolyte supplements mentioned previously (McCubbin, 2021). Although electrolyte replacement is important, athletes should guard against overconsuming sodium, which can trigger fluid imbalances as well as GI disturbances such as nausea, stomach cramps, diarrhea, and vomiting. Athletes who combine high-sodium foods with a sport drink or electrolyte supplement are at greatest risk for overconsumption of sodium.

Supplement Options for Athletes Competing in Hot Environments

Beyond maintaining fluid balance through replacement of sweat losses, there are certain strategies and supplements commonly used by athletes that may have an impact on the pathophysiological processes of exertional heat stroke (EHS). EHS has been determined to be a leading cause of sudden nontraumatic death in all athletes, with male athletes shown to be at higher risk than female athletes (Hosokawa et al., 2021https://www.ncbi.nlm.nih.gov/pmc/articles/PMC9790308/#eph13182-bib-0051). Athletes who are heavy sweaters may benefit from increasing sodium intake prior to hot weather training to help maintain sodium balance and reduce risk of EHS. Regular ingestion of 30 to 90 g/hour of carbohydrate during subclinical exertional heat stress and maintaining optimal carbohydrate availability is another approach that has been shown to consistently dampen pathophysiological features of EHS, thereby providing a protective effect against severe injury (Lee et al., 2022). There is also preliminary evidence showing some benefit of supplementation with glutamine, ginkgo, and antioxidant supplements on EHS risk; however, further research is needed before conclusive recommendations can be made (Lee et al., 2022; Sahib et al., 2021). Furthermore, supplemental use of sodium bicarbonate and dietary nitrates (e.g., beetroot) supplements have been shown to facilitate the development of EHS, and thus may be contraindicated when training and competing in hot and humid environments (Lee et al., 2022).

In addition to protecting against issues of thermoregulation, certain dietary supplements or nutrition ingredients can affect serotonin and dopamine receptors regulating the brain's involvement in the onset of fatigue, especially in hot conditions. Table 4.13 includes a list of potential dietary supplements to consider.

TABLE 4.13 Highlighted Supplement Options for Athletes Competing in Hot and Humid Environments

Supplement	Potential benefit	Recommended dose
Sports drinks	Support euhydration	Preexercise: 16-24 oz (0.47 to 0.59 L) in the 2h before exercise and another 7-12 ounces immediately prior to starting exercise During Exercise: 4-8 ounces every 15-20 minutes. Athletes should be encouraged to calculate sweat rate and work with a sports RD to develop an individualized hydration plan Postexercise: 1.25-1.50 L of fluid per kilogram of body mass (BM)
Calcium	Replaces sweat losses	0-120 mg/L of sweat loss
Carbohydrate	Prevents central nervous system (CNS) fatigue and fuel depletion, promotes fluid uptake	30-90 g/hour of exercise, depending on heat tolerance Maintain 6%-8% carbohydrate concentration, no more than 10% if using more than one sugar type
Chloride	Replaces sweat losses	710-2,840 mg/L of sweat loss
Glycerol	Increases fluid retention, promotes hyperhydration	1.2-1.4 g of glycerol/kg FFM paired with ~25 mL of fluid/kg FFM, consumed 90-180 minutes before exercise
Magnesium	Replaces sweat losses	0-36 mg/L of sweat loss
Potassium	Replaces sweat losses	160-320 mg/L of sweat loss
Sodium (Na+)	Enhances fluid uptake, promotes electrolyte balance	500-700 mg/L of fluid consumed; endurance athletes should aim for >300-600 mg of sodium/hour Loading: 20-40 mg sodium/kg consumed with 10 mL/kg (0.338 ounces/kg) fluid 1-2 hours before exercise *Note that 1 gram of salt provides approximately 400 mg of sodium and 600 mg of chloride *1 tsp of salt equals 2,300 mg of sodium
Tyrosine	May reduce central nervous system (CNS) fatigue	150 mg/kg of L-tyrosine consumed 90 minutes before exercise

Athletes Competing at Altitude

Altitude training was brought to the forefront of sports when Mexico City, at an elevation of 2,240 m (7,300 ft), was chosen to host the 1968 Olympic Games. Altitude can decrease exercise capacity by 3% for every 300 m (982 ft) above 1,500 m (4,921 ft). However, strategic implementation of altitude training at 1,600 to 2,400 m over 2 to 4 weeks can adequately prepare the athlete to perform at peak at higher elevations as well as provide a significant boost to performance at sea level, particularly in endurance-focused sports like distance running and cycling (Chapman et al., 2014a, 2014b). This boost is primarily driven by an erythropoietin (EPO) boost in red blood cells, with secondary benefits being increased buffering capacity, possible improvements in exercise economy, and extensive genetic responses of hypoxia inducible factor 1-alpha (Gore et al., 2007; Stellingwerff et al., 2019). Colorado Springs was chosen as the site of the U.S. Olympic Training Center in 1978 because of its high elevation. Currently, most scientists suggest that living and training lightly at moderate to high elevations and training hard and competing at or near sea level is best for enhancing performance (Millet et al., 2010). Bärtsch and Saltin (2008) established the following parameters for low, moderate, high, and extreme altitude:

- Low altitude: 500 to 2,000 m
- Moderate altitude: 2,000 to 3,000 m
- High altitude: 3,000 to 5,500 m
- Extreme altitude: Over 5,500 m

Athletes training and competing at altitude need to focus on similar performance nutrition attributes as when they are at sea level, though special attention needs to be given to optimizing energy and carbohydrate availability as well as maintaining hydration, particularly at altitudes above 1,600 m. Emerging data has also demonstrated an increased demand for iron to support optimal training adaptations at altitudes above 1,600 m. Increased consumption of antioxidants may be warranted to help offset a possible increase in oxidative stress associated with altitude exposure.

Performance Obstacles for Athletes Competing at Altitude

It has been established that approximately 45 kcal/kg FFM/day is necessary to achieve optimal EA and support long-term health and performance. It should be noted, however, that basal metabolic rate has been shown to increase 10% to 28% at high to extreme altitudes (4,000-6,000 m) as a result of labored breathing and thermoregulation required in the extreme environment as well as the increase in energy expenditure compared to sea level (Viscor et al., 2023; Westerterp et al., 1994). Even at a moderate elevation of 2,200 m, the resting metabolic rates of elite runners increased by 19% over 4 weeks (Woods et al., 2017). Thus, optimal EA is likely to exceed 45 kcal/kg FFM/day for athletes training at moderate to extreme elevations.

When an athlete suffers from low EA (<30 kcal/kg FFM/day), several parameters of health and performance are negatively affected. For the athlete exerting at altitude, the resulting drop in sex hormone levels (estrogen and testosterone) can negatively affect hematological adaptations to altitude, particularly as it relates to iron and hypoxia-induced EPO production. Challenges for achieving EA at altitude may include loss of appetite, altitude sickness, and, at the most extreme altitudes, the energy cost of carrying adequate fuel and supplies and difficulties in melting the required quantity of water for drinking, rehydrating food, or cooking (Viscor et al., 2023).

Nutritional Recommendations for Athletes Competing at Altitude

General recommendations for athletes training or competing at altitude, particularly moderate to high altitudes, include prioritizing carbohydrates to support an increased reliance on anaerobic metabolism while maintaining protein balance and protecting against loss of lean body mass during a noted downregulation of protein synthesis. Consuming the right amount of carbohydrates and protein before, during, and after exercising in hypoxia will help preserve glycogen stores, enhance muscle recovery, and promote optimal immune function. Depending on training volume and intensity, athletes training at sea level are encouraged to consume anywhere from 3 to 12 g of carbohydrate/kg and 1.2 to 2.0 g of protein/kg. With the noted increases in RMR at moderate to high altitudes, increased energy intake from carbohydrate and protein may be achieved by focusing on the higher end of these averages and possibly more in extreme cases—again, dependent on training status (or expedition phase for mountaineering).

In addition, proper timing of fuel before, during, and after training at altitude can help maximize favorable adaptations. Carbohydrate ingestion, at a dose of 1 to 4 g/kg in the 1 to 4 hours leading into simulated hypoxia, helps to maintain oxygen saturation and ventilation. In addition, consumption of carbohydrate at a rate of 30 to 90 g/hour during prolonged activity at high altitude is beneficial to endurance and immune functionality. Gastrointestinal issues and lack of appetite are commonly experienced at high to extreme altitudes and can hinder the athlete's ability to tolerate nutrition. Nonetheless, the goal should be encouraged to get as close to these targets as tolerance allows. Sport gels—particularly hydrogels that can be consumed without additional water and do not freeze as easily—may be an attractive option for athletes at high to extreme elevations where temperatures may drop below freezing. After exertion, glycogen stores can be aggressively restored by consuming 1.2 g/kg/hour or by combining carbohydrate (0.8 g/kg/hour) with protein (0.2-0.4 g/kg/hour).

Fluid Needs of Athletes Competing at Altitude

Hypoxia and low humidity associated with moderate- to high-altitude environments increase fluid loss via diuresis and respiration both at rest and in training, putting athletes at greater risk for dehydration. Daily resting fluid goals at sea level are generally calculated as half an athlete's body mass (in pounds). However, data has shown that at moderate altitudes (up to 4,000 m), respiratory water loss may be increased up to 1,900 mL/day in men and 850 mL/day in women, in addition to an increase in 500 mL/day of urinary water loss, elevating overall fluid demands compared to sea level (Viscor et al, 2023). These losses are likely to be more pronounced at high to extreme altitudes.

Dehydration can have multiple detrimental effects on the athlete, including decreases in physical and cognitive performance and increased risk of injury. As little as 1% to 2% loss of body water can equate to a 5% to 15% drop in performance. It is important that athletes monitor and address their hydration status and be proactive with fluid and electrolyte intake before, during, and after training. In addition to meeting daily fluid demands, guidelines for fluid intake during mountain activities entail drinking 400 to 800 mL/hour with 0.5 to 1 g of sodium/L of water. Glacier water, which is low in minerals and electrolytes, often serves as the primary source for hydration and cooking for long treks at extreme altitudes, thus electrolyte supplementation might be warranted to maintain optimal fluid and electrolyte balance. Electrolytes derived from foods also can be paired with water intake to facilitate hydration. When temperatures drop below freezing, maintaining hydration status becomes important to offset the risk of developing frostbite (as well as hypothermia when paired with carbohydrate). Athletes may also consider drinking hot fluids, like tea, hot cider, or hot cocoa, when temperatures are below freezing. Note that overall fluid strategies while at altitude should be adjusted to meet the athlete's individual sweat rates and urinary control, as well as address symptoms of altitude illness, which can cause fluid retention.

Micronutrient Needs of Athletes Competing at Altitude

During hypoxia, higher intake of certain micronutrients may be warranted to sustain both health and performance, particularly antioxidants and iron. Antioxidants are thought to help minimize oxidative damage caused by increased production of reactive oxygen and nitrogen species at low to moderate altitudes. Increasing iron intake is thought to help accommodate increases in red cell bloods during hypoxia.

Antioxidants

Altitude increases the stress load associated with training and competition due to an uptick in the production of stress hormones and free radicals, and though hypoxia-induced free radical formation may promote acclimatization to altitude, in excess, it can impair muscle function as well as capillary perfusion. These hormonal aberrations may also result in poor sleep patterns and delayed recovery times. Current guidelines suggest integrating ample amounts of antioxidant-rich foods into athletes' daily dietary regimes while training at altitude to help mitigate the impact of altitude-induced oxidative stress. However, as a whole, there is not sufficient evidence to recommend high-dose single antioxidant supplementation to attenuate this stress, especially at low to moderate altitudes.

Iron

To compensate for hypoxia during acclimatization to altitude, there is an increased production of red blood cells. This has been correlated with a decrease in iron and ferritin, which can impair the increase in hemoglobin concentration. Current recommendations are to assess iron status anywhere from 4 to 10 weeks prior to beginning any altitude training camp or competition; assessing closer to 1 month before altitude exposure, however, will provide a more precise ferritin assessment while still allowing adequate time to supplement and correct prior to altitude if warranted (Stellingwerff et al., 2019). Prealtitude ferritin thresholds of at least 30 ng/mL for female athletes and at least 40 ng/mL for male athletes have been indicated to ensure optimal adaptations and whether supplemental iron is appropriate, though these levels require further scientific validation (Bergeron et al., 2012; Stellingwerff et al., 2019).

Supplementation to correct impaired iron and ferritin levels is appropriate and should begin 2 to 3 weeks before beginning and continue throughout any significant training at altitude. In a retrospective analysis of hematological data collected from athletes engaged in altitude training at moderate altitudes (1,350-3,000 m), athletes who did not take an iron supplement reported a 1.2% increase in red blood cell count, versus a 3.3% and 4.0% increase in those athletes who supplemented with 105 mg or 210 mg of ferrous sulfate (Govus et al., 2015). Table 4.14, adapted from guidelines presented by Stellingwerff and colleagues (2019), summarizes supplement recommendations based on an athlete's serum ferritin levels before as well as while training at altitude. It is important to note that excessive hematocrit levels is known to increase the risk of high-altitude thromboembolism and thus, iron supplementation should be monitored closely by a sports physician or a sports dietitian.

TABLE 4.14 Iron Supplementation Guidelines for Athletes Competing at Altitude

Timeline	Supplement guidelines
Prealtitude (4-6 weeks prior)	• If ferritin <35 ng/mL, consider supplementing with 100 mg of elemental iron per day as a single-day dose. • If ferritin <15 ng/mL or iron-deficiency anemia is suspected, consult with a sports physician about parenteral iron (IV).
During altitude (~2 weeks prior and throughout)	• If ferritin <100 ng/mL at prealtitude blood check (not taking iron), start with 100 mg of elemental iron/day as a single-day dose for 2 weeks prior to altitude, then progress to 100-200 mg of elemental iron/day per athlete tolerance throughout the altitude camp as a single-day dose. • If ferritin is between 100-130 ng/mL at prealtitude blood check, supplement with 100 mg elemental iron/day as a single-day dose in the 2 weeks prior to and throughout the altitude camp. • If ferritin >130 ng/mL at prealtitude blood check, supplemental iron is not necessary.

Adapted from T. Stellingwerff, P. Peeling, L.A. Garvican-Lewis, et al., "Nutrition and Altitude: Strategies to Enhance Adaptation, Improve Performance and Maintain Health: A Narrative Review," *Sports Medicine* 49, no. 2 (2019): 169-184. doi: 10.1007/s40279-019-01159-w.

https://pmc.ncbi.nlm.nih.gov/articles/PMC6901429/figure/Fig3/

Supplement Options for Athletes Competing at Altitude

There is an overall shortage of data evaluating the impact ergogenic aids may present to an athlete who is training or competing at altitude, making more research necessary before definite recommendations for supplementation can be made. Nonetheless, there are several ingredients that are hypothesized to provide benefit to the athlete training or competing at altitude, including BCAAs, especially leucine, which can act as a substrate and regulator of protein synthesis; dietary nitrates like beetroot, which promote improvements in exercise economy (Kelly et al., 2014; Masschelein et al., 2012; Muggerridge et al., 2014); buffering agents like sodium bicarbonate or citrate, which lead to extracellular increases in bicarbonate (Deb et al., 2018); and beta-alanine, which leads to increased intracellular muscle carnosine synthesis (Peeling et al., 2018). In addition, there is evidence that N-acetylcysteine ingestion, through its antioxidant effects, may minimize oxidative stress and exercise-induced inflammation (Slattery et al., 2014) as well as modulate EPO production and the hypoxic ventilatory response (Hildebrandt et al., 2002). Finally, use of the herb extract Ginkgo biloba is purported to help athletes training at altitude by reducing tissue hypoxia, increasing vasodilation, and minimizing the risk for mild cases of acute mountain sickness (Moraga et al., 2007; Tsai et al., 2018). More research is required before use of these ergogenic aids can be recommended for altitude exposure in athletes, with factors such as dose, duration of consumption, and the mechanism of action all needing further clarification.

Table 4.15 provides information about a variety of sport supplements that can support these added nutritional needs.

TABLE 4.15 Highlighted Supplement Options for Athletes Competing at Altitude

Supplement	Potential benefit	Recommended dose
Beetroot	Increases vasodilation, enhances exercise economy at altitude	500 mL (~16 oz) of juiced beetroot taken 2.5 hours prior to exercise
Beta-alanine	Increases intracellular muscle carnosine synthesis	3-6 g/day for 6-8 weeks prior to and during altitude training
Calorie replacement shakes and bars	Assists in meeting energy needs, promotes weight gain	Varies depending on diet and calorie needs
Carbohydrate	Meets increased metabolic demand necessary to support performance	Daily needs depend on training but range from 3-12 g/kg Preexercise: 1-4 g/kg BM for every hour prior to starting During exercise: 30-90 g/hour Postexercise: 1.2 g/kg/hour
Ginkgo biloba	Reduces tissue hypoxia, increases vasodilation, lowers risk for mild AMS (acute mountain sickness)	Daily split doses of 80-120 mg consumed before and during exertion at moderate to high altitudes for a total of 3-5 days
Iron	Supports acclimatization with increase in red blood cell production in hypoxic conditions	Varies dependent on athlete's iron status (see table 4.14)
Leucine	Maintains protein balance	0.03-0.045 g/kg/day
N-acetylcysteine (NAC)	Minimizes oxidative stress and inflammatory response, enhances fatigue resistance	600-1,200 mg/day for 5-9 days
Protein (whey, soy, casein, egg)	Supports protein balance during altitude-induced downregulation of protein synthesis	1.2-2.0 g/kg/day Postworkout: 0.2-0.4 g/kg/hour
Sodium	Maintains fluid and electrolyte balance	500-1,000 mg of sodium/L of water consumed during exercise
Sodium bicarbonate or citrate	Helps serve as a buffering agent against metabolic acidosis	~300 mg/kg taken as a single dose 1-2 hours prior to exercise
Vitamin C	Provides antioxidant support; aids uptake of iron	RDA (men): 90 mg/day RDA (women): 75 mg/day
Vitamin E	Provides antioxidant support	RDA: 15 mg/day

Summary

Although general nutritional recommendations can serve as solid framework for a successful sporting season, the power of customized nutrition, including the addition of specific dietary supplements, can be profound. There are a multitude of conditions that may warrant further customization, some of which are described in this chapter. Athletes with specialized concerns are encouraged to work closely with a registered sport dietitian, a certified strength and conditioning specialist (CSCS) or exercise physiologist, and a doctor to develop a nutritional and supplementation plan best suited to their needs.

ABOUT THE AUTHORS

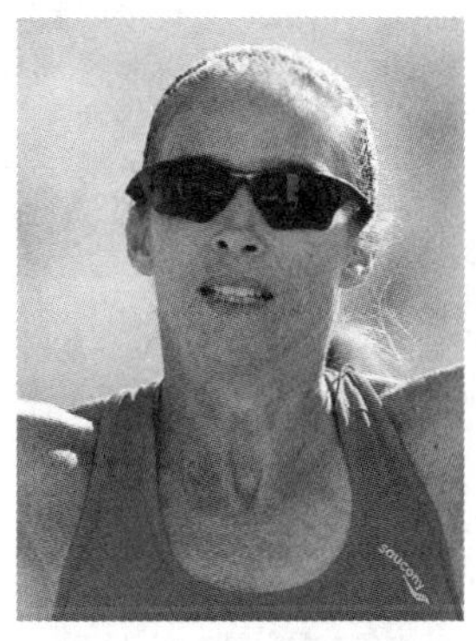

Kimberly Mueller, RD, CSSD, is a registered dietitian and board-certified specialist in sport dietetics with a master's degree in exercise physiology. She has been providing custom menu planning and nutrition coaching to active individuals worldwide for over 25 years through her company, Fuel Factor Nutrition Coaching. She uses her own practical sport experiences and knowledge of nutrition science to help fellow athletes achieve optimal health and peak fitness performance.

Mueller's passion for customized nutrition also led her to help develop and launch Infinit Nutrition, a company that creates custom blends of ingredients to address the performance and health goals of recreational and professional athletes, including those competing in such prestigious events as the Tour de France and the Formula 500 Championship. She is well known for her nutrition clinics and as a contributor to books such as *The Performance Zone*, *The Woman Triathlete*, *Triathlon Revolution*, *Racing Weight*, and *The New Rules of Marathon and Half Marathon Nutrition*. She is also the coauthor of *The Athlete's Guide to Sports Supplements*.

Lonnie Lowery, PhD, LD (ret), FISSN, is the president of Nutrition, Exercise & Wellness (NEW) Associates. He has a long history of supporting scientific research and product development for adult and sport nutrition products across the food and dietary supplement industries. He also has 25 years of experience as a professor of nutrition and exercise physiology, led a Division I university sport nutrition program, and was a finalist in multiple regional bodybuilding competitions.

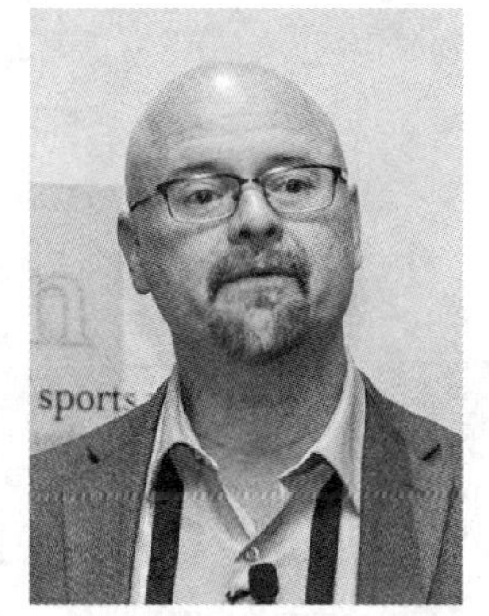

Lowery has researched uncommon lipids and physical stress, very-high-protein diets, and, most recently, bioactive compounds in coffee. This work has resulted in provisional patents, national and international presentations, scientific and popular media articles, books, and book chapters; he was coeditor of the book *Dietary Protein and Resistance Exercise*. Lowery is a member of the American Society for Nutrition and the Institute of Food Technologists; he is also past president of the American Society of Exercise Physiologists and is a fellow of the International Society of Sports Nutrition. Lonnie earned his first two graduate degrees (MA, PhD) in exercise physiology from Kent State University and later obtained his MS in nutrition/dietetics from the same institution.

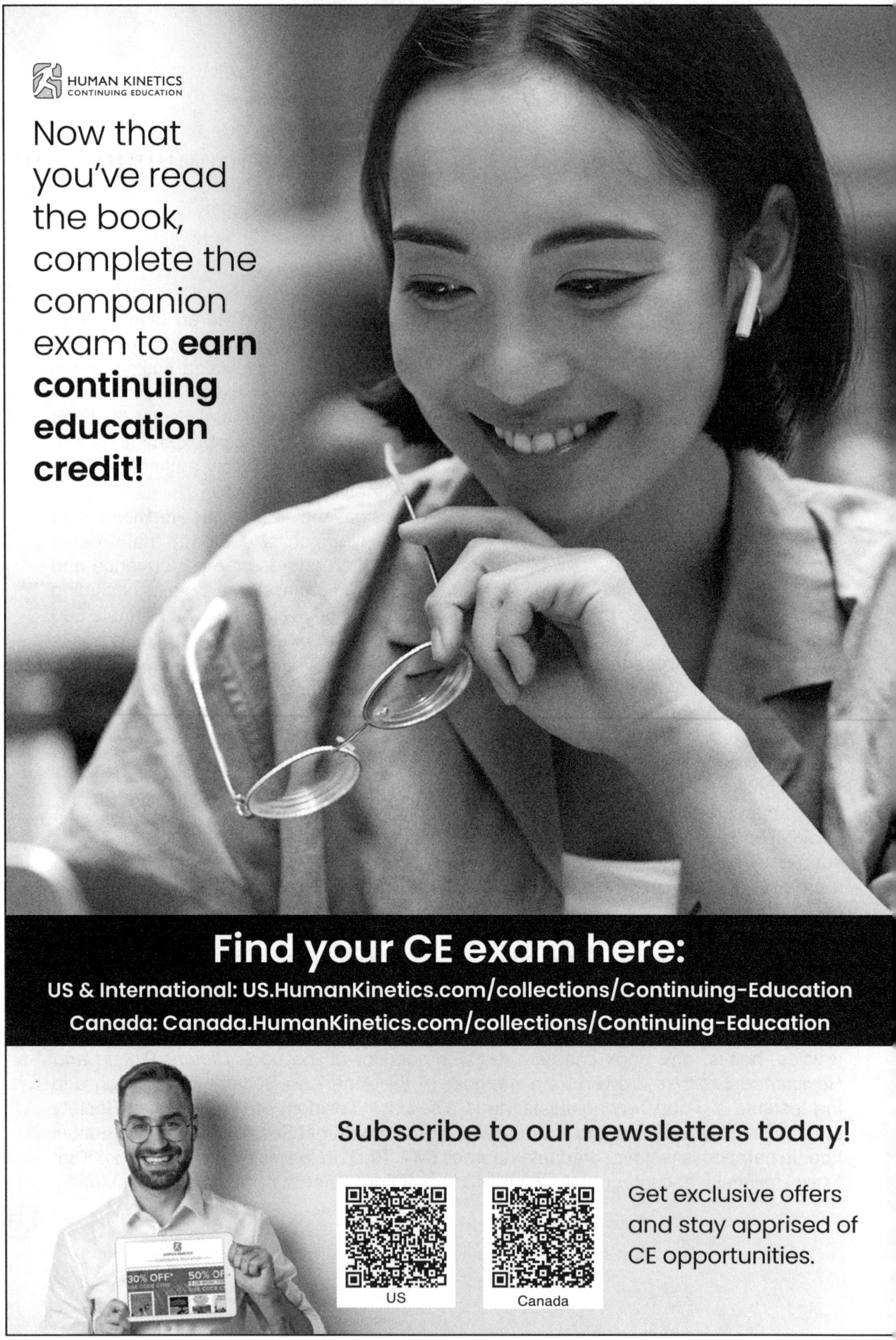

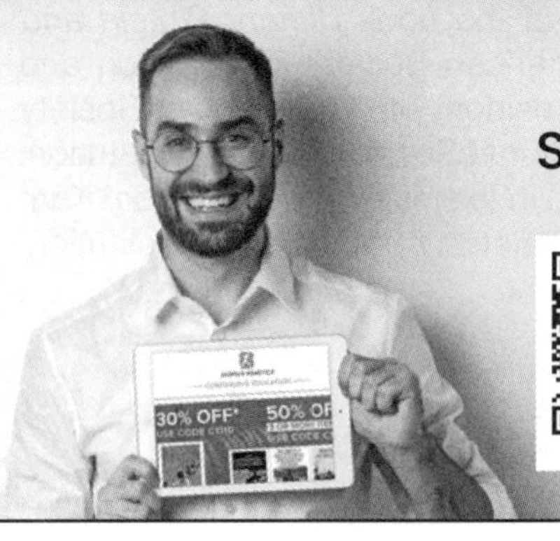

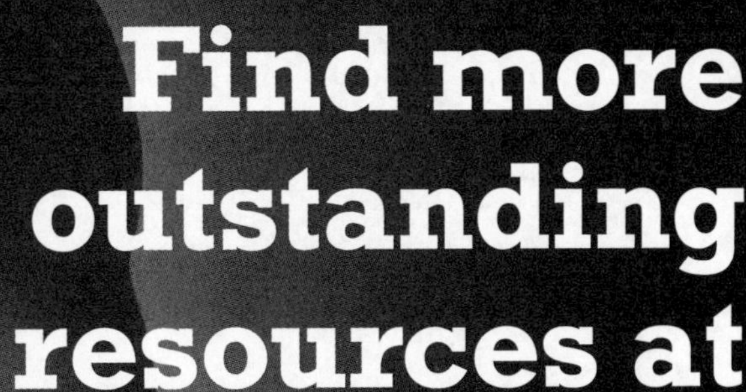

Find more outstanding resources at

US.HumanKinetics.com
Canada.HumanKinetics.com

In the U.S. call 1-800-747-4457
Canada 1-800-465-7301
International 1-217-351-5076

HUMAN KINETICS

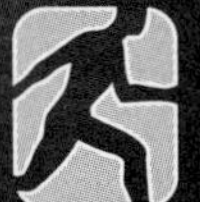

Sign up for our newsletters!

Get the latest insights with regular newsletters, plus
periodic product information and special insider offers
from Human Kinetics.